Respiratory Medicine

Respiratory Medicine offers clinical and research-oriented resources for pulmonologists and other practitioners and researchers interested in respiratory care. Spanning a broad range of clinical and research issues in respiratory medicine, the series covers such topics as COPD, asthma and allergy, pulmonary problems in pregnancy, molecular basis of lung disease, sleep disordered breathing, and others.

The series editors are Sharon Rounds, MD, Professor of Medicine and of Pathology and Laboratory Medicine at the Alpert Medical School at Brown University, Anne Dixon, MD, Professor of Medicine and Director of the Division of Pulmonary and Critical Care at Robert Larner, MD College of Medicine at the University of Vermont, and Lynn M. Schnapp, MD, George R. And Elaine Love Professor and Chair of Medicine at the University of Wisconsin-Madison School of Medicine and Public Health.

Farbod N. Rahaghi • Laszlo Farkas
Oksana A. Shlobin
Editors

The Pulmonary Vasculature in Chronic Lung Disease

Humana Press

ATS American Thoracic Society

Editors
Farbod N. Rahaghi
Division of Pulmonary, Critical Care
Medicine, Clinical Immunology,
and Allergy
Department of Medicine, David Geffen
School of Medicine at the University
of California-Los Angeles
Los Angeles, CA, USA

Oksana A. Shlobin
Advanced Lung Disease and
Transplant Program
Inova Fairfax Hospital
Falls Church, VA, USA

Laszlo Farkas
Davis Heart & Lung Research Institute
The Ohio State University
Columbus, OH, USA

ISSN 2197-7372 ISSN 2197-7380 (electronic)
Respiratory Medicine
ISBN 978-3-032-03580-6 ISBN 978-3-032-03581-3 (eBook)
https://doi.org/10.1007/978-3-032-03581-3

This Humana imprint is published by the registered company Springer Nature Switzerland AG
The registered company address is: Gewerbestrasse 11, 6330 Cham, Switzerland

Introduction

Pulmonary hypertension (PH) in the setting of chronic lung disease is the second most common cause of PH and is a significant cause of morbidity and mortality in this patient population. Most data come from patients with chronic obstructive pulmonary disease (COPD) [1–12] and interstitial lung disease (ILD) [13–24]. While significant progress has been made in the prevention and treatment of lung diseases, the treatment of pulmonary hypertension associated with lung disease remains an important unmet therapeutic target. This is in part due to the complexity of phenotyping lung disease, and in part due to the unique challenges associated with deploying screening, diagnosis, and treatment approaches targeted at pulmonary arterial hypertension (PAH) in PH associated with lung disease.

Timely identification of pulmonary hypertension associated with lung disease is complicated by multiple factors. The most common symptoms of PH are shortness of breath and limited exercise capacity, similar to the underlying lung diseases, which delays an evaluation for PH [25, 26]. The severity of lung disease is poorly correlated with the development of PH [27, 28], and the use of noninvasive tools often used for to screen for PAH is limited by lower performance in the context of lung disease [29–42]. These factors overall contribute to a relatively late diagnosis of PH, particularly in the context of COPD [25, 26, 39, 40].

Prior to the availability of home oxygen, hypoxemia was the most significant driver of PH and right ventricular failure in lung disease. However, with home oxygen therapy becoming available, it is increasingly clear that the development of pulmonary vascular disease can be associated with many factors including inflammation, vascular ablation due to parenchymal destruction, and vascular rarefaction in the areas of preserved parenchyma. Pulmonary vasodilators, which have significantly improved survival and exercise tolerance in PAH, had not historically yielded positive results in PH associated with lung disease. The INCREASE trial recently demonstrated the utility of inhaled treprostinil in patients with PH associated with interstitial lung disease [43–45]. At the same time, in a separate trial, inhaled treprostinil was not successful in the treatment of patients with COPD [46, 47], despite the presence of the theoretical benefit of inhaled pulmonary vasodilator therapy in both circumstances. These results are exciting in that they show that PH associated with lung disease can be treated beyond the use of oxygen. However, they also point to the importance of identifying the specific phenotype of patients in treating their underlying PH, which at its center is driven by differences in biological and pathophysiological mechanisms of lung destruction.

Meanwhile, significant progress has been made in understanding the potential contributions of different pulmonary vascular mural cells, as well as circulating and inflammatory cells [48]. New technologies have enabled the identification of disease-specific subpopulations of vascular cells, including endothelial cells, which may contribute to the complex interactions between the pulmonary vascular bed and lung parenchymal destruction in chronic lung diseases [49, 50].

In this collection of chapters, the authors present the progress in both the understanding of the pathobiology of PH associated with lung disease and the clinical care of this diverse and challenging population. It is our hope that by simultaneously presenting the basic science and clinical frontiers in the treatment of PH in lung disease, we can provide a comprehensive update on this very exciting and challenging topic.

Laszlo Farkas
Oksana Shlobin
Farbod N. Rahaghi

References

1. Torres-Castro R, Gimeno-Santos E, Vilaró J, et al. Effect of pulmonary hypertension on exercise tolerance in patients with COPD: a prognostic systematic review and meta-analysis. Eur Resp Rev. 2021;30.
2. Portillo K, Torralba Y, Blanco I, et al. Pulmonary hemodynamic profile in chronic obstructive pulmonary disease. Int J Chronic Obstruct Pulmon Dis. 2015;10:1313–20.
3. Cuttica MJ, Kalhan R, Shlobin OA, et al. Categorization and impact of pulmonary hypertension in patients with advanced COPD. Resp Med. 2010;104:1877–82.
4. Wells JM, Washko GR, Han MK, et al. Pulmonary arterial enlargement and acute exacerbations of COPD. N Engl J Med. 2012;367:913–21.
5. Hilde JM, Skjørten I, Grøtta OJ, et al. Right ventricular dysfunction and remodeling in chronic obstructive pulmonary disease without pulmonary hypertension. J Am College Cardiol. 2013;62:1103–11.
6. Pistenmaa CL, Nardelli P, Ash SY, et al. Pulmonary arterial pruning and longitudinal change in percent emphysema and lung function: the genetic epidemiology of COPD study. Chest. 2021.
7. Washko GR, Nardelli P, Ash SY, et al. Arterial vascular pruning, right ventricular size, and clinical outcomes in chronic obstructive pulmonary disease. a longitudinal observational study. Am J Respir Crit Care Med. 2019;200:454–61.
8. LaFon DC, Bhatt SP, Labaki WW, et al. Pulmonary artery enlargement and mortality risk in moderate to severe COPD: results from COPDGene. Eur Respir J. 2020;55.

9. Minai OA, Chaouat A, Adnot S. Pulmonary hypertension in COPD: epidemiology, significance, and management: pulmonary vascular disease: the global perspective. Chest. 2010;137:39s–51s.
10. Oswald-Mammosser M, Weitzenblum E, Quoix E, et al. Prognostic factors in COPD patients receiving long-term oxygen therapy. Importance of pulmonary artery pressure. Chest. 1995;107:1193–8.
11. Falk JA, Kadiev S, Criner GJ, Scharf SM, Minai OA, Diaz P. Cardiac disease in chronic obstructive pulmonary disease. Proc Am Thoracic Soc. 2008;5:543–8.
12. Antonelli Incalzi R, Fuso L, De Rosa M, et al. Co-morbidity contributes to predict mortality of patients with chronic obstructive pulmonary disease. Eur Resp J. 1997;10:2794–800.
13. Nathan SD, Shlobin OA, Ahmad S, et al. Serial development of pulmonary hypertension in patients with idiopathic pulmonary fibrosis. Respiration. 2008;76:288–94.
14. Alhamad EH, Cal JG, Alrajhi NN, Alharbi WM. Predictors of mortality in patients with interstitial lung disease-associated pulmonary hypertension. J Clin Med. 2020;9.
15. Raghu G, Nathan SD, Behr J, et al. Pulmonary hypertension in idiopathic pulmonary fibrosis with mild-to-moderate restriction. Eur Respir J. 2015;46:1370–7.
16. King CS, Brown AW, Shlobin OA, et al. Prevalence and impact of WHO group 3 pulmonary hypertension in advanced idiopathic nonspecific interstitial pneumonia. Eur Respir J. 2018;52.
17. Oliveira RK, Pereira CA, Ramos RP, et al. A haemodynamic study of pulmonary hypertension in chronic hypersensitivity pneumonitis. Eur Respir J. 2014;44:415–24.
18. Nadrous HF, Pellikka PA, Krowka MJ, et al. Pulmonary hypertension in patients with idiopathic pulmonary fibrosis. Chest. 2005;128:2393–9.
19. Piccari L, Allwood B, Antoniou K, et al. Pathogenesis, clinical features, and phenotypes of pulmonary hypertension associated with interstitial lung disease: a consensus statement from the Pulmonary Vascular Research Institute's Innovative Drug Development Initiative—Group 3 Pulmonary Hypertension. Pulm Circ. 2023;13:e12213.
20. Lettieri CJ, Nathan SD, Barnett SD, Ahmad S, Shorr AF. Prevalence and outcomes of pulmonary arterial hypertension in advanced idiopathic pulmonary fibrosis. Chest. 2006;129:746–52.
21. Rivera-Lebron BN, Forfia PR, Kreider M, Lee JC, Holmes JH, Kawut SM. Echocardiographic and hemodynamic predictors of mortality in idiopathic pulmonary fibrosis. Chest. 2013;144:564–70.
22. Gall H, Felix JF, Schneck FK, et al. The Giessen Pulmonary Hypertension Registry: survival in pulmonary hypertension subgroups. J Heart Lung Transplant. 2017;36:957–67.
23. Minai OA, Santacruz JF, Alster JM, Budev MM, McCarthy K. Impact of pulmonary hemodynamics on 6-min walk test in idiopathic pulmonary fibrosis. Resp Med. 2012;106:1613–21.

24. Andersen CU, Mellemkjær S, Hilberg O, Nielsen-Kudsk JE, Simonsen U, Bendstrup E. Pulmonary hypertension in interstitial lung disease: prevalence, prognosis and 6 min walk test. Resp Med. 2012;106:875–82.
25. Rutten FH, Broekhuizen BDL. Misclassification of both chronic obstructive pulmonary disease and heart failure. JAMA Netw Open. 2018;1:e185486.
26. Lawson CA, Mamas MA, Jones PW, et al. Association of medication intensity and stages of airflow limitation with the risk of hospitalization or death in patients with heart failure and chronic obstructive pulmonary disease. JAMA Netw Open. 2018;1:e185489–e.
27. Nathan SD, Shlobin OA, Ahmad S, Urbanek S, Barnett SD. Pulmonary hypertension and pulmonary function testing in idiopathic pulmonary fibrosis. Chest. 2007;131:657–63.
28. Zisman DA, Karlamangla AS, Ross DJ, et al. High-resolution chest CT findings do not predict the presence of pulmonary hypertension in advanced idiopathic pulmonary fibrosis. Chest. 2007;132:773–9.
29. Keir GJ, Wort SJ, Kokosi M, et al. Pulmonary hypertension in interstitial lung disease: Limitations of echocardiography compared to cardiac catheterization. Respirology (Carlton, Vic). 2018;23:687–94.
30. Nathan SD, Shlobin OA, Barnett SD, et al. Right ventricular systolic pressure by echocardiography as a predictor of pulmonary hypertension in idiopathic pulmonary fibrosis. Resp Med. 2008;102:1305–10.
31. Swanson KL, Utz JP, Krowka MJ. Doppler echocardiography-right heart catheterization relationships in patients with idiopathic pulmonary fibrosis and suspected pulmonary hypertension. Med Sci Monitor. 2008;14:Cr177–82.
32. Modrykamien AM, Gudavalli R, McCarthy K, Parambil J. Echocardiography, 6-minute walk distance, and distance-saturation product as predictors of pulmonary arterial hypertension in idiopathic pulmonary fibrosis. Resp Care. 2010;55:584–8.
33. Nikkho SM, Richter MJ, Shen E, et al. Clinical significance of pulmonary hypertension in interstitial lung disease: a consensus statement from the Pulmonary Vascular Research Institute's innovative drug development initiative—Group 3 pulmonary hypertension. Pulm Circ. 2022;12:e12127.
34. Behr J, Ryu JH. Pulmonary hypertension in interstitial lung disease. Eur Resp J. 2008;31:1357.
35. Arcasoy SM, Christie JD, Ferrari VA, et al. Echocardiographic assessment of pulmonary hypertension in patients with advanced lung disease. Am J Respir Crit Care Med. 2003;167:735–40.
36. Fakharian A, Hamidi N, Hosseinloo BH, et al. Correlation between the pulmonary artery pressure measured in echocardiography and pulmonary artery diameter in the CT-scan of patients suffering from interstitial lung disease. Tanaffos. 2011;10:37–41.
37. Ratanawatkul P, Oh A, Richards JC, Swigris JJ. Performance of pulmonary artery dimensions measured on high-resolution computed tomography scan for identifying pulmonary hypertension. ERJ Open Res. 2020;6.

38. Alhamad EH, Al-Boukai AA, Al-Kassimi FA, et al. Prediction of pulmonary hypertension in patients with or without interstitial lung disease: reliability of CT findings. Radiology. 2011;260:875–83.
39. Roversi S, Fabbri LM, Sin DD, Hawkins NM, Agusti A. Chronic obstructive pulmonary disease and cardiac diseases. an urgent need for integrated care. Am J Respir Crit Care Med. 2016;194:1319–36.
40. Hawkins NM, Virani S, Ceconi C. Heart failure and chronic obstructive pulmonary disease: the challenges facing physicians and health services. Eur Heart J. 2013;34:2795–803.
41. Fisher MR, Forfia PR, Chamera E, et al. Accuracy of Doppler echocardiography in the hemodynamic assessment of pulmonary hypertension. Am J Respir Crit Care Med. 2009;179:615–21.
42. Fisher MR, Criner GJ, Fishman AP, et al. Estimating pulmonary artery pressures by echocardiography in patients with emphysema. Eur Resp J. 2007;30:914–21.
43. Waxman A, Restrepo-Jaramillo R, Thenappan T, et al. Inhaled treprostinil in pulmonary hypertension due to interstitial lung disease. N Engl J Med. 2021;384:325–34.
44. Waxman A, Restrepo-Jaramillo R, Thenappan T, et al. Long-term inhaled treprostinil for pulmonary hypertension due to interstitial lung disease: INCREASE open-label extension study. Eur Respir J. 2023;61.
45. Nathan SD, Tapson VF, Elwing J, et al. Efficacy of inhaled treprostinil on multiple disease progression events in patients with pulmonary hypertension due to parenchymal lung disease in the INCREASE trial. Am J Respir Crit Care Med. 2022;205:198–207.
46. Nathan SD, Argula R, Trivieri MG, et al. Inhaled treprostinil in pulmonary hypertension associated with COPD: PERFECT study results. Eur Respir J. 2024;63.
47. Nathan SD, Lacasse V, Bell H, et al. COPD associated pulmonary hypertension: a post hoc analysis of the PERFECT study. Pulm Circ. 2024;14:e12430.
48. Borek I, Birnhuber A, Voelkel NF, Marsh LM, Kwapiszewska G. The vascular perspective on acute and chronic lung disease. J Clin Investig. 2023;133.
49. Adams TS, Schupp JC, Poli S, et al. Single-cell RNA-seq reveals ectopic and aberrant lung-resident cell populations in idiopathic pulmonary fibrosis. Sci Adv. 2020;6:eaba1983.
50. Schupp JC, Manning EP, Chioccioli M, et al. Alveolar vascular remodeling in nonspecific interstitial pneumonia: replacement of normal lung capillaries with COL15A1-positive endothelial cells. Am J Respir Crit Care Med. 2023;208:819–22.

Contents

Contributors

B. W. Allwood Division of Pulmonology, Department of Medicine, Stellenbosch University & Tygerberg Hospital, Cape Town, South Africa

Aparna Balasubramanian Division of Pulmonary and Critical Care Medicine, Department of Medicine, Johns Hopkins University School of Medicine, Baltimore, MD, USA

A. Buckley Division of Pulmonology, Department of Medicine, Stellenbosch University, Cape Town, South Africa

Vaughn Craddock Division of Pulmonary, Critical Care and Sleep Medicine, Department of Internal Medicine, University of Kansas Medical Center, Kansas City, Kansas, KS, USA

Navneet Kaur Dhillon Division of Pulmonary, Critical Care and Sleep Medicine, Department of Internal Medicine, University of Kansas Medical Center, Kansas City, Kansas, KS, USA

Laszlo Farkas Division of Pulmonary, Critical Care and Sleep Medicine, Department of Internal Medicine, College of Medicine, The Ohio State University, Columbus, OH, USA
Davis Heart and Lung Research Institute, College of Medicine, The Ohio State University, Columbus, OH, USA

Lindsay M. Forbes Division of Pulmonary, Allergy and Critical Care Medicine, University of Colorado, Denver, CO, USA

Paul M. Heerdt Department of Anesthesiology, Yale School of Medicine, New Haven, CT, USA

Anna R. Hemnes Department of Anesthesiology, Vanderbilt University Medical Center, Nashville, TN, USA

Cheng-Jun Hu Department of Craniofacial Biology, University of Colorado School of Dental Medicine, Denver, CO, USA

Karys Khilzi Department of Pulmonology, Hospital del Mar, Barcelona, Spain
Hospital del Mar Research Institute, Barcelona, Spain

Yunhye Kim Division of Pulmonary Medicine, Boston Children's Hospital, Harvard Medical School, Boston, MA, USA

Christopher S. King Advanced Lung Disease and Lung Transplant Program, Inova Fairfax Medical Center, Falls Church, VA, USA

Timothy Klouda Division of Pulmonary Medicine, Boston Children's Hospital, Harvard Medical School, Boston, MA, USA

Martin R. J. Kolb Firestone Institute for Respiratory Health, Research Institute at St. Joseph's Healthcare, Department of Medicine, McMaster University, Hamilton, ON, Canada

Vasilis Kouranos Interstitial Lung Disease Team, Royal Brompton Hospital, Part of Guy's and St Thomas' NHS Foundation Trust, London, UK
National Heart and Lung Institute, Imperial College London, London, UK

Mona Lichtblau Department of Pulmonology, University Hospital Zürich, Zürich, Switzerland
University of Zürich, Zürich, Switzerland

Min Li Cardiovascular Pulmonary Research Laboratories, Department of Pediatrics and Medicine, University of Colorado School of Medicine, Denver, CO, USA

Alexander Liu Department of Cardiology, Royal Brompton Hospital, Part of Guy's and St Thomas' NHS Foundation Trust, London, UK

E. H. Louw Division of Pulmonology, Department of Medicine, Stellenbosch University, Cape Town, South Africa
Department of Medicine, Karl Bremer Hospital, Cape Town, South Africa

Geoffrey Newcomb Division of Pulmonary, Critical Care and Sleep Medicine, Department of Internal Medicine, College of Medicine, The Ohio State University, Columbus, OH, USA
Davis Heart and Lung Research Institute, College of Medicine, The Ohio State University, Columbus, OH, USA

Kohei Otsubo Department of Respiratory Medicine, Graduate School of Medical Sciences, Kyushu University, Fukuoka, Japan

Sahil Pandya Division of Pulmonary, Critical Care and Sleep Medicine, Department of Internal Medicine, University of Kansas Medical Center, Kansas City, Kansas, KS, USA

Lucilla Piccari Department of Pulmonology, Hospital del Mar, Barcelona, Spain
Hospital del Mar Research Institute, Barcelona, Spain

Laura C. Price National Heart and Lung Institute, Imperial College London, London, UK
National Pulmonary Hypertension Service, Royal Brompton Hospital, Part of Guy's and St Thomas' NHS Foundation Trust, London, UK

Farbod N. Rahaghi Division of Pulmonary, Critical Care Medicine, Clinical Immunology, and Allergy, Department of Medicine, David Geffen School of Medicine at the University of California-Los Angeles, Los Angeles, CA, USA

Diego A. Rodríguez Chiaradía Department of Pulmonology, Hospital del Mar, Barcelona, Spain
Hospital del Mar Research Institute, Barcelona, Spain
Department of Medicine and Life Sciences (MELIS), Universitat Pompeu Fabra (UPF), Barcelona, Spain
Centro de Investigación en Red de Enfermedades Respiratorias (CIBERES), Instituto de Salud Carlos III (ISCIII), Madrid, Spain

Kevin Schwalbach Division of Allergy, Pulmonary and Critical Care Medicine, Vanderbilt University Medical Center, Nashville, TN, USA

Inderjit Singh Division of Pulmonary, Critical Care, and Sleep Medicine, Department of Internal Medicine, Yale School of Medicine, New Haven, CT, USA

Leslie Spikes Division of Pulmonary, Critical Care and Sleep Medicine, Department of Internal Medicine, University of Kansas Medical Center, Kansas City, Kansas, KS, USA

Kurt R. Stenmark Cardiovascular and Pulmonary Research Laboratory, Departments of Pediatrics and Medicine, University of Colorado School of Medicine, Denver, CO, USA

Andrew J. Synn Division of Pulmonary, Critical Care, and Sleep Medicine, Beth Israel Deaconess Medical Center, Harvard Medical School, Boston, MA, USA

Christopher Thomas Advanced Lung Disease and Lung Transplant Program, Inova Fairfax Medical Center, Falls Church, VA, USA

J. K. van Heerden Department of Paediatrics, Medical Sciences Division, University of Oxford, Oxford, UK

Toyoshi Yanagihara Department of Respiratory Medicine, Fukuoka University Hospital, Fukuoka, Japan

Ke Yuan Division of Pulmonary Medicine, Boston Children's Hospital, Harvard Medical School, Boston, MA, USA

Fatima Zeba Division of Pulmonary, Critical Care, and Sleep Medicine, Department of Internal Medicine, Yale School of Medicine, New Haven, CT, USA

Hui Zhang Cardiovascular Pulmonary Research Laboratories, Department of Pediatrics and Medicine, University of Colorado School of Medicine, Denver, CO, USA

Chapter 1
Lung Endothelial Cells and Their Heterogeneity in Chronic Lung Diseases

Geoffrey Newcomb and Laszlo Farkas

Introduction

In recent decades, researchers have focused on understanding the changes in the pulmonary vascular system during chronic lung diseases. Studies have shown that both the structure and function of vascular cells play a significant role in the development of conditions like idiopathic pulmonary fibrosis (IPF) and emphysema [1–7]. These diseases exhibit changes at both the microvascular and capillary levels and the macrovascular levels in the lungs. While the structural changes have been recognized, we have only recently gained a more comprehensive understanding of functional changes in different pulmonary vascular cell types. This is due to the advent of single-cell omics technologies, such as single-cell RNA sequencing (scRNA-Seq), which has provided invaluable insights into the diversity of lung vascular cells [8, 9]. This chapter specifically focuses on the heterogeneity of endothelial cells (ECs) in the lung, which are critical cell types lining the vasculature across all anatomic compartments. ECs play a pivotal role in regulating various vascular functions, including inflammatory cell accumulation, vasotonus, hemostasis, and gas exchange [10, 11]. While prior knowledge hinted at distinct entities within the pulmonary endothelium, applying scRNA-seq has revealed heterogeneity in pulmonary ECs that was not previously identified.

G. Newcomb · L. Farkas (✉)
Division of Pulmonary, Critical Care and Sleep Medicine, Department of Internal Medicine, College of Medicine, The Ohio State University, Columbus, OH, USA

Davis Heart and Lung Research Institute, College of Medicine, The Ohio State University, Columbus, OH, USA
e-mail: Laszlo.Farkas@osumc.edu

F. N. Rahaghi et al. (eds.), *The Pulmonary Vasculature in Chronic Lung Disease*, Respiratory Medicine, https://doi.org/10.1007/978-3-032-03581-3_1

Heterogeneity of the Lung Endothelium

The traditional classification of endothelial cells (ECs) in the lung has historically relied on anatomical location, including pulmonary arteries, alveolar capillaries, pulmonary veins, and the lung lymphatic system. Studies have shown functional differences between microvascular capillary ECs and pulmonary artery ECs, with the former demonstrating a higher rate of proliferation in rat lungs [12]. In addition, previous research on the stem and progenitor cell populations responsible for repairing the lungs has encountered challenges due to the varying definitions of these cells [13]. Techniques such as flow cytometry and isolation methods, often relying on surface markers, have been employed to identify these cells. While CD34 and VEGFR2 were used as criteria to identify endothelial progenitor cells in the systemic circulation, different markers such as CD133 and c-kit (CD117) have been identified in patients with pulmonary arterial hypertension [14–17]. In particular, c-kit expression has been found to delineate primitive endothelial progenitor or stem cells in the developing human lung and adult murine lung [16, 17]. Our group has demonstrated that isolating highly proliferative c-kit-expressing ECs from rat lungs leads to a stem-like EC population that promotes pulmonary artery remodeling and pulmonary hypertension (PH) [18]. Recently, CD157 has been identified as another marker of tissue-resident endothelial stem cells [19].

In addition to flow cytometry markers, it is important to distinguish between different types of endothelial populations using various isolation methods. For instance, early and late outgrowth ECs are two types of ECs that can be differentiated based on these methods. Asahara cells and early outgrowth ECs share similarities with hematopoietic cells with angiogenic properties but appear unable to engraft into blood vessels persistently [20, 21]. Some endothelial-protective effects were ascribed to these early-outgrowth ECs by paracrine secretion of EC-protective factors, including interleukin-10 [21]. In contrast, late-outgrowth ECs express endothelial markers but not hematopoietic markers and can engraft into vasculature [22–24]. Similar isolation techniques were also used to obtain endothelial colony-forming cells (ECFCs) from human and rat lungs, and these ECFCs exhibit vascular regenerative potential in animal experiments [25, 26]. It is worth noting that the origin of these progenitor cell populations continues to be studied, sometimes with contradictory results. Whereas bone marrow-derived cells have been suggested as a source for endothelial progenitor cells, recent work identified using lineage tracing that circulating ECs are derived from the blood vessel wall [27, 28]. This would have important implications for lung circulation as well.

The emergence of single-cell omics, particularly scRNA-Seq, has revolutionized our understanding of lung EC heterogeneity and its adaptation to diseases. Although subpopulations of ECs in the pulmonary arteries, veins, and lymphatic system have been identified, their roles remain unclear. They may depend on their functional states and diseases associated with [29, 30]. In contrast, populations in the microvascular/alveolar capillary endothelium, specifically aerocytes (aCap) and generally capillary (gCap) ECs, have been more precisely defined based on their expression of markers and anatomical position in the alveolar walls [8, 31–35]. Differences in marker expression and anatomical distribution in the alveolar walls have identified these two subpopulations. Aerocytes are located throughout the alveolar walls close to type I alveolar epithelial cells and have multiple pores that appear to facilitate gas exchange in the lung alveoli [31]. Aerocytes express complementary patterns of growth factors and their receptors to the gCap ECs. For instance, aerocytes express stem cell factor, the ligand for c-kit, which is expressed in gCap ECs [31]. The current understanding suggests that aCap ECs function as the endothelial side of the alveolocapillary unit and facilitate gas exchange, similar to the role of type I alveolar epithelial cells on the epithelial side [31]. In contrast, gCap ECs represent a stem/progenitor cell population that accounts for the high regenerative potential of the pulmonary capillary endothelial network [36]. The expression of stem/progenitor cell markers such as c-kit in gCap ECs supports this concept [17, 18, 37]. Figure 1.1 summarizes the endothelial heterogeneity in the lung. Table 1.1 provides an overview of the markers used to distinguish the different EC populations in the lung. The critical question remains how these EC populations are regulated in

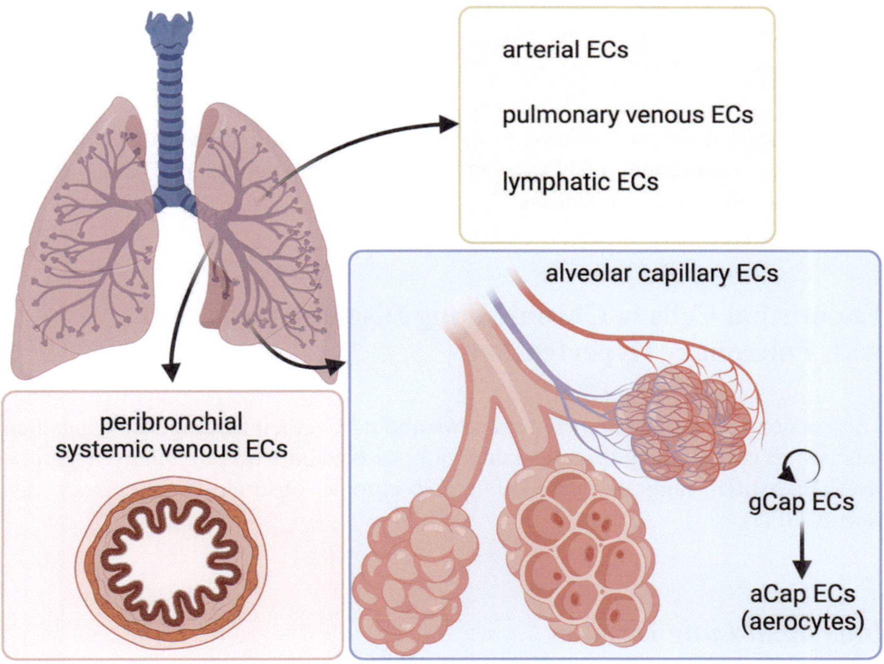

Fig. 1.1 Summary of the heterogeneity of the lung endothelium. Throughout the lungs, arterial and pulmonary venous endothelial cells (ECs) are found, as well as lymphatic ECs. Around the airways, systemic venous ECs are found, and the alveolar-capillary ECs comprise two types of ECs: aCap ECs ("aerocytes") are mainly responsible for gas exchange. General capillary ECs (gCap ECs) are a stem cell population that gives rise to aCap ECs and renews the gCap population. Created with BioRender.com

Table 1.1 Markers for endothelial subpopulations in the lung identified using scRNAseq

EC subpopulation	Marker pattern	Publication
aCap (aerocyte)	*CAR4, EDNRB, APLN, KITL, EMCN, EDNRB, TBX2, FOXP2, CLEC4E, SPON2, PRKG, CHRM2, S100A4, EDA*	Gillich et al. [31]; Schupp et al. [8]; Villa Ellis et al. [33]; Kalucka et al. [35]
gCap	*APLNR, PTPRB, TEK, KIT, vWF, EDN1, GPI-HBP1, CD36, FCN3, BTNL9, BTNL8, CD14, IL7R, IL18R1*	Gillich et al. [31]; Schupp et al. [8]; Villa Ellis et al. [33]; Kalucka et al. [35]
Arterial	*EFNB2, SOX17, BMX, SEMA3G, HEY1, LTBP4, FBLN5, GJA5, GJA4, CLDN10, FBLIM1, FBLN2, MGP, BGN, LTBP1, FN1, SERPINE2, CPAMD8, CXCL12, VEGFA, NOS1, PDE3A, PDE4D, DKK2, DLL4, SOX5, SOX17, HES4, PRDM16*	Schupp et al. [8]
Pulmonary venous	*EBF1, EBF3, MEOX1, MEOX2, ZNF385D, TACR1, ROBO1, CYSLTR1, CPXM2, MMP16, PDE7B, PDE2A, SPRY1, CPE, DKK3, EFEMP1, CDH11*	Schupp et al. [8]
Systemic venous (peribronchial)	*COL15A1, vWA1, PLVAP*	Schupp et al. [8]
Lymphatic	*PROX1, LYVE1, FLT4, PDPN, CCL21, SEMA3A, SEMA3D, TBX1, HOXD3, NR2F1, NRF2F2, GPR182*	Schupp et al. [8]

chronic lung diseases and whether disease-specific subpopulations can be identified for therapeutic targeting. scRNA-seq offers promise for uncovering disease-specific alterations in lung EC populations.

Endothelial Cells in Chronic Lung Diseases Associated with Pulmonary Hypertension

This section will summarize what is known about ECs, their heterogeneity, and their function in chronic lung diseases commonly associated with pulmonary hypertension, interstitial lung disease (ILD), and chronic obstructive pulmonary disease (COPD).

Interstitial Lung Diseases

ILDs are chronic lung conditions that involve the gradual buildup of an abnormal fibrotic extracellular matrix (ECM) [38–40]. This process damages the structure of the lung tissue, which causes symptoms such as shortness of breath and exercise intolerance and can ultimately result in premature death. Specific types of ILDs include idiopathic pulmonary fibrosis (IPF) and systemic sclerosis (SSc) associated with ILD. The morphological correlate of IPF is usual interstitial pneumonia (UIP) [38]. ECs, despite their close relationship with epithelial cells in the lung alveoli, have yet to be extensively studied in the context of ILDs. In conditions such as IPF/UIP, there is a discrepancy between reduced density and dysregulation of capillaries within the fibrotic areas and the increased density of immature capillaries at the border zone between fibrotic and non-fibrotic tissue [41, 42]. Studies using a model that overexpresses active transforming growth factor-β (TGF-β), a protein involved in cell growth, differentiation, and fibrosis, have confirmed these findings. This work found that angiogenesis protected from endothelial apoptosis and reduced associated PH [2], whereas pulmonary fibrosis was enhanced with endothelial dysfunction and pulmonary vascular remodeling [43]. Recent work has highlighted the protective role of pro-angiogenic signaling and endothelial repair in reducing the underlying fibrotic condition [7]. Growth factors like hepatocyte growth factor and transcription factors like the ETS-related gene play crucial roles in maintaining pulmonary vascular homeostasis and protecting against pulmonary fibrosis [44, 45]. EC function is also notably reduced in the advanced fibrotic lung zones of patients with fibrotic hypersensitivity pneumonitis, one of the most common forms of ILD with histologic features similar to IPF [46]. This indicates that vascular cells, particularly ECs, are not just bystanders but active participants in interstitial remodeling in ILD.

The Asahara cells are important in maintaining vascular homeostasis [14]. Although they seem unable to engraft into blood vessels [20], they have been linked to systemic vascular diseases and related ILDs [47, 48]. Circulating EPCs increase in active systemic vascular diseases, such as rheumatoid arthritis (RA) and SSc, as a compensatory response to microvascular injury and inflammation [49–51]. The levels of EPCs are higher in the peripheral circulation of patients with rheumatoid arthritis (RA)-related and SSc-related forms of ILD compared to patients with RA and SSc without ILD [52, 53]. Thus, monitoring circulating EPC levels has been proposed as a biomarker for monitoring progression toward ILD. ECFCs show enhanced procoagulant and proliferative, but also pro-apoptotic, senescent, and pro-inflammatory phenotypes in ILD, which have all the potential to contribute to pulmonary vascular disease [54–56]. However, experimental evidence in animal models that ECFCs promote pulmonary fibrosis has so far been elusive [57].

Endothelial-to-mesenchymal transition (EndMT) is a potential fate of ECs that has received attention in pulmonary vascular pathophysiology. This transition process, where ECs change to a fibroblast/smooth muscle cell-like phenotype, is driven by mechanisms similar to pulmonary fibrosis [58–67]. This mechanism involves an imbalance of bone morphogenic protein (BMP) and TGF-β signaling. EndMT has been observed in models of ILD, such as pulmonary fibrosis, and it may contribute to the accumulation of myofibroblasts and the dysregulation of the endothelial network. This can cause endothelial dysfunction and pulmonary vascular remodeling and contribute to fibrosis [68–70]. Explanted lung tissue from patients with SSc-related ILD has also shown an increased occurrence of EndMT [71].

Two major findings have been made regarding endothelial subpopulations in IPF using single-cell RNA sequencing (scRNA-seq): First, there is a reduction in the endothelial subpopulations in the lungs of IPF patients, including aerocytes and gCap ECs in the lung alveoli. This reduction aligns with a previously suggested decrease in the microvascular density [1, 41, 42, 72]. A decline in gCap ECs indicates a lower progenitor density within the capillary endothelium [31]. Given the senescent (aging) nature of the adjacent alveolar epithelium, it is possible that the capillary endothelium could adopt a senescent characteristic due to the influence of the alveolar epithelial cells' secretory pattern [73, 74]. The second potentially even more relevant finding was the increase in collagen 15A1 (COL15A1) expressing ECs within IPF-affected lungs [72]. In healthy human lungs, these COL15A1$^+$ ECs are primarily found in the peribronchial region, albeit at lower numbers. However, there appears to be a replacement of alveolar-capillary ECs by COL15A1$^+$ peribronchial ECs during alveolar vascular remodeling observed in patients' lungs with nonspecific interstitial pneumonia (NSIP). This shift could be responsible for distorted lung capillary structures, reduced gas exchange efficiency, and increased permeability observed in fibrotic regions of ILDs [75]. Targeting COL15A1$^+$ ECs might offer a therapeutic approach to enhance EC function and restore pulmonary vascular homeostasis.

Chronic Obstructive Pulmonary Disease

COPD represents a group of diseases that includes chronic obstructive bronchitis and emphysema. It is characterized by a spectrum of structural alterations in the airways and lung parenchyma that cause a gradual reduction in airflow [76]. Since the discovery that inhibition of VEGF receptors induces emphysema, a potential key role has been shown for microvascular EC apoptosis in animal models of emphysema [3, 5, 6, 77–80]. However, more recent work has failed to identify a shift between the different EC subpopulations, namely aerocytes, gCap, arterial, venous, lymphatic, and peribronchial ECs in the lungs of COPD patients and those without the condition [81]. Nonetheless, the data showed significant differences in gene expression between the two groups. Gene ontology (GO) pathways for cellular responses to cytokines, cellular responses to stress, and cytokine signaling pathways were universally found in all lung ECs. Moreover, specific differential gene expression was also found according to anatomical and functional subsets, such as enhanced inflammatory signaling and cellular responses to stress and reduced endothelial repair in capillary ECs.

The gene expression profile is more affected by COPD than the relative abundance of different EC subpopulations in the lung. This suggests that the functional alteration of the lung endothelium is a critical component of COPD-associated pulmonary vascular disease. Endothelial dysfunction is an early feature of COPD and can even be seen in smokers who have not yet developed COPD. Patients with varying stages of COPD, including those with mild COPD, have reduced nitric oxide-mediated relaxation of pulmonary artery (PA) rings. This is associated with an increase in intima diameter in patients with COPD and smokers without COPD compared to nonsmokers. All these findings suggest that endothelial dysfunction plays a vital role in the early development of COPD [82, 83].

There have been various suggested mechanisms for the endothelial dysfunction seen in COPD. Among them, the most significant and well-researched is the connection between smoking and the development of EC dysfunction and COPD. CS causes the death of ECs [84] and increases lung EC permeability, making the lungs more prone to acute lung injury. This occurs due to the inactivation of protein kinase B (Akt) through oxidative stress-induced and the subsequent activation of glycogen synthase kinase-3β (GSK-3β) [85]. CS also contains reactive oxygen species (ROS) and reactive nitrogen species (RNS) [86, 87]. ECs, in turn, produce ROS via xanthine oxidase, NADH/NADPH oxidase, and uncoupled eNOS, leading to vascular dysfunction [88]. Furthermore, circulating inflammatory cells generate additional ROS and RNS, which cause intravascular micro-thrombosis and reduced blood flow through dysfunctional endothelium [89, 90].

In addition to endothelial dysfunction, hypoxic vasoconstriction has been suggested to cause pulmonary vascular remodeling, whereas endothelial drop-out via apoptosis leads to rarefaction of airways and pulmonary arteries [10]. The importance of ECs in lung parenchymal homeostasis is further supported by the findings that supplementation of ECs reverses experimental emphysema [4]. Conversely, induction of endothelial senescence has been linked to emphysema [91]. At the same time, the loss of the lung tissue homeostatic microRNA-126 has been associated with endothelial senescence and pulmonary vascular remodeling in COPD [92, 93].

The combination of pulmonary fibrosis and emphysema leads to an elevated risk of developing severe pulmonary hypertension in patients [94, 95]. Although the pathobiology of this rare clinical entity is not yet fully understood, we propose that structural and functional alteration of the lung endothelium, including dysregulation of specific subpopulations, may play a role in the vascular phenotype of this combined condition.

Summary and Conclusions

Advanced techniques, particularly scRNA-seq, have expanded our understanding of the various types of ECs present in the lungs. The findings demonstrate that the lung microvascular endothelium is specialized, similar to the alveolar epithelium. In chronic lung diseases that frequently result in associated with pulmonary hypertension, there is a subtype switch in IPF but not in COPD. However, both diseases share altered transcriptomics and endothelial dysfunction as common features. The use of advanced Omics technologies will allow us to examine further the role of ECs in the development of chronic lung diseases and their potential treatments.

References

1. Farkas L, et al. Pulmonary hypertension and idiopathic pulmonary fibrosis: a tale of angiogenesis, apoptosis, and growth factors. Am J Respir Cell Mol Biol. 2011;45(1):1–15.
2. Farkas L, et al. VEGF ameliorates pulmonary hypertension through inhibition of endothelial apoptosis in experimental lung fibrosis in rats. J Clin Invest. 2009;119(5):1298–311.
3. Kasahara Y, et al. Inhibition of VEGF receptors causes lung cell apoptosis and emphysema. J Clin Invest. 2000;106(11):1311–9.
4. Hisata S, et al. Reversal of emphysema by restoration of pulmonary endothelial cells. J Exp Med. 2021;218(8)
5. Pasupneti S, et al. Endothelial HIF-2α as a key endogenous mediator preventing emphysema. Am J Respir Crit Care Med. 2020;202(7):983–95.
6. Clauss M, et al. Lung endothelial monocyte-activating protein 2 is a mediator of cigarette smoke-induced emphysema in mice. J Clin Invest. 2011;121(6):2470–9.
7. Bian F, et al. Lung endothelial cells regulate pulmonary fibrosis through FOXF1/R-Ras signaling. Nat Commun. 2023;14(1):2560.
8. Schupp JC, et al. Integrated single-cell atlas of endothelial cells of the human lung. Circulation. 2021;144(4):286–302.
9. Travaglini KJ, et al. A molecular cell atlas of the human lung from single-cell RNA sequencing. Nature. 2020;587(7835):619–25.
10. Borek I, et al. The vascular perspective on acute and chronic lung disease. J Clin Invest. 2023;133(16)
11. Evans CE, et al. Endothelial cells in the pathogenesis of pulmonary arterial hypertension. Eur Respir J. 2021;58(3):2003957.
12. Alvarez D, et al. Lung microvascular endothelium is enriched with progenitor cells that exhibit vasculogenic capacity. Am J Phys Lung Cell Mol Phys. 2008;294(3):L419–30.
13. Medina RJ, et al. Endothelial progenitors: a consensus statement on nomenclature. Stem Cells Transl Med. 2017;6(5):1316–20.
14. Asahara T, et al. Isolation of putative progenitor endothelial cells for angiogenesis. Science. 1997;275(5302):964–7.
15. Toshner M, et al. Evidence of dysfunction of endothelial progenitors in pulmonary arterial hypertension. Am J Respir Crit Care Med. 2009;180(8):780–7.
16. Suzuki T, et al. c-Kit immunoexpression delineates a putative endothelial progenitor cell population in developing human lungs. Am J Phys Lung Cell Mol Phys. 2014;306(9):L855–65.
17. Fang S, et al. Generation of functional blood vessels from a single c-kit+ adult vascular endothelial stem cell. PLoS Biol. 2012;10:e1001407.
18. Bhagwani A, et al. Clonally selected primitive endothelial cells promote occlusive pulmonary arteriopathy and severe pulmonary hypertension in rats exposed to chronic hypoxia. Sci Rep. 2020;10(1):1136.
19. Wakabayashi T, et al. CD157 marks tissue-resident endothelial stem cells with homeostatic and regenerative properties. Cell Stem Cell. 2018;22(3):384–397.e6.
20. Case J, et al. Human CD34+AC133+VEGFR-2+ cells are not endothelial progenitor cells but distinct, primitive hematopoietic progenitors. Exp Hematol. 2007;35(7):1109–18.
21. Ormiston M, et al. Innate immunity in the therapeutic actions of endothelial progenitor cells in pulmonary hypertension. Am J Respir Cell Mol Biol. 2010;43(5):546–54.
22. Aday S, et al. Synthetic microparticles conjugated with VEGF(165) improve the survival of endothelial progenitor cells via microRNA-17 inhibition. Nat Commun. 2017;8(1):747.
23. Baker CD, et al. Endothelial colony-forming cell conditioned media promote angiogenesis in vitro and prevent pulmonary hypertension in experimental bronchopulmonary dysplasia. Am J Phys Lung Cell Mol Phys. 2013;305(1):L73–81.
24. Minami Y, et al. Angiogenic potential of early and late outgrowth endothelial progenitor cells is dependent on the time of emergence. Int J Cardiol. 2015;186:305–14.

25. Alphonse RS, et al. Existence, functional impairment, and lung repair potential of endothelial colony-forming cells in oxygen-induced arrested alveolar growth. Circulation. 2014;129(21):2144–57.
26. Alphonse RS, et al. The isolation and culture of endothelial colony-forming cells from human and rat lungs. Nat Protoc. 2015;10(11):1697–708.
27. Aliotta J, et al. Bone marrow endothelial progenitor cells are the cellular mediators of pulmonary hypertension in the murine monocrotaline injury model. Stem Cells Transl Med. 2017;6(7):1595–606.
28. Lin Y, et al. Origin, prospective identification, and function of circulating endothelial colony-forming cells in mice and humans. JCI Insight. 2023;8(5)
29. Crnkovic S, et al. Single-cell transcriptomics reveals skewed cellular communication and phenotypic shift in pulmonary artery remodeling. JCI Insight. 2022;7(20)
30. Asosingh K, et al. Single-cell transcriptomic profile of human pulmonary artery endothelial cells in health and pulmonary arterial hypertension. Sci Rep. 2021;11(1):14714.
31. Gillich A, et al. Capillary cell-type specialization in the alveolus. Nature. 2020;586(7831):785–9.
32. Niethamer T, et al. Defining the role of pulmonary endothelial cell heterogeneity in the response to acute lung injury. elife. 2020:9.
33. Vila Ellis L, et al. Epithelial vegfa specifies a distinct endothelial population in the mouse lung. Dev Cell. 2020;52(5):617–30.e6.
34. Zhang L, et al. Single-cell transcriptomic profiling of lung endothelial cells identifies dynamic inflammatory and regenerative subpopulations. JCI Insight. 2022;7(11)
35. Kalucka J, et al. Single-cell transcriptome atlas of murine endothelial cells. Cell. 2020;180(4):764–79.e20.
36. Godoy RS, et al. Single cell transcriptomic atlas of lung microvascular regeneration after targeted endothelial cell ablation. elife. 2023:12.
37. Ren X, et al. Postnatal alveologenesis depends on FOXF1 signaling in c-KIT(+) endothelial progenitor cells. Am J Respir Crit Care Med. 2019;200(9):1164–76.
38. Lederer DJ, Martinez FJ. Idiopathic pulmonary fibrosis. N Engl J Med. 2018;378(19):1811–23.
39. McCarthy C, Keane MP. Contemporary Concise Review 2021: interstitial lung disease. Respirology. 2022;27(7):539–48.
40. Wijsenbeek M, Cottin V. Spectrum of fibrotic lung diseases. N Engl J Med. 2020;383(10):958–68.
41. Ebina M, et al. Heterogeneous increase in CD34-positive alveolar capillaries in idiopathic pulmonary fibrosis. Am J Respir Crit Care Med. 2004;169(11):1203–8.
42. Cosgrove GP, et al. Pigment epithelium-derived factor in idiopathic pulmonary fibrosis: a role in aberrant angiogenesis. Am J Respir Crit Care Med. 2004;170(3):242–51.
43. Yanagihara T, et al. Vascular-parenchymal cross-talk promotes lung fibrosis through BMPR2 signaling. Am J Respir Crit Care Med. 2023;207(11):1498–514.
44. Cao Z, et al. Targeting the vascular and perivascular niches as a regenerative therapy for lung and liver fibrosis. Sci Transl Med. 2017;9(405)
45. Caporarello N, et al. Dysfunctional ERG signaling drives pulmonary vascular aging and persistent fibrosis. Nat Commun. 2022;13(1):4170.
46. De Sadeleer LJ, et al. Lung microenvironments and disease progression in fibrotic hypersensitivity pneumonitis. Am J Respir Crit Care Med. 2022;205(1):60–74.
47. Ferrante A, et al. Endothelial progenitor cells: are they displaying a function in autoimmune disorders? Mech Ageing Dev. 2016;159:44–8.
48. Distler JH, et al. Endothelial progenitor cells: novel players in the pathogenesis of rheumatic diseases. Arthritis Rheum. 2009;60(11):3168–79.
49. Distler JH, et al. EULAR Scleroderma Trials and Research group statement and recommendations on endothelial precursor cells. Ann Rheum Dis. 2009;68(2):163–8.
50. Jodon de Villeroche V, et al. Enhanced late-outgrowth circulating endothelial progenitor cell levels in rheumatoid arthritis and correlation with disease activity. Arthritis Res Ther. 2010;12(1):R27.

51. Rodriguez-Carrio J, et al. Circulating endothelial cells and their progenitors in systemic lupus erythematosus and early rheumatoid arthritis patients. Rheumatology (Oxford). 2012;51(10):1775–84.
52. Pulito-Cueto V, et al. Endothelial progenitor cells as a potential biomarker in interstitial lung disease associated with rheumatoid arthritis. J Clin Med. 2020;9(12)
53. Pulito-Cueto V, et al. Endothelial progenitor cells: relevant players in the vasculopathy and lung fibrosis associated with the presence of interstitial lung disease in systemic sclerosis patients. Biomedicine. 2021;9(7)
54. Billoir P, et al. Endothelial colony-forming cells from idiopathic pulmonary fibrosis patients have a high procoagulant potential. Stem Cell Rev Rep. 2021;17(2):694–9.
55. Blandinières A, et al. Interleukin-8 release by endothelial colony-forming cells isolated from idiopathic pulmonary fibrosis patients might contribute to their pathogenicity. Angiogenesis. 2019;22(2):325–39.
56. Smadja DM, et al. Imbalance of circulating endothelial cells and progenitors in idiopathic pulmonary fibrosis. Angiogenesis. 2013;16(1):147–57.
57. Blandinières A, et al. Endothelial colony-forming cells do not participate to fibrogenesis in a bleomycin-induced pulmonary fibrosis model in nude mice. Stem Cell Rev Rep. 2018;14(6):812–22.
58. Hopper R, et al. In pulmonary arterial hypertension, reduced BMPR2 promotes endothelial-to-mesenchymal transition via HMGA1 and its target slug. Circulation. 2016;133(18):1783–94.
59. Machado R, et al. BMPR2 haploinsufficiency as the inherited molecular mechanism for primary pulmonary hypertension. Am J Hum Genet. 2001;68(1):92–102.
60. Mammoto T, et al. Twist1 in hypoxia-induced pulmonary hypertension through transforming growth factor-β-smad signaling. Am J Respir Cell Mol Biol. 2018;58(2):194–207.
61. Jonigk D, et al. Plexiform lesions in pulmonary arterial hypertension composition, architecture, and microenvironment. Am J Pathol. 2011;179(1):167–79.
62. Sime PJ, et al. Adenovector-mediated gene transfer of active transforming growth factor-beta1 induces prolonged severe fibrosis in rat lung. J Clin Invest. 1997;100(4):768–76.
63. Koli K, et al. Bone morphogenetic protein-4 inhibitor gremlin is overexpressed in idiopathic pulmonary fibrosis. Am J Pathol. 2006;169(1):61–71.
64. Myllärniemi M, et al. Gremlin-mediated decrease in bone morphogenetic protein signaling promotes pulmonary fibrosis. Am J Respir Crit Care Med. 2008;177(3):321–9.
65. Farkas L, et al. Transient overexpression of Gremlin results in epithelial activation and reversible fibrosis in rat lungs. Am J Respir Cell Mol Biol. 2011;44(6):870–8.
66. Arciniegas E, et al. Perspectives on endothelial-to-mesenchymal transition: potential contribution to vascular remodeling in chronic pulmonary hypertension. Am J Phys Lung Cell Mol Phys. 2007;293(1):L1–8.
67. Good RB, et al. Endothelial to mesenchymal transition contributes to endothelial dysfunction in pulmonary arterial hypertension. Am J Pathol. 2015;185(7):1850–8.
68. Hashimoto N, et al. Endothelial-mesenchymal transition in bleomycin-induced pulmonary fibrosis. Am J Respir Cell Mol Biol. 2009;
69. Gaikwad AV, et al. Endothelial-to-mesenchymal transition: a precursor to pulmonary arterial remodelling in patients with idiopathic pulmonary fibrosis. ERJ Open Res. 2023;9(2)
70. Singh S, et al. Endothelial-specific loss of IFT88 promotes endothelial-to-mesenchymal transition and exacerbates bleomycin-induced pulmonary fibrosis. Sci Rep. 2020;10(1):4466.
71. Mendoza FA, et al. Endothelial cells expressing endothelial and mesenchymal cell gene products in lung tissue from patients with systemic sclerosis-associated interstitial lung disease. Arthritis Rheumatol. 2016;68(1):210–7.
72. Adams TS, et al. Single-cell RNA-seq reveals ectopic and aberrant lung-resident cell populations in idiopathic pulmonary fibrosis. Sci Adv. 2020;6(28):eaba1983.
73. Schafer MJ, et al. Cellular senescence mediates fibrotic pulmonary disease. Nat Commun. 2017;8:14532.

74. Yao C, et al. Senescence of alveolar type 2 cells drives progressive pulmonary fibrosis. Am J Respir Crit Care Med. 2021;203(6):707–17.
75. Schupp JC, et al. Alveolar vascular remodeling in nonspecific interstitial pneumonia: replacement of normal lung capillaries with COL15A1-positive endothelial cells. Am J Respir Crit Care Med. 2023;208(7):819–22.
76. Olsson KM, et al. Pulmonary hypertension associated with lung disease: new insights into pathomechanisms, diagnosis, and management. Lancet Respir Med. 2023;11(9):820–35.
77. Giordano RJ, et al. Targeted induction of lung endothelial cell apoptosis causes emphysema-like changes in the mouse. J Biol Chem. 2008;283(43):29447–60.
78. Koike K, et al. Role of glucosylceramide in lung endothelial cell fate and emphysema. Am J Respir Crit Care Med. 2019;200(9):1113–25.
79. Petrache I, et al. Ceramide upregulation causes pulmonary cell apoptosis and emphysema-like disease in mice. Nat Med. 2005;11(5):491–8.
80. Sakhatskyy P, et al. Cigarette smoke-induced lung endothelial apoptosis and emphysema are associated with impairment of FAK and eIF2α. Microvasc Res. 2014;94:80–9.
81. Sauler M, et al. Characterization of the COPD alveolar niche using single-cell RNA sequencing. Nat Commun. 2022;13(1):494.
82. Peinado VI, et al. Endothelial dysfunction in pulmonary arteries of patients with mild COPD. Am J Phys. 1998;274(6):L908–13.
83. Dinh-Xuan AT, et al. Impairment of endothelium-dependent pulmonary-artery relaxation in chronic obstructive lung disease. N Engl J Med. 1991;324(22):1539–47.
84. Lu Q, Gottlieb E, Rounds S. Effects of cigarette smoke on pulmonary endothelial cells. Am J Phys Lung Cell Mol Phys. 2018;314(5):L743–56.
85. Borgas D, et al. Cigarette smoke disrupted lung endothelial barrier integrity and increased susceptibility to acute lung injury via histone deacetylase 6. Am J Respir Cell Mol Biol. 2016;54(5):683–96.
86. Valavanidis A, Vlachogianni T, Fiotakis K. Tobacco smoke: involvement of reactive oxygen species and stable free radicals in mechanisms of oxidative damage, carcinogenesis and synergistic effects with other respirable particles. Int J Environ Res Public Health. 2009;6(2):445–62.
87. Pryor WA, Stone K. Oxidants in cigarette smoke. Radicals, hydrogen peroxide, peroxynitrate, and peroxynitrite. Ann N Y Acad Sci. 1993;686:12–27; discussion 27–8
88. Cai H, Harrison DG. Endothelial dysfunction in cardiovascular diseases: the role of oxidant stress. Circ Res. 2000;87(10):840–4.
89. Pober JS, Sessa WC. Evolving functions of endothelial cells in inflammation. Nat Rev Immunol. 2007;7(10):803–15.
90. Bombeli T, et al. Apoptotic vascular endothelial cells become procoagulant. Blood. 1997;89(7):2429–42.
91. Beaulieu D, et al. Phospholipase A2 receptor 1 promotes lung cell senescence and emphysema in obstructive lung disease. Eur Respir J. 2021;58(2)
92. Alique M, et al. MicroRNA-126 regulates Hypoxia-Inducible Factor-1α which inhibited migration, proliferation, and angiogenesis in replicative endothelial senescence. Sci Rep. 2019;9(1):7381.
93. Musri MM, et al. MicroRNA dysregulation in pulmonary arteries from chronic obstructive pulmonary disease. relationships with vascular remodeling. Am J Respir Cell Mol Biol. 2018;59(4):490–9.
94. Nemoto M, et al. Combined pulmonary fibrosis and emphysema: a narrative review. Mayo Clin Proc. 2023;98(11):1685–96.
95. Ni H, et al. An increased risk of pulmonary hypertension in patients with combined pulmonary fibrosis and emphysema: a meta-analysis. BMC Pulm Med. 2023;23(1):221.

Chapter 2
Pericytes and Smooth Muscle Cells in the Pathogenesis of Pulmonary Arterial Hypertension

Timothy Klouda, Yunhye Kim, and Ke Yuan

Introduction

The lung comprises various cell populations that closely interact to facilitate essential physiological processes, including gas exchange, immune surveillance, and the removal of harmful environmental toxins. At the distal level of the lung, capillary endothelial cells (ECs) form a thin and delicate network (with a diameter of approximately 10 μm) that covers alveolar epithelial cells, facilitating efficient gas exchange. Perivascular mural cell populations, including pericytes (PCs) and smooth muscle cells (SMCs), provide crucial structural support to ECs within the microvasculature. PCs are mesenchymal-derived mural cells embedded in the basement membrane of the capillaries [1, 2]. They play essential roles in maintaining capillary homeostasis by regulating vascular tone and angiogenesis, providing structural support to the capillaries, and participating in repair processes responding to stimuli such as inflammation, infection, and hypoxia (Hx) [3, 4]. Due to their pivotal role in regulating and maintaining the integrity of the microvasculature, the absence or aberrant function of PCs may be associated with numerous chronic respiratory diseases. Dysfunction or a loss of PCs can lead to a miscommunication between PCs and the microvasculature, dedifferentiation of PCs into other mural cell populations, and the upregulation of pro-inflammatory pathways. These factors have been implicated in the pathogenesis of several pulmonary diseases, including

---

Authors Timothy Klouda and Yunhye Kim have contributed equally to this chapter.

T. Klouda · Y. Kim · K. Yuan (✉)
Division of Pulmonary Medicine, Boston Children's Hospital, Harvard Medical School, Boston, MA, USA
e-mail: Timothy.Klouda@childrens.harvard.edu; Yunhye.Kim@childrens.harvard.edu; ke.yuan@childrens.harvard.edu

F. N. Rahaghi et al. (eds.), *The Pulmonary Vasculature in Chronic Lung Disease*, Respiratory Medicine, https://doi.org/10.1007/978-3-032-03581-3_2

asthma, chronic obstructive pulmonary disease, and pulmonary arterial hypertension (PAH) [5, 6].

Pulmonary SMCs are organized into anatomical structures in arterioles, arteries, venules, and veins, each with diverse architectures reflecting its varied physiological functions. SMCs are crucial in regulating vascular tone and maintaining vessel integrity in response to external stimuli [7–9]. In the middle layer of vessels, SMCs surround ECs, regulating vessel stability, diameter, and blood flow through cell-to-cell communication between ECs and adventitial fibroblasts. SMCs demonstrate a remarkable capacity for context-dependent phenotypic changes, transitioning from non-synthetic contractile to synthetic proliferative states, with other cell characteristics such as fibroblast-like, macrophage-like, or adipogenic-like cells [10, 11]. This unique physiological plasticity and heterogeneity across different vascular beds have profound implications for the roles of SMCs in disease development and have been widely studied in injury response and the pathogenesis of cardiovascular diseases, including PAH.

Key pathological features in the lungs of patients with PAH are the obliteration and loss of the distal vasculature, thickening of the intima and media layers of blood vessels, increased extracellular matrix (ECM) deposition, and immune cell infiltration [12, 13]. These complex vascular lesions are characterized by an excessive accumulation of SMCs, ECs, fibroblasts, and various immune cells. The underlying molecular pathways and cell populations responsible for these vascular lesions are primarily proposed in a single-cell population. Developing effective therapeutic strategies requires a better understanding of the cell-to-cell interactions that drive vascular remodeling. Due to their common embryonic lineage (similarity to mesenchymal cells) and proximity to ECs, SMCs and PCs have been suggested to contribute to vascular remodeling and the development of PAH. In this section, we will review and examine the evidence supporting the involvement of PCs and SMCs in the development of PAH. Additionally, we will discuss future directions and current limitations in investigating the role of perivascular mural cells in PAH.

Pericytes in PAH

Abnormal Endothelial Cell and Pericyte Communication in PAH

The pulmonary capillaries comprise a thin layer of ECs that interact directly with epithelial cells to form the alveolar membrane. PCs are abundant in the lung's microvasculature (the EC to PC ratio is roughly 8:1) and interact with capillary ECs through direct contact and the release of various cytokines and growth factors. This communication between PCs and ECs is crucial for the microvasculature's formation, stabilization, and function [14]. While developing new blood vessels, PCs exert an anti-angiogenic effect, stabilizing newly formed vessels and limiting further proliferation and migration of ECs [15]. Signaling molecules and growth factors, including platelet-derived growth factor (PDGF), transforming growth factor beta (TGF-β), and angiopoietin-1 (ANG-1), play vital roles in regulating EC-pericyte interactions during homeostasis and have been implicated in regulating angiogenesis [16, 17]. Abnormal communication between PCs and capillary ECs can lead to the progression of various disease processes, including tumor angiogenesis, stoke, and PAH [18]. Table 2.1 summarizes the key literature relevant to PCs and the development of PAH discussed in this chapter.

In healthy lungs, PCs are abundant in pre-capillary, capillary, and post-capillary networks [19]. With their long, thin branches protruding from oval-shaped cell bodies, a single PC can support and interact with numerous ECs. However, examination of vascular lesions from patients with PAH reveals an accumulation of PCs in the medial and adventitial layers of blood vessels, in contrast to their almost exclusive presence in the intima of healthy vessels. The absence of PC-capillary communication can lead to EC dysfunction, loss of vessel integrity, inflammation, and ultimately, the loss of distal vasculature. While the Wnt signaling pathway is known to play a role in angiogenesis, its relationship to PC recruitment is unclear. Studies have shown that ECs isolated from patients with PAH exhibit an inability to recruit healthy PCs due to defective Wnt5a signaling, resulting in decreased PC coverage of the microvasculature [20]. Furthermore, PCs from patients with PAH, when seeded with healthy human microvascular ECs, demonstrate abnormal polarization toward the endothelium through abnormal signaling of the Wnt/planar cell polarity (PCP) pathway, forming a smaller vascular network. However, the restoration of the Wnt signaling in PAH PCs through upregulation of frizzled 7 (FZD7) and CDC42, two downstream genes crucial to the Wnt/PCP pathway that are reduced in PAH PCs, results in the formation of larger and improved vascular beds [21]. These studies suggest that Wnt5a production from microvascular ECs is essential for PC recruitment, and both PCs and ECs from patients with PAH exhibit abnormal signaling through the Wnt/PCP pathway, leading to a loss of distal vasculature and abnormal angiogenesis. Moreover, EC knock-out of Wnt5a in transgenic mice (Wnt5a$^{EC\text{-}KO}$) leads to irreversible Hx-induced PH and a reduced accumulation of PCs in microvasculature [20]. Although mice exposed to Hx did not develop exacerbated signs of PH compared to hypoxic wildtypes, Wnt5a$^{EC\text{-}KO}$ mice demonstrated persistent PH and RV dysfunction when returned to normoxic conditions, which correlated with reduced PC coverage in the microvessels [20]. Taken together, restoration of the Wnt pathway in PCs and ECs may stabilize the microvasculature and protect against the development of PAH.

The hypoxia-inducible factor (HIF) prolyl 4-hydroxylase-2 (PHD2) dysfunction has played a crucial role in developing PAH. Specifically, PHD2 deletion in ECs using an endothelial-specific PHD2 knock-out mouse model promotes the accumulation of PCs in the pulmonary arteries, leading to increased arterial media size and exacerbated pulmonary artery pressures [22]. The accumulation of PCs within arteries following PHD2 deletion in ECs is mediated by abnormal Ang1/Notch3 signaling. Deletion of PHD2 in transgenic mice results in higher levels of Ang1, leading to increased levels of Notch3. Notch signaling is highly conserved and has diverse functions across multiple organ systems, including stabilizing angiogenesis,

Table 2.1 Role of pericytes in the development of pulmonary arterial hypertension and associated pathways

Authors	Pathway	Key finding	References
Yuan et al., *Am J Respir Cell Mol Biol* (2020)	SDF1	NG2+ mural cells from patients with PAH demonstrate a genetic profile similar to PASMCs SDF1 knockout mice have reduced vascular remodeling SDF1 knockout in PAH PCs results in reduced contractility	[4]
Yuan et al., *Circulation* (2019)	Wnt5a	Wnt5a is a key mediator for healthy EC-PC interactions Loss of Wnt5a reduces the ability to form new vessels Wnt5a knockout mice demonstrate persistent PH and RV failure after exposure to Hx	[20]
Yuan et al., *Am J Pathol* (2015)	Wnt/PCP	Reduced expression of Wnt/PCP pathway genes (*Fzd7*, *cdc42*) causes reduced angiogenesis, motility and PC polarization toward PMVECs	[21]
Wang et al., *Oncotarget* (2016)	PHD2	EC PHD2 knockout in mice results in upregulated TGF-b and Notch3 expression and increased PC coverage on distal arterioles	[22]
Kim et al., *EMBO* (2024)	HIF2α	HIF2α overexpression in PCs increases cell contractility and impairs EC-PC interactions PC overexpression of HIF2α in mice results in exacerbated PH and RVH	[30]
Bordenave et al., *Cardiovascular Research* (2019)	Cxcl12/ Cxcr4	MCT and SU/Hx rats treated with Cxcl12 antagonist result in ameliorated PH and decreased PCs coverage on vasculature. Cxcl12 neutralization in PC and SMCs inhibits cell migration	[35]
Farkas et al., *PLoS One* (2014)	Cxcl12/ Cxcr4	Cxcl12 is upregulated in SU/Hx rats Cxcr4 inhibition decreases severity of PH in SU/Hx rats	[36]

(continued)

Table 2.1 (continued)

Authors	Pathway	Key finding	References
Bordenave et al., *Arterioscler Thromb Vasc Biol* (2020)	Cxcl12/ Cxcr4/ Cxcr7 TGF-βRII	PAH PCs overexpress Cxcr7 and TGF-βRII and have increased proliferation and differentiation into SMCs. The CXCL12/CXCR4/CXCR7 axis is required for PC accumulation in lungs in response to Hx The TGF-β/TGF-βRII axis plays a central role in PC differentiation into contractile cells	[37]
Ricard et al., *Circulation* (2014)	FGF-2 and IL-6	PAH PCs have increased proliferation and migration FGF-2 and IL-6 increase PC coverage of vasculature in retina TGF–β overexpression promotes PC differentiation into contractile SMCs	[38]
Yuan et al., *Am J Pathol* (2016)	PDK4	PDK4 expression is elevated in PAH PCs and associated with increased proliferation Reduced PDK4 expression in PAH PCs improves EC-PC interactions	[39]
Klouda et al., *Am J Respir Cell Mol Biol* (2023)	Cxcl12	In response to left pneumonectomy, NG2+ PC from mice upregulate Cxcl12 expression	[40]
Pienkos et al., *Front Med* (2021)	TNIP2 and TRAF2	Knockdown of TNIP2 and TRAF2 increases NF-κB activity and proliferation in healthy PCs	[42]

EC endothelial cells, *Hx* hypoxia, *MCT* monocrotaline, *PAH* pulmonary arterial hypertension, *PASMCs* pulmonary artery smooth muscle cells, *PC* pericytes, *PH* pulmonary hypertension, *PMVEC* pulmonary microvascular endothelial cells, *RVH* right ventricle hypertrophy, *SMC* smooth muscle cells, *SU* Sugen-5416

promoting neuronal development, and expanding hematopoietic stem cells [23]. Activation of Notch receptors in perivascular cells results in PC maturation, as evidenced by increased expression of α-SMA. Studies have shown that deletion of Notch1 and Notch3 in mice results in a global loss of PCs and increased vascular leakage, indicating that Notch signaling is crucial for proper PC-EC formation [24]. In humans, Notch3 expression is concentrated in distal pulmonary arterioles and highly expressed in SMCs, making it a potential target for future PAH treatments focusing on SMCs and PCs [24, 25].

Pericyte Differentiation into SMC-Like Cells in Vascular Remodeling

A key pathological feature of the distal pulmonary arterioles of patients with PAH is the excessive accumulation of SMCs. The potential for PCs to differentiate into other mural cell populations, including SMCs, makes them an attractive target for potential disease-modifying therapies [26, 27]. Because SMCs and PCs exhibit similar cell markers and both closely interact with ECs in the pulmonary vasculature, the transformation of PCs into SMC-like cells is suspected to play a role in vascular remodeling and disease progression. Bulk RNA-seq analysis of human lungs obtained from patients with PAH has revealed that PCs and SMCs share a similar transcriptional pattern, and PCs expressing α-SMA have increased contractility [4]. This data suggests that PCs in the lung may represent a contractile, α-SMA expressing cell similar to myofibroblasts, contributing to vascular remodeling in PAH. Further analyses of single-cell RNA sequence (scRNA-seq) revealed an increase of oxygen-sensing mural cells located in close proximity to remodeled vessels, with a notable increase in *NDUFA4L2*, a gene with functions in the electron chain of mitochondria and associated with the development of Hx-induced PH [28, 29]. Using scRNAseq from patients with idiopathic pulmonary arterial hypertension (IPAH) and Hx-induced pulmonary hypertension (PH) mouse models, *EPAS1*(gene name for HIF2α) was identified as a major molecular regulator for the transformation of pericytes into SMC-like cells. PC-selective HIF2α overexpression in mice exacerbates PH and right ventricular hypertrophy [30]. While human and rodent studies have provided insight into the potential of PCs to transition into other mural cells and contribute to the development of PAH, the underlying mechanisms and pathways responsible for such transition still need investigation.

SDF-1 (Cxcl12) is a pro-angiogenic chemokine with roles promoting angiogenesis, inflammation, and cell migration [32, 33]. It is upregulated in both SMCs and PCs from patients with PAH, and elevated serum levels are associated with increased mean right atrial pressures, serving as an independent risk factor for mortality [4. 28, 34]. Furthermore, knock-out of SDF-1 in NG2+ mural cells is protective against the development of Hx-induced PH, and SDF-1 stimulation results in proliferation and increased contractility of healthy PCs [4]AMD3100 inhibits CXCR4, a receptor for SDF-1, leading to amelioration of PH in Hx-induced mice and the SU-5416 and MCT-rat models of PAH [4, 35, 36]. Despite substantial evidence implicating SDF-1 in the development of PAH, the downstream molecules resulting in disease development and the stimuli resulting in SDF-1 upregulation remain unknown. CXCR7, a receptor specific for SDF-1, is required to accumulate PCs in Hx-induced vascular remodeling, while the TGF-β/TGF-βRII pathway differentiates PCs into contractile SMCs [37]. Further evidence for the role of TGF-β in PC-mediated vascular remodeling in PAH is provided by cultured PCs from patients with PAH, which, when treated with TGF-β1, differentiated into contractile SMC-like cells [38]. A hyperproliferative phenotype observed in PAH PCs is associated with upregulated pyruvate dehydrogenase kinase 4 (PDK4), an enzyme that prevents the conversion of pyruvate to acetyl-CoA, promoting glycolysis. Reducing levels of PDK4 in PCs restores mitochondrial activity and improves EC-PC interactions [39]. Furthermore, PDK isoforms are overexpressed in SMCs from the lungs of patients with PAH, promoting cell longevity by suppressing apoptosis [39].

Given the transcriptomic and phenotypic similarities between PCs and SMCs in patients with PAH, mural cells may exhibit similar responses to inflammatory stimuli, leading to remodeling of the distal vasculature. Additionally, shear stress of the vasculature can result in PC overexpression of SDF-1 and other pathways, which contributes to vascular remodeling and the development of PH, as seen in the left pneumonectomy mouse model [40]. To better understand the relationship between SDF-1, inflammation, and angiogenesis, it is necessary to identify the exogenous stimuli and downstream molecules that result in pericyte overexpression of SDF-1.

Alongside impaired endothelium and PC communication promoting vascular remodeling, an enhanced and increased inflammatory response can also contribute to the development of PAH. The accumulation of inflammatory cells, including macrophages, dendritic cells, monocytes, and T cell subsets (CD3+, CD8+, CD4+), are found near the vascular lesions of patients with PAH [41]. Whole genome sequencing on patients with PAH from two families revealed deficits in TNIP2 and TRAF2, proteins that regulate the activity of NF-kβ [42]. NF-kβ is a transcription factor that targets numerous genes associated with inflammation, which can also directly increase the production of proinflammatory chemokines, including IL-6, TNF-α, and IL-2 [43]. Knockdown of these genes (TNIP2 and TRAF2) in healthy lung PCs increased NF-kβ and promoted cell proliferation, proving that PCs can respond to inflammation and contribute to vascular remodeling [42]. IL-6 and FGF-2 released from ECs promote the migration of PCs from the microvasculature to distal arterioles. Treatment with TGF-β1 further increases their proliferation, migration, and differentiation into SMC-like cells [38]. Altered PDGF-β signaling in the lung has been shown to protect against Hx-induced vascular remodeling. PDGF-β $^{ret/ret}$ mice, with downregulated PDGF-β activity, exhibit highly disorganized and less severe vascular remodeling than wild type (WT) mice, resulting in ameliorated PH hemodynamics [44]. While PDGFRβ blockade is possible with medications such as imatinib, the global and widespread expression of this cell marker results in damaging side effects when used as a medication for PAH. This highlights the need for more cell-targeted therapies aimed at specific cell types [45].

SMCs in PAH

Genetic Mechanisms

Mutations in bone morphogenetic receptor 2 (BMPR2) are present in 70% of patients with familial PAH and 20% of hereditary PAH [46]. PAH pulmonary artery smooth muscle cells (PASMC) with abnormal BMPR2 exhibit their hyper-proliferative state and hence contribute to lesion formation and progressive obliteration of the pulmonary circulation due to abnormal metabolism, DNA damage, impaired activation of PPARγ, and an increase in aldehyde dehydrogenase 1 family member A3 (ALDH1A3) [47–49]. Other PAH-related genes, including *ACVRL1*, *ENG*, *GDF2*, *BMP10*, and *KCNK3*, have been associated with SMC depolarization, proliferation, resistance to apoptosis, and contraction.

Loss of BMPR2 impairs PASMC motility [50]. Impaired contractility due to reduced BMPR2 increases pERK1/2-pP38-pSMAD2/3, upregulating ARRB2 and pAKT causing GSK3β inactivation and CTNNB1 mediated heightened proliferation, as well as reduced RHOA and RAC1 signaling [51]. By modulating the post-translational modifications of the BMP/TGF-β pathway via the ALK2-Smad1/5/9-PPARγ axis, BRCC3 acts as an antagonist for SMURF3. It may play a role in preventing pulmonary vascular remodeling, thereby inhibiting the pathogenesis of PAH [52]. Other studies have emphasized dysfunctional SMAD signaling, impaired contractile gene expression, and amplification of abnormalities with endothelin-1 [53–55].

The imbalance of TGF-β and BMP signaling pathways in SMC has emerged as a significant factor in the pathogenesis of PAH. Accumulating evidence suggests a shift toward TGF-β–activating signaling in human PAH, even in the absence of mutations in members of the TGF-β superfamily. This shift increases the risk of developing PAH and is strongly suspected of contributing to disease pathogenesis by modulating cell survival, metabolism, inflammation, genome instability, migration, and cell differentiation [56, 57]. While the focus has predominantly been on BMPR2 in pulmonary artery endothelial cells (PAECs), the functional and molecular connection between loss of BMPR2 and TGF-β signaling and the development of PAH requires further investigation. IPAH patients had higher serum and pulmonary TGF-β levels, and PAH PASMC are highly proliferative and apoptosis-resistant [58]. These hyperproliferative phenotypes in PAH PASMCs are mediated by Smad1/5/8 phosphorylation and the production of fibroblast growth factor 2 (FGF2) and PDGF-β. Conversely, BMP-2/BMP receptor type II (BMP-RII) signaling confers protective effects against PAH by inhibiting proliferation and fibrosis of PASMCs. However, loss of BMPR2 in SMCs contributes to pathological arterial remodeling in PAH. The underlying mechanisms involve multiple signaling pathways, including disruption of peroxisome proliferator-activated receptor gamma (PPARγ) signaling or the upregulation of phosphorylated extracellular signal-regulated kinase 1/2 (pERK1/2), phosphorylated p38 (pP38), phosphorylated Smad2/3 (pSMAD2/3), and β-arrestin2 (ARRB2) [59–61]. PPARγ serves as a molecular link between BMP-2 and TGF-β pathways in SMCs by inhibiting TGF-β/STAT3 and TGF-β/Smad3 pathways [62]. Functional evidence further supports the role of BMP signaling: BMPR2 knockdown by small interference RNA in both healthy PASMC and PASMC from patients with PAH significantly reduced SMC proliferation. Thus, these finding suggest that selectively targeting TGF-β with enhancement of BMP signaling may offer a promising approach for treating PAH.

Noncoding RNAs in PAH

There is a growing amount of evidence suggesting that epigenetic mechanisms play a crucial role in mediating gene-environment interactions associated with PAH. Epigenetics refers to heritable changes in gene activity that do not alter the primary DNA sequence or genotypes. These modifications involve DNA methylation, histone acetylation, methylation, and noncoding RNAs (ncRNAs).

ncRNAs are emerging as promising biomarkers for risk stratification in PH due to their stability, ease of collection, and detectability at low levels via amplification [63, 64]. The miR-130/301 family has been identified as a master regulator for cell proliferation through STAT3-signaling and can activate vasoconstriction in PASMC [65, 66]. This family of micro-RNAs (miRNAs) is induced by Hx and affects gene expression through PPARγ, regulating endothelin-1 (ET-1) expression [65]. The miR-130/301 axis is a central pathway involving multiple genes associated with heritable PAH, perivascular remodeling, and arterial stiffening [67, 68]. Other Hx-stimulated pathways, such as HIF-1α, upregulate miR-9, which promotes PASMC differentiation by suppressing contractile genes and enhancing proliferation [69]. RPS4L also mediates PASMC proliferation via ILF3/HIF-1α [70]. Additionally, the miR-200 cluster is a central regulator of SMC quiescence and is significantly downregulated after SMC dedifferentiation induced by PDGF-β. Dysregulated expression of BMPR2 is regulated by miR-17/92 [71]. MiR-204 directly targets SHP2, and its downregulation correlates with PAH severity and accounts for the proliferative and anti-apoptotic phenotypes of PAH PASMCs [72]. MiR-21 also plays a significant role in Hx-induced pulmonary vascular SMC proliferation and migration by targeting programmed cell death protein 4 (PDCD4), Sprouty 2 (SPRY2), and peroxisome proliferator-activated receptor-α (PPARα) [73].

Long noncoding RNAs (LncRNAs) regulate mRNA expression primarily by interacting with miRNAs, forming complex lncRNA-miRNA-mRNA coregulatory networks. Among them, metastasis-associated lung adenocarcinoma transcript 1 (MALAT1) is consistently upregulated in pulmonary arteries, PASMCs, and plasma derived from PAH patients. Increased expression of MALAT1 promotes PASMC proliferation, migration, and cell cycle progression, while inhibiting apoptosis through the miR-124-3p.1/KLF5 and miR-503/TLR4 axis [74]. Beyond MALAT1, other lncRNAs have also been implicated in PAH pathogenesis. LncRNA TUG1 expression was increased in hypoxic PASMCs and total lung tissues from PAH patients, acting through interactions with multiple miRNAs and their target mRNAs. Similarly, overexpression of H19 induced cell proliferation through the let-7b/AT1R axis, whereas knockout of H19 protected against the development of PH [75]. As detection methods for ncRNAs become more accessible, larger studies to validate their potential as biomarkers for disease severity and therapeutic response.

Hypoxia and Metabolism

Metabolic abnormalities are commonly observed in human PAH and animal models of PH. These abnormalities are characterized by a shift to glycolysis, increased glutamine utilization, one-carbon metabolism, and decreased fatty acid oxidation [76, 77]. The increased generation of reactive oxygen species (ROS) and changes in tricarboxylic acid (TCA) cycle intermediates may contribute to the stabilization of HIF, driving the observed metabolic changes. Arginine metabolism, which links nitric oxide (NO) production and the TCA cycle, plays a key role in connecting the vasoconstrictive phenotype of the disease with metabolic abnormalities. The metabolic phenotype of PAH resembles that of proliferative cells, such as those found in cancer. Therefore, therapies targeting metabolism in cancer may also be relevant in addressing the hyperproliferation seen in PAH SMCs.

SMCs are functionally classified as either contractile or synthetic. Contractile SMCs are regarded as differentiated and quiescent cells under physiological conditions, expressing a panel of typical contractile proteins crucial to maintaining vascular tension. ScRNA-seq analyses consistently identified contractile SMCs as the predominant cell type within the healthy vessel wall, characterized by the transcriptomic profile delineated [78]. However, through the integration of extensive lineage tracing studies, additional SMC subpopulations exhibiting distinct gene expression signatures have been identified [28]. During the development of PAH, PASMCs undergo phenotypic and functional alterations characterized by enhanced proliferation, increased migratory capacities, and metabolic reprogramming. Notably, IPAH SMCs exhibit upregulation of ADGRG6/GPR126, an adhesion G protein-coupled receptor (GPCR), compared to control PASMCs [79]. Genes associated with proliferation, such as cyclin B1 (CCNB1), cyclin-dependent kinase 1 (CDK1), and the transcription factor forkhead box protein M1 (FOXM1), are also significantly increased in IPAH-PASMCs [80, 81].

Metabolic adaptations play a crucial role in driving PASMC proliferation. Increased expression of histone methylase family (JMJC) and aldehyde dehydrogenase family 1 member 3 (ALDH1A3) in response to Hx-induced PH promotes PASMC proliferation through glycolysis flux [82, 83]. Contrary to the Warburg effect which is characterized by increased glycolytic metabolism, augmented NADPH oxidase (Nox) activity and enhanced pentose phosphate pathway (PPP) flux have been identified as independent mechanisms supporting PASMC proliferation [82]. These metabolic adaptations underscore the complex interplay between cellular metabolism and proliferative responses in PASMCs during PAH pathogenesis.

A subset of SMCs expressing the pluripotency factor Kruppel-like factor 4 (KLF4) has been identified at the muscular-nonmuscular border of pulmonary arterioles in Hx-induced PH [84]. These KLF4-expressing SMC serve as progenitor cells for the muscularization of distal arterioles. They express the mesenchymal marker PDGFR-β and migrate into distal sites, where they undergo dedifferentiation and clonal expansion. They ultimately contribute to the pool of distal SMCs in a HIF1-α-dependent manner [84, 85]. Moreover, KLF4 expression is also observed in proliferating SMCs from PAH patients [84]. This underscores the pivotal role of KLF4 as an initiator of phenotypic switching and neointimal thickening [86–88]. The induction of KLF4 expression contributes to hyperproliferation and drives phenotypic switching towards a fibroblast-like state in lung tissue and promotes collagen synthesis in other tissues [89, 90]. This dual impact suggests potential therapeutic targets for mitigating the pathological processes associated with vascular remodeling in PAH. Further studies into the mechanisms by which Hx drives SMCs dedifferentiation into synthetic and proliferative states will provide valuable insights for developing targeted therapies.

Other Pathways to Affect SMC in Vascular Remodeling During PAH Development

Ion channels, exchangers, and pumps play an important role in systemic and pulmonary vasculature by controlling Ca2+ homeostasis, vascular tone, angiogenesis, cellular proliferation/apoptosis, and diverse cellular processes. The resting membrane potential of PASMC mainly regulates pulmonary arterial tone and, hence, arterial diameter. Resting membrane potential, intracellular ion homeostasis, and cell volume are controlled by membrane permeability to cations Na^+, Ca^{2+}, K^+, and anions Cl^- and bicarbonate. Ion channels are ubiquitous and constitutively active or modulated by several stimuli, such as signaling molecules or membrane potential changes. Identified mutations or polymorphisms in ion channels demonstrate their crucial role in PAH. In 2013, six mutations were identified in the *KCNK3* gene (Potassium Channel, Subfamily K, Member 3) in PAH patients [91]. Moreover, single-nucleotide polymorphisms (SNPs) in the *KCNA5* gene (Potassium Voltage-Gated Channel Subfamily A Member 5) and in the promoter region of *TRPC6* (Transient Receptor Potential Canonical 6) have been associated with increased susceptibility to IPAH [92–94].

Common SMC molecular hallmarks are well-established, such as smooth muscle protein 22-alpha (SM22α/TAGLN), calponin (CNN1), smooth muscle actin (ACTA2), and smooth muscle myosin heavy chain (MYH11). The latter two are regulated by the transcription factor serum responsive factor (SRF) and its coactivator myocardin (MYOCD) [78, 95–99]. Under pathophysiological conditions, exposure to soluble factors such as PDGF-BB, TGF-β, activin, or TNF-α, promotes PASMCs to undergo dedifferentiation into synthetic SMCs, accompanied by downregulation of most contractile markers. scRNA-seq analyses have further confirmed SMCs phenotypic switching toward a synthetic state in PAH arteries. Moreover, ECM remodeling, such as collagen accumulation contributes to vascular fibrosis and decreased compliance of pulmonary arteries in PAH. Patients with PAH exhibit increased expression of genes encoding fibril-associated collagen (COL14A1), network-forming collagen (COL4A5), and endostatin-producing collagen (COL18A1) in the intima and media of the pulmonary arteries [100]. Aberrant endothelial and SMC interaction and cross-talk, including communication via cellular injunctions and extracellular vesicles, also play important roles in regulating cell phenotypes [101].

Current Limitations and Future Direction

Despite the evidence describing PCs' contribution to the development of PAH, a significant limitation in studying PCs is the inability to distinguish them from other mural cell populations due to the lack of a universal and specific cell marker. Commonly used PC markers in the lung including *CSPG4* (gene name for NG2) and *PDGFRB*, are expressed in other mural cell populations [102]. Therefore, current lineage tracing studies cannot precisely determine the roles of PCs during disease progress. Moreover, the heterogeneity of PC markers across various organ systems poses challenges in investigating their function and contribution to disease development. Currently, the identification of pulmonary PCs depends on using shared cell markers with other mural cells and relying on their location in the capillary network and distinct appearance, such as an oval-shaped cell body with multiple processes partially encircling the endothelium [103]. However, until unique markers are identified, their propensity to migrate and differentiate into other cell populations in response to stimuli makes interpreting cell-lineage studies and the identification of PCs in human histological and transcriptomic studies, most of which focus on end-stage disease, challenging. A recent scRNA-seq analysis has identified *HIGD1B* as a potential pericyte-specific cell marker in the heart and lungs of humans and mice, making it a promising cell maker for future studies [104]. Recent advances in bioinformatics techniques, including scRNA-seq, spatial transcriptomic, proteomics, metabolomics, network analysis, systems biology, and gene-modifiable mice, will allow for a deeper understanding of discerning the role of PCs in the development of PAH. Big data and computational modeling will also provide tools by which we can address the questions of how mural cells in PAH develop and determine which pathways are ideal therapeutic targets.

There is much to learn about PCs and their contribution to PAH and vascular remodeling through genetic and epigenetic mechanistic studies. While their ability to differentiate into other cell types and key roles regulating angiogenesis and microvascular stability make them an ideal target for regenerative therapeutics, it is first essential to identify the underlying molecular pathways contributing to disease development. Future work is needed to elucidate these pathways and determine if morphological and genetic changes in PCs contribute to disease development or are a physiological response to injury and inflammation. Although current therapies predominantly focus on vasodilation by targeting dysregulated pathways in PAH—such as inhibiting endothelin-1 signaling or boosting downstream mediators of the prostacyclin and NO pathways—the recent approval of Sotatercept by the U.S Food and Drug Administration (FDA) presents a novel approach. Sotatercept, an

IgG–activin receptor type IIA (ActRIIA) fusion protein, acts by sequestering activin and other TGFβ ligands, thereby dampening this signaling cascade. Since ActRIIA signaling negatively regulates BMPR2 signaling, Sotatercept holds potential therapeutic benefits for PAH treatment. However, despite clinically meaningful improvements, further investigations are required to evaluate these treatments' long-term efficacy and safety.

Understanding the context-specific nature of PC and SMC biology in the pathogenesis of PAH will be crucial for guiding the development of novel therapeutic approaches targeting one specific cell type at one time. Given the lack of disease-modifying therapies for patients with PAH and the associated morbidity and mortality with disease progression, expanding our knowledge of PC and SMC biology in physiological and pathological conditions will provide new and exciting information that can be applied to improve patient outcomes. Thus, continued research efforts to unravel the mechanisms underlying PC and SMC involvement in disease pathophysiology are warranted.

References

1. Warren E, Gerecht S. Beyond the endothelium: the role of mural cells in vascular biology: in vitro systems to study endothelial/pericyte cell interactions. Vasc Biol. 2023;5.
2. Yuan K, Agarwal S, Chakraborty A, Condon DF, Patel H, Zhang S, Huang F, Mello SA, Kirk OI, Vasquez R, de Jesus Perez VA. Lung pericytes in pulmonary vascular physiology and pathophysiology. Compr Physiol. 2021;11:2227–47.
3. Hellström M, Gerhardt H, Kalén M, Li X, Eriksson U, Wolburg H, Betsholtz C. Lack of pericytes leads to endothelial hyperplasia and abnormal vascular morphogenesis. J Cell Biol. 2001;153:543–53.
4. Yuan K, Liu Y, Zhang Y, Nathan A, Tian W, Yu J, Sweatt AJ, Shamshou EA, Condon D, Chakraborty A, Agarwal S, Auer N, Zhang S, Wu JC, Zamanian RT, Nicolls MR, de Jesus Perez VA. Mural cell SDF1 signaling is associated with the pathogenesis of pulmonary arterial hypertension. Am J Respir Cell Mol Biol. 2020;62:747–59. https://doi.org/10.1165/rcmb.2019-0401OC.
5. Garrison AT, Bignold RE, Wu X, Johnson JR. Pericytes: the lung-forgotten cell type. Front Physiol. 2023;14:1150028.
6. Joulia R, Puttur F, Stolting H, Traves WJ, Entwistle LJ, Voitovich A, Garcia Martin M, Al-Sahaf M, Bonner K, Scotney E, Molyneaux PL, Hewitt RJ, Walker SA, Yates L, Saglani S, Lloyd CM. Mast cell activation disrupts interactions between endothelial cells and pericytes during early life allergic asthma. J Clin Invest. 2024;134.
7. Galie N, Manes A, Branzi A. The endothelin system in pulmonary arterial hypertension. Cardiovasc Res. 2004;61:227–37.
8. Quyyumi AA, Dakak N, Andrews NP, Gilligan DM, Panza JA, Cannon RO 3rd. Contribution of nitric oxide to metabolic coronary vasodilation in the human heart. Circulation. 1995;92:320–6.
9. Brozovich FV, Nicholson CJ, Degen CV, Gao YZ, Aggarwal M, Morgan KG. Mechanisms of vascular smooth muscle contraction and the basis for pharmacologic treatment of smooth muscle disorders. Pharmacol Rev. 2016;68:476–532.
10. Bennett MR, Sinha S, Owens GK. Vascular smooth muscle cells in atherosclerosis. Circ Res. 2016;118:692–702.

11. Yap C, Mieremet A, de Vries CJM, Micha D, de Waard V. Six shades of vascular smooth muscle cells illuminated by KLF4 (Kruppel-Like Factor 4). Arterioscler Thromb Vasc Biol. 2021;41:2693–707.
12. Stacher E, Graham BB, Hunt JM, Gandjeva A, Groshong SD, McLaughlin VV, Jessup M, Grizzle WE, Aldred MA, Cool CD, Tuder RM. Modern age pathology of pulmonary arterial hypertension. Am J Respir Crit Care Med. 2012;186:261–72.
13. Tuder RM, Marecki JC, Richter A, Fijalkowska I, Flores S. Pathology of pulmonary hypertension. Clin Chest Med. 2007;28(23-42):vii.
14. Li G, Gao J, Ding P, Gao Y. The role of endothelial cell–pericyte interactions in vascularization and diseases. J Adv Res. 2024.
15. Sweeney M, Foldes G. It takes two: endothelial-perivascular cell cross-talk in vascular development and disease. Front Cardiovasc Med. 2018;5:154.
16. Lee S, Elaskandrany M, Lau LF, Lazzaro D, Grant MB, Chaqour B. Interplay between CCN1 and Wnt5a in endothelial cells and pericytes determines the angiogenic outcome in a model of ischemic retinopathy. Sci Rep. 2017;7:1405.
17. Ribatti D, Nico B, Crivellato E. The role of pericytes in angiogenesis. Int J Dev Biol. 2011;55:261–8.
18. Armulik A, Abramsson A, Betsholtz C. Endothelial/pericyte interactions. Circ Res. 2005;97:512–23.
19. Wu Y, Fu J, Huang Y, Duan R, Zhang W, Wang C, Wang S, Hu X, Zhao H, Wang L, Liu J, Gao G, Yuan P. Biology and function of pericytes in the vascular microcirculation. Anim Models Exp Med. 2023;6:337–45.
20. Yuan K, Shamskhou EA, Orcholski ME, Nathan A, Reddy S, Honda H, Mani V, Zeng Y, Ozen MO, Wang L, Demirci U, Tian W, Nicolls MR, de Jesus Perez VA. Loss of endothelium-derived Wnt5a is associated with reduced pericyte recruitment and small vessel loss in pulmonary arterial hypertension. Circulation. 2019;139:1710–24.
21. Yuan K, Orcholski ME, Panaroni C, Shuffle EM, Huang NF, Jiang X, Tian W, Vladar EK, Wang L, Nicolls MR, Wu JY, de Jesus Perez VA. Activation of the Wnt/planar cell polarity pathway is required for pericyte recruitment during pulmonary angiogenesis. Am J Pathol. 2015;185:69–84.
22. Wang S, Zeng H, Xie XJ, Tao YK, He X, Roman RJ, Aschner JL, Chen JX. Loss of prolyl hydroxylase domain protein 2 in vascular endothelium increases pericyte coverage and promotes pulmonary arterial remodeling. Oncotarget. 2016;7:58848–61.
23. Kopan R. Notch signaling. Cold Spring Harb Perspect Biol. 2012;4.
24. Kofler NM, Cuervo H, Uh MK, Murtomäki A, Kitajewski J. Combined deficiency of Notch1 and Notch3 causes pericyte dysfunction, models CADASIL, and results in arteriovenous malformations. Sci Rep. 2015 Nov 13;5:16449. https://doi.org/10.1038/srep16449. PMID: 26563570; PMCID: PMC4643246.
25. Li X, Zhang X, Leathers R, Makino A, Huang C, Parsa P. et al. (2009) Notch3 signaling promotes the development of pulmonary arterial hypertension. Nat. Med. 15, 1289–1297 https://doi.org/10.1038/nm.2021.
26. Hosaka K, Yang Y, Seki T, Fischer C, Dubey O, Fredlund E, Hartman J, Religa P, Morikawa H, Ishii Y, Sasahara M, Larsson O, Cossu G, Cao R, Lim S, Cao Y. Pericyte-fibroblast transition promotes tumor growth and metastasis. Proc Natl Acad Sci USA. 2016;113:E5618–27.
27. Volz KS, Jacobs AH, Chen HI, Poduri A, McKay AS, Riordan DP, Kofler N, Kitajewski J, Weissman I, Red-Horse K. Pericytes are progenitors for coronary artery smooth muscle. elife. 2015;4:e10036.
28. Crnkovic S, Valzano F, Fließer E, Gindlhuber J, Thekkekara Puthenparampil H, Basil M, Morley MP, Katzen J, Gschwandtner E, Klepetko W, Cantu E, Wolinski H, Olschewski H, Lindenmann J, Zhao YY, Morrisey EE, Marsh LM, Kwapiszewska G. Single-cell transcriptomics reveals skewed cellular communication and phenotypic shift in pulmonary artery remodeling. JCI Insight. 2022;7.

29. Liu Y, Nie X, Zhu J, Wang T, Li Y, Wang Q, Sun Z. NDUFA4L2 in smooth muscle promotes vascular remodeling in hypoxic pulmonary arterial hypertension. J Cell Mol Med. 2021;25:1221–37.
30. Kim H, Liu Y, Kim J, Kim Y, Klouda T, Fisch S, Baek SH, Liu T, Dahlberg S, Hu CJ, Tian W, Jiang X, Kosmas K, Christou HA, Korman BD, Vargas SO, Wu JC, Stenmark KR, Perez VJ, Nicolls MR, Raby BA, Yuan K. Pericytes contribute to pulmonary vascular remodeling via HIF2α signaling. EMBO Rep. 2024;25:616–45.
31. Liao D, Corle C, Seagroves TN, Johnson RS. Hypoxia-inducible factor-1alpha is a key regulator of metastasis in a transgenic model of cancer initiation and progression. Cancer Res. 2007;67:563–72.
32. Zhang M, Qiu L, Zhang Y, Xu D, Zheng JC, Jiang L. CXCL12 enhances angiogenesis through CXCR7 activation in human umbilical vein endothelial cells. Sci Rep. 2017;7:8289.
33. Cambier S, Gouwy M, Proost P. The chemokines CXCL8 and CXCL12: molecular and functional properties, role in disease and efforts towards pharmacological intervention. Cell Mol Immunol. 2023;20:217–51.
34. McCullagh BN, Costello CM, Li L, O'Connell C, Codd M, Lawrie A, Morton A, Kiely DG, Condliffe R, Elliot C, McLoughlin P, Gaine S. Elevated plasma CXCL12α is associated with a poorer prognosis in pulmonary arterial hypertension. PLoS One. 2015;10:e0123709.
35. Bordenave J, Thuillet R, Tu L, Phan C, Cumont A, Marsol C, Huertas A, Savale L, Hibert M, Galzi J-L, Bonnet D, Humbert M, Frossard N, Guignabert C. Neutralization of CXCL12 attenuates established pulmonary hypertension in rats. Cardiovasc Res. 2019;116:686–97.
36. Farkas D, Kraskauskas D, Drake JI, Alhussaini AA, Kraskauskiene V, Bogaard HJ, Cool CD, Voelkel NF, Farkas L. CXCR4 inhibition ameliorates severe obliterative pulmonary hypertension and accumulation of C-kit$^+$ cells in rats. PLoS One. 2014;9:e89810.
37. Bordenave J, Tu L, Berrebeh N, Thuillet R, Cumont A, Le Vely B, Fadel E, Nadaud S, Savale L, Humbert M, Huertas A, Guignabert C. Lineage tracing reveals the dynamic contribution of pericytes to the blood vessel remodeling in pulmonary hypertension. Arterioscler Thromb Vasc Biol. 2020;40:766–82.
38. Ricard N, Tu L, Le Hiress M, Huertas A, Phan C, Thuillet R, Sattler C, Fadel E, Seferian A, Montani D, Dorfmüller P, Humbert M, Guignabert C. Increased pericyte coverage mediated by endothelial-derived fibroblast growth factor-2 and interleukin-6 is a source of smooth muscle-like cells in pulmonary hypertension. Circulation. 2014;129:1586–97.
39. Yuan K, Shao NY, Hennigs JK, Discipulo M, Orcholski ME, Shamskhou E, Richter A, Hu X, Wu JC, de Jesus Perez VA. Increased pyruvate dehydrogenase kinase 4 expression in lung pericytes is associated with reduced endothelial-pericyte interactions and small vessel loss in pulmonary arterial hypertension. Am J Pathol. 2016;186:2500–14.
40. Klouda T, Tsikis ST, Kim H, Liu T, Visner G, Fernandez-Gonzalez A, Kourembanas S, Puder M, Raby B, Yuan K. Pericytes contribute to flow-induced pulmonary hypertension. Am J Respir Cell Mol Biol. 2023;68:705–8.
41. Savai R, Pullamsetti SS, Kolbe J, Bieniek E, Voswinckel R, Fink L, Scheed A, Ritter C, Dahal BK, Vater A, Klussmann S, Ghofrani HA, Weissmann N, Klepetko W, Banat GA, Seeger W, Grimminger F, Schermuly RT. Immune and inflammatory cell involvement in the pathology of idiopathic pulmonary arterial hypertension. Am J Respir Crit Care Med. 2012;186:897–908.
42. Pienkos S, Gallego N, Condon DF, Cruz-Utrilla A, Ochoa N, Nevado J, Arias P, Agarwal S, Patel H, Chakraborty A, Lapunzina P, Escribano P, Tenorio-Castaño J, de Jesús Pérez VA. Novel TNIP2 and TRAF2 variants are implicated in the pathogenesis of pulmonary arterial hypertension. Front Med (Lausanne). 2021;8:625763.
43. Liu T, Zhang L, Joo D, Sun S-C. NF-κB signaling in inflammation. Sign Transduct Target Ther. 2017;2:17023.
44. Tannenberg P, Chang YT, Muhl L, Laviña B, Gladh H, Genové G, Betsholtz C, Folestad E, Tran-Lundmark K. Extracellular retention of PDGF-B directs vascular remodel-

ing in mouse hypoxia-induced pulmonary hypertension. Am J Phys Lung Cell Mol Phys. 2018;314:L593–l605.
45. Hoeper MM, Barst RJ, Bourge RC, Feldman J, Frost AE, Galié N, Gómez-Sánchez MA, Grimminger F, Grünig E, Hassoun PM, Morrell NW, Peacock AJ, Satoh T, Simonneau G, Tapson VF, Torres F, Lawrence D, Quinn DA, Ghofrani HA. Imatinib mesylate as add-on therapy for pulmonary arterial hypertension: results of the randomized IMPRES study. Circulation. 2013;127:1128–38.
46. International PPHC, Lane KB, Machado RD, Pauciulo MW, Thomson JR, Phillips JA 3rd, Loyd JE, Nichols WC, Trembath RC. Heterozygous germline mutations in BMPR2, encoding a TGF-beta receptor, cause familial primary pulmonary hypertension. Nat Genet. 2000;26:81–4.
47. Sutendra G, Bonnet S, Rochefort G, Haromy A, Folmes KD, Lopaschuk GD, Dyck JR, Michelakis ED. Fatty acid oxidation and malonyl-CoA decarboxylase in the vascular remodeling of pulmonary hypertension. Sci Transl Med. 2010;2:44ra58.
48. Meloche J, Pflieger A, Vaillancourt M, Paulin R, Potus F, Zervopoulos S, Graydon C, Courboulin A, Breuils-Bonnet S, Tremblay E, Couture C, Michelakis ED, Provencher S, Bonnet S. Role for DNA damage signaling in pulmonary arterial hypertension. Circulation. 2014;129:786–97.
49. Hansmann G, de Jesus Perez VA, Alastalo TP, Alvira CM, Guignabert C, Bekker JM, Schellong S, Urashima T, Wang L, Morrell NW, Rabinovitch M. An antiproliferative BMP-2/PPARgamma/apoE axis in human and murine SMCs and its role in pulmonary hypertension. J Clin Invest. 2008;118:1846–57.
50. Spiekerkoetter E, Guignabert C, de Jesus Perez V, Alastalo TP, Powers JM, Wang L, Lawrie A, Ambartsumian N, Schmidt AM, Berryman M, Ashley RH, Rabinovitch M. S100A4 and bone morphogenetic protein-2 codependently induce vascular smooth muscle cell migration via phospho-extracellular signal-regulated kinase and chloride intracellular channel 4. Circ Res. 2009;105:639–47, 13 p following 47.
51. Perez VA, Ali Z, Alastalo TP, Ikeno F, Sawada H, Lai YJ, Kleisli T, Spiekerkoetter E, Qu X, Rubinos LH, Ashley E, Amieva M, Dedhar S, Rabinovitch M. BMP promotes motility and represses growth of smooth muscle cells by activation of tandem Wnt pathways. J Cell Biol. 2011;192:171–88.
52. Shen H, Gao Y, Ge D, Tan M, Yin Q, Wei TW, He F, Lee TY, Li Z, Chen Y, Yang Q, Liu Z, Li X, Chen Z, Yang Y, Zhang Z, Thistlethwaite PA, Wang J, Malhotra A, Yuan JX, Shyy JY, Gong K. BRCC3 regulation of ALK2 in vascular smooth muscle cells: implication in pulmonary hypertension. Circulation. 2024.
53. Yang X, Long L, Southwood M, Rudarakanchana N, Upton PD, Jeffery TK, Atkinson C, Chen H, Trembath RC, Morrell NW. Dysfunctional Smad signaling contributes to abnormal smooth muscle cell proliferation in familial pulmonary arterial hypertension. Circ Res. 2005;96:1053–63.
54. Tada Y, Majka S, Carr M, Harral J, Crona D, Kuriyama T, West J. Molecular effects of loss of BMPR2 signaling in smooth muscle in a transgenic mouse model of PAH. Am J Phys Lung Cell Mol Phys. 2007;292:L1556–63.
55. Yao C, Yu J, Taylor L, Polgar P, McComb ME, Costello CE. Protein expression by human pulmonary artery smooth muscle cells containing a BMPR2 mutation and the action of ET-1 as determined by proteomic mass spectrometry. Int J Mass Spectrom. 2015;378:347–59.
56. Gore B, Izikki M, Mercier O, Dewachter L, Fadel E, Humbert M, Dartevelle P, Simonneau G, Naeije R, Lebrin F, Eddahibi S. Key role of the endothelial TGF-beta/ALK1/endoglin signaling pathway in humans and rodents pulmonary hypertension. PLoS One. 2014;9:e100310.
57. Upton PD, Davies RJ, Tajsic T, Morrell NW. Transforming growth factor-beta(1) represses bone morphogenetic protein-mediated Smad signaling in pulmonary artery smooth muscle cells via Smad3. Am J Respir Cell Mol Biol. 2013;49:1135–45.
58. Selimovic N, Bergh CH, Andersson B, Sakiniene E, Carlsten H, Rundqvist B. Growth factors and interleukin-6 across the lung circulation in pulmonary hypertension. Eur Respir J. 2009;34:662–8.

59. Wang L, Moonen JR, Cao A, Isobe S, Li CG, Tojais NF, Taylor S, Marciano DP, Chen PI, Gu M, Li D, Harper RL, El-Bizri N, Kim YM, Stankunas K, Rabinovitch M. Dysregulated smooth muscle cell BMPR2-ARRB2 axis causes pulmonary hypertension. Circ Res. 2023;132:545–64.
60. Atkinson C, Stewart S, Upton PD, Machado R, Thomson JR, Trembath RC, Morrell NW. Primary pulmonary hypertension is associated with reduced pulmonary vascular expression of type II bone morphogenetic protein receptor. Circulation. 2002;105:1672–8.
61. Zhang Q, Feng W, Wang Q, Wang J, Chai L, Chen Y, Wang Y, Liu J, Li M, Xie X. PPARgamma activation inhibits PDGF-induced pulmonary artery smooth muscle cell proliferation and migration by modulating TERT. Biomed Pharmacother. 2022;152:113233.
62. Calvier L, Chouvarine P, Legchenko E, Hoffmann N, Geldner J, Borchert P, Jonigk D, Mozes MM, Hansmann G. PPARgamma links BMP2 and TGFbeta1 pathways in vascular smooth muscle cells, regulating cell proliferation and glucose metabolism. Cell Metab. 2017;25:1118–34 e7.
63. Zen K, Zhang CY. Circulating microRNAs: a novel class of biomarkers to diagnose and monitor human cancers. Med Res Rev. 2012;32:326–48.
64. Schlosser K, White RJ, Stewart DJ. miR-26a linked to pulmonary hypertension by global assessment of circulating extracellular microRNAs. Am J Respir Crit Care Med. 2013;188:1472–5.
65. Bertero T, Lu Y, Annis S, Hale A, Bhat B, Saggar R, Saggar R, Wallace WD, Ross DJ, Vargas SO, Graham BB, Kumar R, Black SM, Fratz S, Fineman JR, West JD, Haley KJ, Waxman AB, Chau BN, Cottrill KA, Chan SY. Systems-level regulation of microRNA networks by miR-130/301 promotes pulmonary hypertension. J Clin Invest. 2014;124:3514–28.
66. Bertero T, Cottrill K, Krauszman A, Lu Y, Annis S, Hale A, Bhat B, Waxman AB, Chau BN, Kuebler WM, Chan SY. The microRNA-130/301 family controls vasoconstriction in pulmonary hypertension. J Biol Chem. 2015;290:2069–85.
67. Bertero T, Cottrill KA, Lu Y, Haeger CM, Dieffenbach P, Annis S, Hale A, Bhat B, Kaimal V, Zhang YY, Graham BB, Kumar R, Saggar R, Saggar R, Wallace WD, Ross DJ, Black SM, Fratz S, Fineman JR, Vargas SO, Haley KJ, Waxman AB, Chau BN, Fredenburgh LE, Chan SY. Matrix remodeling promotes pulmonary hypertension through feedback mechanoactivation of the YAP/TAZ-miR-130/301 circuit. Cell Rep. 2015;13:1016–32.
68. Bertero T, Handen AL, Chan SY. Factors associated with heritable pulmonary arterial hypertension exert convergent actions on the miR-130/301-vascular matrix feedback loop. Int J Mol Sci. 2018;19.
69. Shan F, Li J, Huang QY. HIF-1 alpha-induced up-regulation of miR-9 contributes to phenotypic modulation in pulmonary artery smooth muscle cells during hypoxia. J Cell Physiol. 2014;229:1511–20.
70. Liu Y, Zhang H, Li Y, Yan L, Du W, Wang S, Zheng X, Zhang M, Zhang J, Qi J, Sun H, Zhang L, Li G, Zhu D. Long noncoding RNA Rps4l mediates the proliferation of hypoxic pulmonary artery smooth muscle cells. Hypertension. 2020;76:1124–33.
71. Brock M, Trenkmann M, Gay RE, Michel BA, Gay S, Fischler M, Ulrich S, Speich R, Huber LC. Interleukin-6 modulates the expression of the bone morphogenic protein receptor type II through a novel STAT3-microRNA cluster 17/92 pathway. Circ Res. 2009;104:1184–91.
72. Courboulin A, Paulin R, Giguere NJ, Saksouk N, Perreault T, Meloche J, Paquet ER, Biardel S, Provencher S, Cote J, Simard MJ, Bonnet S. Role for miR-204 in human pulmonary arterial hypertension. J Exp Med. 2011;208:535–48.
73. Sarkar J, Gou D, Turaka P, Viktorova E, Ramchandran R, Raj JU. MicroRNA-21 plays a role in hypoxia-mediated pulmonary artery smooth muscle cell proliferation and migration. Am J Phys Lung Cell Mol Phys. 2010;299:L861–71.
74. Brock M, Schuoler C, Leuenberger C, Buhlmann C, Haider TJ, Vogel J, Ulrich S, Gassmann M, Kohler M, Huber LC. Analysis of hypoxia-induced noncoding RNAs reveals metastasis-associated lung adenocarcinoma transcript 1 as an important regulator of vascular smooth muscle cell proliferation. Exp Biol Med (Maywood). 2017;242:487–96.

75. Lv Z, Jiang R, Hu X, Zhao Q, Sun Y, Wang L, Li J, Miao Y, Wu W, Yuan P. Dysregulated lncRNA TUG1 in different pulmonary artery cells under hypoxia. Ann Transl Med. 2021;9:879.
76. Xu W, Janocha AJ, Erzurum SC. Metabolism in pulmonary hypertension. Annu Rev Physiol. 2021;83:551–76.
77. Chan SY, Rubin LJ. Metabolic dysfunction in pulmonary hypertension: from basic science to clinical practice. Eur Respir Rev. 2017;26.
78. Muhl L, Mocci G, Pietila R, Liu J, He L, Genove G, Leptidis S, Gustafsson S, Buyandelger B, Raschperger E, Hansson EM, Bjorkegren JLM, Vanlandewijck M, Lendahl U, Betsholtz C. A single-cell transcriptomic inventory of murine smooth muscle cells. Dev Cell. 2022;57:2426–43 e6.
79. Gorr MW, Sriram K, Muthusamy A, Insel PA. Transcriptomic analysis of pulmonary artery smooth muscle cells identifies new potential therapeutic targets for idiopathic pulmonary arterial hypertension. Br J Pharmacol. 2020;177:3505–18.
80. Wilson JL, Wang L, Zhang Z, Hill NS, Polgar P. Participation of PLK1 and FOXM1 in the hyperplastic proliferation of pulmonary artery smooth muscle cells in pulmonary arterial hypertension. PLoS One. 2019;14:e0221728.
81. Dai Z, Zhu MM, Peng Y, Jin H, Machireddy N, Qian Z, Zhang X, Zhao YY. Endothelial and smooth muscle cell interaction via FoxM1 signaling mediates vascular remodeling and pulmonary hypertension. Am J Respir Crit Care Med. 2018;198:788–802.
82. Zhang C, Sun Y, Guo Y, Xu J, Zhao H. JMJD1C promotes smooth muscle cell proliferation by activating glycolysis in pulmonary arterial hypertension. Cell Death Dis. 2023;9:98.
83. Li D, Shao NY, Moonen JR, Zhao Z, Shi M, Otsuki S, Wang L, Nguyen T, Yan E, Marciano DP, Contrepois K, Li CG, Wu JC, Snyder MP, Rabinovitch M. ALDH1A3 coordinates metabolism with gene regulation in pulmonary arterial hypertension. Circulation. 2021;143:2074–90.
84. Sheikh AQ, Misra A, Rosas IO, Adams RH, Greif DM. Smooth muscle cell progenitors are primed to muscularize in pulmonary hypertension. Sci Transl Med. 2015;7:308ra159.
85. Sheikh AQ, Saddouk FZ, Ntokou A, Mazurek R, Greif DM. Cell autonomous and non-cell autonomous regulation of SMC progenitors in pulmonary hypertension. Cell Rep. 2018;23:1152–65.
86. Shankman LS, Gomez D, Cherepanova OA, Salmon M, Alencar GF, Haskins RM, Swiatlowska P, Newman AA, Greene ES, Straub AC, Isakson B, Randolph GJ, Owens GK. KLF4-dependent phenotypic modulation of smooth muscle cells has a key role in atherosclerotic plaque pathogenesis. Nat Med. 2015;21:628–37.
87. Chen PY, Qin L, Li G, Malagon-Lopez J, Wang Z, Bergaya S, Gujja S, Caulk AW, Murtada SI, Zhang X, Zhuang ZW, Rao DA, Wang G, Tobiasova Z, Jiang B, Montgomery RR, Sun L, Sun H, Fisher EA, Gulcher JR, Fernandez-Hernando C, Humphrey JD, Tellides G, Chittenden TW, Simons M. Smooth muscle cell reprogramming in aortic aneurysms. Cell Stem Cell. 2020;26:542–57 e11.
88. Alencar GF, Owsiany KM, Karnewar S, Sukhavasi K, Mocci G, Nguyen AT, Williams CM, Shamsuzzaman S, Mokry M, Henderson CA, Haskins R, Baylis RA, Finn AV, McNamara CA, Zunder ER, Venkata V, Pasterkamp G, Bjorkegren J, Bekiranov S, Owens GK. Stem cell pluripotency genes Klf4 and Oct4 regulate complex SMC phenotypic changes critical in late-stage atherosclerotic lesion pathogenesis. Circulation. 2020;142:2045–59.
89. Penke LR, Speth JM, Huang SK, Fortier SM, Baas J, Peters-Golden M. KLF4 is a therapeutically tractable brake on fibroblast activation that promotes resolution of pulmonary fibrosis JCI Insight. 2022;7.
90. Wang C, Jiang D. Exogenous PRAS40 reduces KLF4 expression and alleviates hypertrophic scar fibrosis and collagen deposition through inhibiting mTORC1. Burns. 2024.
91. Ma L, Roman-Campos D, Austin ED, Eyries M, Sampson KS, Soubrier F, Germain M, Tregouet DA, Borczuk A, Rosenzweig EB, Girerd B, Montani D, Humbert M, Loyd JE, Kass RS, Chung WK. A novel channelopathy in pulmonary arterial hypertension. N Engl J Med. 2013;369:351–61.

92. Remillard CV, Tigno DD, Platoshyn O, Burg ED, Brevnova EE, Conger D, Nicholson A, Rana BK, Channick RN, Rubin LJ, O'Connor DT, Yuan JX. Function of Kv1.5 channels and genetic variations of KCNA5 in patients with idiopathic pulmonary arterial hypertension. Am J Phys Cell Physiol. 2007;292:C1837–53.
93. Wipff J, Dieude P, Guedj M, Ruiz B, Riemekasten G, Cracowski JL, Matucci-Cerinic M, Melchers I, Humbert M, Hachulla E, Airo P, Diot E, Hunzelmann N, Caramaschi P, Sibilia J, Valentini G, Tiev K, Girerd B, Mouthon L, Riccieri V, Carpentier PH, Distler J, Amoura Z, Tarner I, Degano B, Avouac J, Meyer O, Kahan A, Boileau C, Allanore Y. Association of a KCNA5 gene polymorphism with systemic sclerosis-associated pulmonary arterial hypertension in the European Caucasian population. Arthritis Rheum. 2010;62:3093–100.
94. Yu Y, Keller SH, Remillard CV, Safrina O, Nicholson A, Zhang SL, Jiang W, Vangala N, Landsberg JW, Wang JY, Thistlethwaite PA, Channick RN, Robbins IM, Loyd JE, Ghofrani HA, Grimminger F, Schermuly RT, Cahalan MD, Rubin LJ, Yuan JX. A functional single-nucleotide polymorphism in the TRPC6 gene promoter associated with idiopathic pulmonary arterial hypertension. Circulation. 2009;119:2313–22.
95. Duong TE, Wu Y, Sos BC, Dong W, Limaye S, Rivier LH, Myers G, Hagood JS, Zhang K. A single-cell regulatory map of postnatal lung alveologenesis in humans and mice. Cell Genom. 2022;2.
96. Long X, Bell RD, Gerthoffer WT, Zlokovic BV, Miano JM. Myocardin is sufficient for a smooth muscle-like contractile phenotype. Arterioscler Thromb Vasc Biol. 2008;28:1505–10.
97. Fisher SA. Vascular smooth muscle phenotypic diversity and function. Physiol Genomics. 2010;42A:169–87.
98. Owens GK, Kumar MS, Wamhoff BR. Molecular regulation of vascular smooth muscle cell differentiation in development and disease. Physiol Rev. 2004;84:767–801.
99. Rensen SS, Doevendans PA, van Eys GJ. Regulation and characteristics of vascular smooth muscle cell phenotypic diversity. Neth Hear J. 2007;15:100–8.
100. Hoffmann J, Marsh LM, Pieper M, Stacher E, Ghanim B, Kovacs G, Konig P, Wilkens H, Haitchi HM, Hoefler G, Klepetko W, Olschewski H, Olschewski A, Kwapiszewska G. Compartment-specific expression of collagens and their processing enzymes in intrapulmonary arteries of IPAH patients. Am J Phys Lung Cell Mol Phys. 2015;308:L1002–13.
101. Gao Y, Chen T, Raj JU. Endothelial and smooth muscle cell interactions in the pathobiology of pulmonary hypertension. Am J Respir Cell Mol Biol. 2016;54:451–60.
102. van Splunder H, Villacampa P, Martínez-Romero A, Graupera M. Pericytes in the disease spotlight. Trends Cell Biol. 2024;34:58–71.
103. Armulik A, Genové G, Betsholtz C. Pericytes: developmental, physiological, and pathological perspectives, problems, and promises. Dev Cell. 2011;21:193–215.
104. Baek SH, Maiorino E, Kim H, Glass K, Raby BA, Yuan K. Single cell transcriptomic analysis reveals organ specific pericyte markers and identities. Front Cardiovasc Med. 2022;9:876591.

Chapter 3
Fibroblasts in Pulmonary Vascular Disease

Hui Zhang, Min Li, Cheng-Jun Hu, and Kurt R. Stenmark

Pulmonary hypertension (PH) is a devastating syndrome with high mortality, affecting both pediatric and adult patients across a wide array of disorders [1]. The pulmonary vasculature in these patients undergoes significant cellular and structural alterations within the intima, media, and adventitia, characterized by augmented proliferation, resistance to apoptosis, and increased production of inflammatory mediators and extracellular matrix proteins [2]. These changes find parallels in various animal models of PH [3] and are particularly pronounced in the pulmonary artery adventitia, marked by robust proliferation of fibroblasts and accumulation of macrophages and lymphocytes [4–7]. These phenotypic changes in adventitial fibroblasts, sustained over multiple passages in culture ex vivo, are partly governed through epigenetic mechanisms [4, 5, 7–9]. This evidence collectively supports the notion that fibroblasts may be important participants in the pathophysiology of PH.

Fibroblasts, first identified in 1858 by Rudolf Virchow as cells within connective tissue [10], constitute a primary cellular component of the fibrous connective tissues dispersed throughout our organs [11–13]. Along with endothelial and blood cells, fibroblasts rank among the most common and widespread cell types in the human body [12]. They are known for their pivotal role in producing collagens and a

Authors Hui Zhang and Min Li have contributed equally to this chapter.

H. Zhang · M. Li · K. R. Stenmark (✉)
Cardiovascular and Pulmonary Research Laboratory, Departments of Pediatrics and Medicine, University of Colorado School of Medicine, Denver, CO, USA
e-mail: hui.zhang@cuanschutz.edu; min.li@cuanschutz.edu; kurt.stenmark@cuanschutz.edu

C.-J. Hu
Department of Craniofacial Biology, University of Colorado School of Dental Medicine, Denver, CO, USA
e-mail: cheng-jun.hu@cuanschutz.edu

F. N. Rahaghi et al. (eds.), *The Pulmonary Vasculature in Chronic Lung Disease*, Respiratory Medicine, https://doi.org/10.1007/978-3-032-03581-3_3

myriad of other proteins that form the extracellular matrix (ECM) of fibrous connective tissues. Notably, collagen type 1, a quintessential product of fibroblasts, stands as the most abundant protein in the human body [14]. The ECM is composed of over 300 core proteins, along with numerous bridging proteins and matrix-modifying enzymes, collectively termed the matrisome [15]. The unique ECM composition of each tissue and the recognition, based on both morphological and molecular criteria including gene expression profiling, that fibroblasts from different anatomical locations exhibit variability [16, 17], underscore their diversity. By regulating ECM production, fibroblasts are instrumental in wound contraction. Gabbiani et al., in 1971, revealed that fibroblasts adapt a contractile, myofibroblast phenotype in response to tissue injury [18], a transformation also implicated in fibrosis, which is essentially chronic, unresolved repair following tissue damage [19]. In the realm of disease, particularly cancer, fibroblasts contribute significantly to the tumor stroma, depositing ECM of varied molecular compositions. Beyond ECM, fibroblasts also secret other diverse growth factors and cytokines that modulate resident cell growth and metastasis [20, 21]. Moreover, their secretion of soluble extracellular signaling molecules is crucial during development and in injury responses, providing paracrine signals essential for the differentiation of various cell types [22–27].

Fibroblasts exhibit heterogeneity both between and within organs. Initial insights into the transcriptional heterogeneity of fibroblasts across organs were gleaned from studies utilizing bulk mRNA isolates from multiple cells, offering molecular perspectives at the organ level [28–30]. These studies proposed specific molecular markers to differentiate fibroblasts from other cell types, including VIM, PDGFRA (Pdgfra), FAP (Fap), FSP1, and CD90 (Thy1). Subsequent single-cell RNA sequencing (scRNA-seq) datasets have cataloged fibroblasts from virtually all major organs in both mice and humans. Within broader atlas projects, fibroblasts were sometimes referred to by other names such as stromal cells, mesenchymal stem cells, myofibroblasts [31], and unknown mesenchymal cells [32], reflecting ongoing ambiguities in cell marker identification and nomenclature. Several studies have specifically focused on fibroblasts' roles in cancer [33], fibrotic diseases [34], inflammatory diseases [35, 36], and development [37]. Muhl et al. conducted comparisons of fibroblasts across healthy adult mouse organs [38], while other research has explored multi-organ comparisons between mice and humans [39]. Notably, the human lung hosts at least four distinct fibroblast populations under normal conditions, compared to three in mice.

The phenotype of fibroblasts significantly alters in response to injury, playing a critical role in pathological tissue fibrosis as the primary fibrogenic cell type. Five decades ago, it was shown that fibroblasts transdifferentiate into myofibroblasts, marked by the expression of certain smooth muscle cell markers such as Acta2, upon activation by tissue injury or stress [18]. Although this transition is a component of the normal wound-healing process, it may lead to persistent fibrosis, severely compromising the function of vital organs like the kidney, lung, liver, and heart. A defining feature of fibrosis is the proliferation of myofibroblasts and the excessive deposition of ECM, culminating in the development of abnormal fibrous connective tissue [20, 40]. It's noteworthy that besides quiescent resident fibroblasts, several other cell origins for myofibroblasts have been identified, including endothelial cells (via endothelial mesenchymal transition), macrophages, and pericytes, among others [40–42].

What about fibroblasts in PH. Work over the last 10 years supports the concept that the vascular adventitia acts as a biological processing center for the retrieval, integration, storage, and release of key regulators of vessel wall function. It is the most complex compartment of the vessel wall and comprises a variety of cells including fibroblasts, immunomodulatory cells, resident progenitor cells, vasa vasorum endothelial cells, and adrenergic nerves. Adventitial fibroblasts have been described to exhibit the earliest, most dramatic, and most sustained proliferative, fibrotic, and inflammatory responses to vascular stress and thus to play a key role in the PH process [43–47]. Failure of activated fibroblasts to deactivate contributes to chronic inflammatory and fibrotic diseases [44, 48]. Thus, it is important to define the mechanisms contributing to sustained activation of vascular adventitial fibroblasts in PH. Numerous studies have shown that miRNAs are pivotal in the gene regulation process, playing important roles in controlling development, tissue-specific cell differentiation, cell proliferation and migration, apoptosis, and stress responses [49–52]. Thus, it was important to determine whether changes in miRNA expression directly control the activated phenotype of pulmonary fibroblasts in PH. The following paragraphs provide insight into mechanisms governing the expression of one of the miRNAs, miRNA124, and its contribution to the emergence of a persistently activated fibroblast in PH and how they directly contribute to chronic inflammation and remodeling.

Based on bulk RNA seq data showing that fibroblasts derived from the remodeled pulmonary arteries of hypoxia-induced PH calves (bovine PH-Fibs) exhibit striking resemblance to glioblastoma cells which have decreased miR-124, Wang et al studied PH-Fibs from hypoxic calves and humans with idiopathic pulmonary arterial hypertension (IPAH) and provided compelling evidence that loss of miR-124 is directly involved in the development of activated PH-Fibs, leading to PH [9]. It was thus important to determine the mechanisms contributing to stable decreases of miR-124 in bovine and human PH-Fibs. The ability of an initial stimulus, such as hypoxia, to engage a miRNA circuit could potentially result in stable changes in pulmonary fibroblasts in animals in vivo, which persist even after the hypoxic stimulus is removed. However, in contrast to a recent report where acute hypoxia led to an immediate reduction in miR-124 in vitro, we did not detect an ability of even prolonged exposure to hypoxia to drive a stable change in the control fibroblast (CO-Fibs) phenotype toward the activated PH-Fibs phenotype or a reduction in miR-124 expression in these cells in vitro, indicating targeting HIF pathway in PH-Fibs, is insufficient to restore miR-124 expression and inactivate PH-Fibs [9]. Thus, the acquisition of stable, functional phenotypic changes likely requires the involvement of epigenetic processes such as might occur in response to altered histone modification, DNA methylation, and changes in miRNA expression profiles. Histone-dependent packaging of genomic DNA into chromatin is a central mechanism for gene regulation. Expression of miRNA genes, as well as other genes such as inflammatory genes,

DNA repair genes, and proliferation genes is controlled by the degree of acetylation of histone and nonhistone proteins produced by histone acetyltransferase (HATs) and histone deacetylases (HDACs) [53–55]. Several reports have documented such changes in HDAC activity in fibroblasts in rheumatoid arthritis and juvenile idiopathic arthritis, with specific increase in HDAC-1 activity [55, 56]. The Wang study demonstrated that HDAC inhibitors can restore miR-124 levels toward normal and reverse characteristics of the activated phenotype. Furthermore, using miR-124 expression in human PH-Fibs as a model, we determined that reduced miR-124 gene transcription, not decreased expression of miRNA processing genes, is responsible for reduced levels of mature miR-124 in human PH-Fibs. More condensed chromatin structure was observed in miR-124-1 gene in human PH-Fibs, compared to CO-Fibs. HDACi relaxed miR-124-1 chromatin structure, evidenced by active chromatin probed by DNAseI-sensitivity assay as well as increased levels of the open chromatin mark H3K27Ac, but decreased levels of closed chromatin mark H3K27Me3. Further, direct delivery of histone acetylase (HAT) to miR-124-1 gene regulatory regions using dCAS9-HAT system increases the activation of miR-124 chromatin structure and gene expression [57]. These findings thus begin to explain the molecular basis for the constitutively activated fibroblast phenotype, which is critical in many aspects of the pulmonary vascular disease process. Importantly, it was demonstrated that apicidin, which selectively inhibits class I HDACs, led to significant increases in miR-124 and decreases in its direct target PTBP1 expression. This is consistent with our previous reports that PH-Fibs exhibited significantly elevated catalytic activity of class I HDACs (HDAC-1, -2, and -3) and that selective inhibition of class I HDACs is sufficient to suppress pulmonary vascular remodeling and hypoxic PH [7, 58, 59].

To better understand the role of miR-124 in PH-Fibs, we performed a series of studies to determine the impact of the reduced expression of miR-124 on PH-Fib phenotype. In PH-Fibs with decreased miR-124 expression, the increased expression of HIF-2α and RNA-binding protein PTBP1 was observed. PTBP1 in turn inhibits cell-cycle regulators Notch1/PTEN/FOXO3/p21 and p27, which ultimately leads to an increase in cell proliferation and migration. Additionally, inhibition of miR-124 increases MCP-1 expression, the key chemokines that regulate migration and infiltration of monocytes/macrophages, resulting in increased inflammation. On the other hand, as an RNA-binding protein, PTBP1 controlled alternative splicing of pyruvate kinase muscle isoforms 1 and 2 (PKM1 and PKM2) resulting in an increased PKM2/PKM1 ratio which promotes glycolysis and proliferation in PH-Fibs. Further, normalizing the PKM2/PKM1 ratio in PH-Fibs by miR-124 overexpression or PTBP1 knockdown reversed the glycolytic phenotype (decreased the production of glycolytic intermediates and byproducts, i.e., lactate), rescued mitochondrial reprogramming, and decreased cell proliferation. Pharmacological manipulation of PKM2 activity with TEPP-46 and Shikonin, or treatment with histone deacetylase inhibitors (HDACi), produced similar results [60].

The low PK enzymatic activity, as would occur when PKM2 is preponderant, has been proposed to divert glycolytic intermediates toward biosynthetic pathways such as the pentose phosphate pathway and serine biosynthesis [61]. Consistent with these studies, steady state and U-13C-glucose tracing metabolomics analyses in

PH-Fibs (having increased PKM2/PKM1 ratio) indicated increased pentose phosphate pathway activation, serine biosynthesis, and significantly increased purine synthesis [62]. Importantly, we found that promoting PKM activity through pharmacological treatment with TEPP-46 or HDACi decreases the subtracts of purine de novo synthesis (serine and ribose) and purines in PH-Fibs. The synergic therapeutic effect was observed when HDACi was combined with a well-known vasodilator and a mainstay in the treatment of PH, sildenafil, in correcting metabolic reprogramming and inhibiting PH-Fibs proliferation.

The studies by Wang et al. and Zhang et al. reveal multiple targets for the development of therapeutic strategies (e.g., HDAC inhibitors, miR-124 mimics, PTBP1 inhibitors, or PKM2 activators) for the treatment of patients with IPAH, which is summarized in Fig. 3.1 [9, 57, 60, 62].

Our research has demonstrated that adventitial fibroblasts in the PH pathogenesis exhibit metabolic reprogramming, favoring increased aerobic glycolysis over oxidative phosphorylation. These findings not only corroborate our prior observations regarding anomalous mitochondrial metabolism in PH but also underscore the critical role of metabolic adaptations in promoting fibroblast proliferation and inflammatory activation [63]. In the following section, we will discuss the role of the transcriptional co-repressor CtBP1 in regulating the activated phenotype of PH-Fib as we have identified an upsurge in the expression of the transcriptional co-repressor CtBP1 in the lungs of experimental PH models induced by hypoxia in bovine and mouse models, as well as in patients with IPAH, linking this expression to the disease pathogenesis. Distinct from other transcriptional co-repressors, CtBP1 is uniquely sensitive to increases in free NADH concentrations, a byproduct of glycolytic reprogramming [64, 65]. Investigations by our team and others have revealed that alterations in the cellular reducing environment modify CtBP1's interaction with DNA-binding transcriptional repressors [65–68], positioning CtBP1 as an adversary of multiple tumor suppressors and a mediator between transcriptional regulation and cellular metabolic status [69]. Consistent with the hypothesis that elevated free NADH concentrations enhance CtBP1 activity, treating PH-Fibs with 2-DG or pyruvate—aimed at disrupting aerobic glycolysis or facilitating NADH oxidation to NAD+, respectively—resulted in diminished CtBP1 activity. This reduction in CtBP1 activity led to decreased PH-Fib proliferation and dampened inflammatory activation, alongside normalization of aberrant metabolic phenotypes and increased expression of the anti-inflammatory HMOX1. Notably, this elevation in CtBP1 activity persisted in PH-Fibs (both bovine and human) in the absence of a hypoxic stimulus, suggesting a stable metabolic reprogramming akin to cancer cells that propels the activity of transcriptional repressors like CtBP1. The knockdown of CtBP1 using siRNA or inhibition of CtBP1 dehydrogenase activity via MTOB treatment notably reduced the proliferation of PH-Fibs, akin to observations in cancer cells where CtBP1 inhibition led to heightened expression of cyclin-dependent kinase inhibitors (p15 and p21) and proapoptotic genes (NOXA and PERP) [70].

While inflammation plays a critical role in PH pathogenesis, its relationship or regulation by metabolic reprogramming remains unclear [71]. Given its significance in PH pathogenesis, our focus on the anti-inflammatory gene heme oxygenase 1

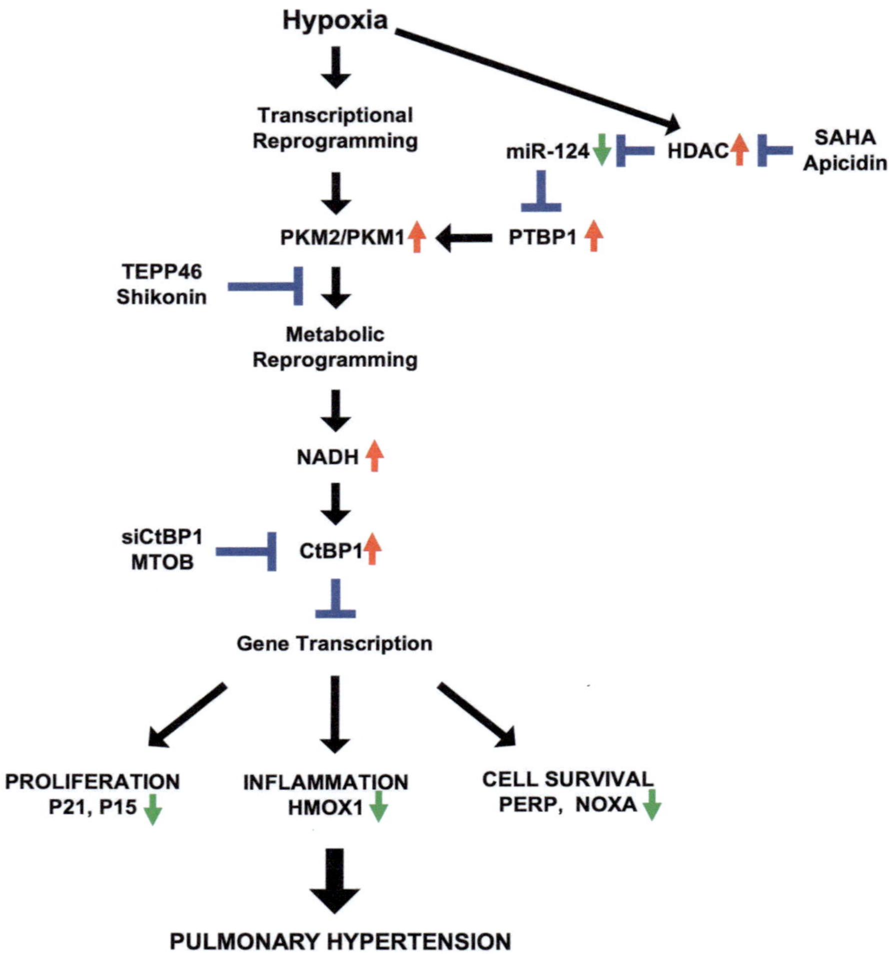

Fig. 3.1 Schematic presentation of reviewed mechanisms concerning how HDAC-miR-124-PTBP1/PKM axis controls metabolic reprogramming and the subsequent regulation of phenotypes by the sensor and regulator of glycolysis CtBP1 in PH-Fibs

(HMOX1, commonly HO-1) in PH-Fibs revealed that inhibition of aerobic glycolysis significantly elevates HMOX1 expression, marking HMOX1 as a direct target of CtBP1. The enzymatic activity of HO, which catalyzes the conversion of heme to carbon monoxide and biliverdin—subsequently converted to bilirubin by biliverdin reductase—offers protection against vasoconstriction and vascular remodeling induced by hypoxia in vitro [72–74]. HO-1's central role in safeguarding the right ventricle from hypoxic pulmonary pressure-induced injury is suggested by studies using an HO-1-null mouse model [75], while transgenic mice with lung-specific over-expression of HO-1 show resistance to early inflammatory changes and protection against PH under prolonged hypoxia exposure [76]. This evidence led us to explore whether targeting CtBP1 at the RNA level via siRNA or at the activity level through

MTOB or by modulating NADH levels with 2-DG or pyruvate could mitigate the proliferative and enhance the anti-inflammatory phenotype of PH-Fibs. These findings suggest that small molecules like MTOB or NSC9539 (a CDC25 inhibitor that impedes the CtBP1-adenovirus E1A protein interaction), known for their anticancer properties, could serve as therapeutic agents for treating hypoxia-induced PH [77, 78]. In a preliminary investigation of this hypothesis, treating hypoxic mice with MTOB (currently a prohibitively expensive drug) successfully ameliorated vascular remodeling induced by hypoxia, including cell proliferation, metabolic reprogramming, macrophage accumulation, and ECM production. Therefore, it is reasonable to speculate that in certain forms or stages of PH, particularly hypoxia (group 3), targeting the transcriptional repressor CtBP1, which bridges metabolic alterations to an activated cellular phenotype, may confer therapeutic benefits. Our findings suggest a more integrated view of vascular cell metabolism, which may open unique therapeutic prospects in targeting the dynamic metabolic reprogramming to attenuate other activated phenotypes of the vascular cells in PH (Fig. 3.1).

The cellular landscape in PH adventitial fibroblasts also encompasses significant mitochondrial alterations. Our findings indicate that persistent changes in mitochondrial metabolism, especially in complex I, characterize the hyperproliferative, apoptosis-resistant, and proinflammatory phenotype of adventitial fibroblasts derived from the remodeled pulmonary arteries of hypoxic calves and humans with IPAH. The compromised mitochondrial energy metabolism in PH-Fibs, coupled with the downregulation of complex I, culminates in augmented mitochondrial superoxide production. Notably, complex I emerges as one of the primary superoxide-generating sites within the mitochondria [79], with the resulting ROS production likely localized to the mitochondrial matrix, predominantly due to NOX4. Crucially, our data functionally connect these metabolic shifts to cellular functionality, as evidenced by the significantly reduced proliferation of PH-Fibs following treatment with the ROS scavenger, tempol. These findings thus underscore the heightened pro-oxidative properties of mitochondria in PH-Fibs. Moreover, the dysfunction of complex I in humans, stemming from a diminished level or the absence of fully assembled complex I, has been implicated in inducing mitochondrial ROS formation [80]. We also observed considerable fragmentation within the mitochondrial network of PH-Fibs, alongside alterations in the expression of mitochondrial fusion proteins, OPA1 and MFN2. The observed mitochondrial fragmentation in PH-Fibs mirrors findings in other cells within the pulmonary hypertensive vessel wall [81]. Besides the altered expression of these proteins, the dynamics of mitochondrial fusion/fission are further regulated by post-translational modifications of the aforementioned proteins, their recruitment to mitochondria, the presence of cofactors, and the composition of membrane lipids [82]. The impact of a fragmented mitochondrial network in PH-Fibs, characterized by suppressed oxidative phosphorylation and a pro-oxidative metabolic state, warrants further investigation.

Our studies have additionally revealed that mitochondrial respiratory parameters are diminished in PH-Fibs, even under normoxic conditions. This decrease in mitochondrial respiration could potentially be attributed to the enhanced phosphorylation of PDH, leading to its inhibition. PDH serves as a pivotal enzyme, regulating the entry of glycolysis-produced pyruvate into the mitochondrial tricarboxylic acid (TCA) cycle by converting it to acetyl-CoA, thereby governing mitochondrial metabolism. The regulation of PDH phosphorylation by hypoxia, through HIF1-mediated upregulation of PDH kinase activity, which in turn increases PDH phosphorylation, has been documented [83]. Interestingly, our research suggests that hypoxia alone, and the HIF1 signaling activated by hypoxia, might not account for the observed metabolic alteration in PH-Fibs. Subjecting CO-Fibs to hypoxia ex vivo sufficed to diminish mitochondrial respiratory parameters via enhanced PDH phosphorylation, yet it did not induce the severe metabolic reprogramming seen in normoxic PH-Fibs, nor did it result in a persistent complex I deficiency [63]. These findings imply that hypoxia alone and elevated HIF1 signaling in response to hypoxia are insufficient to elicit the activated PH-Fib phenotype, aligning with the hypothesis regarding cellular activation of inflammatory macrophages displaying similar metabolic alterations [84]. Current evidence suggests that microenvironmental signals, such as lactate, cytokines, and danger signals, either individually or in combination with hypoxia—but likely not hypoxia alone—are critical regulators of cellular metabolic programs facilitating inflammatory activation [85]. Hence, it is probable that microenvironmental signals within the adventitia, beyond hypoxia, are instrumental in shaping the PH-Fib phenotype. A pivotal observation across human PH cases and various small and large animal PH models is that macrophage accumulation predominantly occurs within the adventitial/perivascular compartment of the vessel wall, underscoring the significant role of the adventitia and adventitial macrophages in the vascular remodeling process integral to PH pathophysiology [86–88]. To determine the cell type(s) and mechanism(s) responsible for adventitial macrophage activation, we exposed naïve primary bone marrow derived macrophages (BMDMs) in vitro to intact whole distal pulmonary artery (dPA) explants, or removal of adventitia from the dPA explant, or adventitia alone, or conditioned media (CM) generated by ex vivo-cultured dPA adventitial fibroblasts from calves and humans. We found that whole dPA explants from calves with hypoxia-induced PH significantly increased transcription of macrophage activation markers Cd163, Cd206, Il4ra, and Socs3 in BMDM. Removal of adventitia from the dPA explant resulted in marked decrease of these genes in BMDMs. However, the adventitia alone and CM from both bovine and human PH-Fibs significantly increased transcription of Cd163, Cd206, Socs3, and Il4rα in BMDM and THP-monocytes. These results indicated that PA adventitia and the adventitial fibroblasts were the cellular source to induce a distinct pro-inflammatory/profibrotic macrophage phenotype in PH [5].

It is acknowledged that the local tissue microenvironment's composition, including the relative concentrations of metabolites, cytokines, growth factors, oxygen, etc., encompassing signals from proximate cell types, are decisive factors in determining macrophage metabolism and functionality [5, 89–92]. In alignment with this concept, our analysis of transcriptomic and metabolomic profiles in naïve mouse bone marrow-derived macrophages (BMDMs) treated with media conditioned by adventitial fibroblasts isolated from pulmonary hypertensive (PH) or age-matched control (CO) animals revealed that: (1) PH-conditioned media (PH-CM) and CO-conditioned media (CO-CM) actively yet differentially influence macrophage transcriptomic landscapes, with PH-CM triggering inflammation, immune response, and metabolic canonical pathways in BMDMs, whereas CO-CM suppresses these pathways; (2) the upstream regulators identified in BMDMs treated with PH-CM or

CO-CM are distinct, with differences attributable to the receptors expressed on BMDMs, as well as activated or inhibited transcriptional regulators and signaling pathways; (3) PH-CM induces metabolic reprogramming in BMDMs, characterized by increased aerobic glycolysis, enhanced pentose phosphate pathway (PPP) activity, an altered TCA cycle marked by heightened glutamine utilization, and accumulation of amino acids, nucleotides, amino-sugars, gamma-glutamyl compounds, and fatty acids [93]. Importantly, our findings also indicate that: (1) elevated glycolysis/free NADH/CtBP1 levels are common attributes in PH-Fibs and BMDMs treated with PH-CM; (2) modulating the adventitial microenvironment by targeting this shared mechanism with MTOB, a pharmacologic CtBP1 inhibitor, results in a reduction of metabolite production and significant inhibition of inflammatory and pro-remodeling gene expression in BMDMs treated with PH-CM in vitro, alongside a marked attenuation of hypoxia-induced inflammation and vascular remodeling in vivo. Specifically, treating hypoxic mice with MTOB led to decreased inflammatory cell accumulation and reduced expression of Tenascin C, an early marker of vascular remodeling, in the lung perivascular area, consistent with prior observations [70]. Flow-sorted macrophages from MTOB-treated hypoxic mice exhibited significant reductions in markers associated with metabolism, inflammation, and extracellular matrix, supporting the notion that targeting metabolism in cell types driving chronic inflammation could effectively mitigate inflammatory responses, thereby influencing PH development. Insights from other organs suggest that activated fibroblasts can influence not only cells of the innate immune system but also cells of the adaptive immune system [94].

Observational studies have documented a variety of T-cell subsets and dendritic cells within the adventitia of pulmonary hypertensive vessel walls. Altered CD4+/CD8+ ratios have been implicated in PH pathology, contributing to abnormal vascular remodeling of the pulmonary vasculature, indicating the involvement of T-cells in PH [95]. Furthermore, it has been established that T-helper cells, particularly Th1 and Th17, elicit an inflammatory response through the production of interleukin-6 (IL6), IL2, IL21, interferon-gamma (IFNg), and tumor necrosis factor (TNFa) in PH [96, 97]. The impact of these T-helper cells can be exacerbated by Th2 dysregulation, dependent on IL4 and IL13 production. It is also becoming increasingly apparent that, for reasons yet to be elucidated, there exists a deficiency in the T-regulatory cell (Tregs) population within the hypertensive vessel wall [98]. Notably, Tregs, which act to limit the immune response in healthy individuals, account for approximately 5–10% of peripheral CD4+ T-cells [99]. FoxP3 Tregs, known for their potent immunosuppressive functions [98], are capable of secreting IL10 and TGF-a, thereby inhibiting the proliferation of immune-associated cells, including CD4+, CD8+ T-cells, natural killer (NK) cells, and antigen-presenting cells. An imbalance in the Treg/Th17 ratio has been observed to influence the progression of PH and correlates with the severity and prognosis of the condition [100, 101]. Prompted by these observations, we sought to examine the effects of activated fibroblasts from the PH vessel wall on T-cell subset numbers and activation status. This investigation is deemed crucial for gaining a comprehensive understanding of the immune dysfunction within the adventitial microenvironment associated with PH. Our studies demonstrated that CD4+ T-cells located in the distal pulmonary artery of PH calves exhibit a reprogramming of their expression profile toward inflammation, evidenced by increased expression of

IFNg and decreased expression of IL4, TGFb, and the absence of the Tregs marker, FOXP3. In vitro experiments exposing isolated bovine/human T-cells to conditioned media from IPAH/PH Fibs (CM-(h)PH Fibs) confirmed the increased inflammatory polarization observed in situ. Human/bovine T-cells differentiated toward a proinflammatory Th1 phenotype, whereas polarization toward Th2 and suppressive regulatory Tregs and gd+ T subsets was diminished in CM-(h)PH Fibs. Intriguingly, the production of immunosuppressive cytokines by Tregs (FOXP3) was also reduced [102]. Previous research has shown that HDAC class I inhibitors can reverse the metabolic abnormalities observed in PH Fibs and, consequently, reduce hypoxia-induced PH in calves [59, 103] partly through the miR-124/PTBP1/PKM pathway [60]. Therefore, we aimed to determine whether restoring normal fibroblast metabolism using the HDAC inhibitor SAHA could inhibit the polarization of T-cells toward proinflammatory signaling. Treating bovine CO and PH Fibs cells with SAHA for 72 h and utilizing the resulting media (CM-CO/PH Fibs+SAHA) to culture bovine T-cells for up to 24 h yielded significant findings. We discovered that CM-PH Fibs+SAHA significantly suppressed proinflammatory T-cell differentiation, as evidenced by a decreased number of IFNg-producing CD4+ T-cells and an increased number of CD4+ T-cells positive for IL4, IL10, and TGFb at both time points, achieving levels comparable to those observed with CM-CO Fibs. The recovery in the abundance of IL10+ and TGFb+ T-cells corresponded to their upregulated expression following exposure to CM-PH Fibs+SAHA compared with CM-PH Fibs, indicating an increase in Treg cell population. When bovine T-cells were cultured in CM-PH Fibs+SAHA, the number of FOXP3 T-cells fully recovered. Additionally, culturing FOXP3 T-cells in CM-PH Fibs+SAHA led to a complete restoration of cytokine levels (IL10, TGFb, and IL4) to those observed when exposed to CM-CO Fibs, underscoring the beneficial impact of CM-PH Fibs+SAHA on reducing T-cell inflammation [102].

In summary, our previous and current findings indicate that pulmonary fibroblasts within the adventitia of pulmonary arteries play an active role in modulating the immune response, specifically the proinflammatory polarization of monocytes and T-cells, through the secretion of cytokines, chemokines, and other molecules. These fibroblasts may thus contribute to local immunomodulation and vessel remodeling in PH, highlighting the complex interplay between metabolic, inflammatory, and immune mechanisms in the disease's pathophysiology.

Our future direction is to explore the mechanism(s) responsible for the persistently activated phenotype of PA adventitial fibroblasts focusing on how gene expression is controlled. We believe examining chromatin structure, activation/binding of TF and epigenetic regulators, with aberrantly expressed genes in pulmonary vascular cells in chronic PH, may uncover new PH therapeutic targets. We propose that the high expression of genes involved in the persistently activated phenotype of PH vascular cells is perpetuated by an open chromatin structure and multiple transcription factors (TFs) via the recruitment of high levels of epigenetic regulators including the histone acetylases P300/CBP, histone acetylation readers including BRDs, the Mediator complex and the positive transcription elongation factor [104](Fig. 3.2). Our most recent findings of integrated analysis of single-cell RNA-seq and single-nuclei ATAC-seq data in distal PAs will provide the opportunities of chromatin mechanism-based therapeutic strategy for PH, which will be updated in the near future.

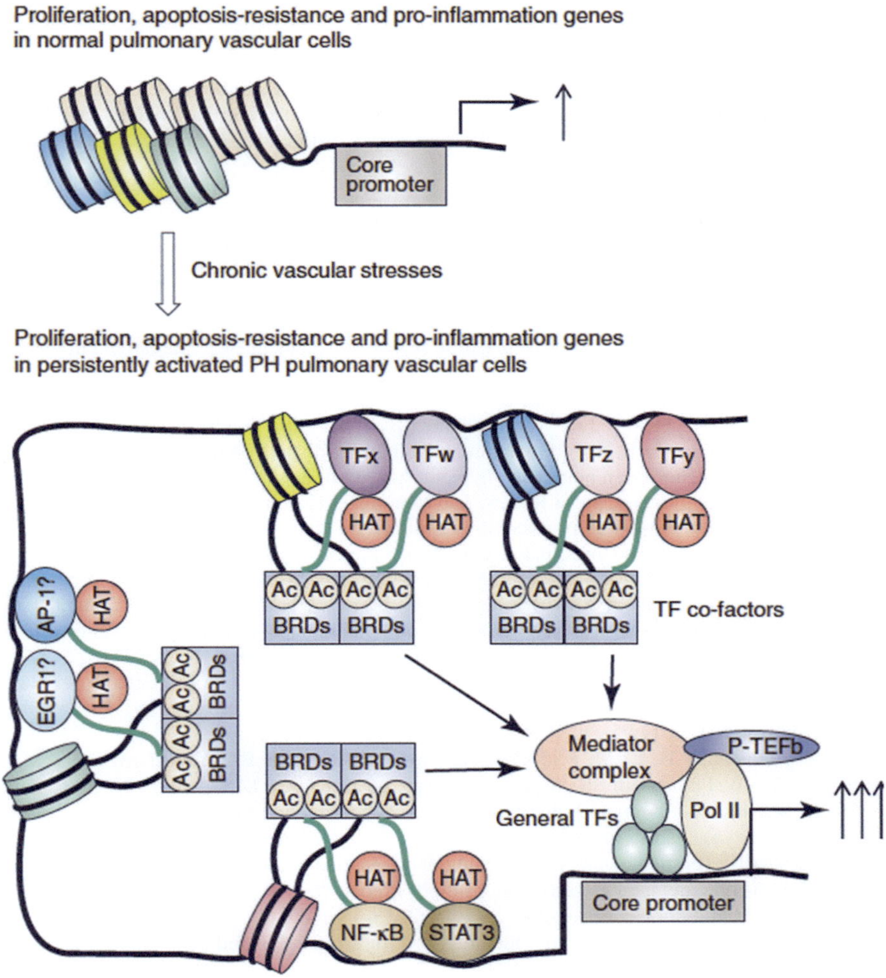

Fig. 3.2 Hypothetical representation of chromatin structure, transcription factors (TFs) and TF co-regulators in normal (top panel), and persistently "activated" PH vascular cells (lower panel) of genes involved in proliferation, apoptosis-resistance, and pro-inflammation. We posit that the persistently high expression of these genes in PH vascular cells is due to their "open" chromatin structure, allowing binding of multiple stress-related TFs and pioneer TF(s), which help maintain an active chromatin structure and high levels of gene expression by recruiting and maintaining high levels of TF co-factors including epigenetic regulators such as HATs, BRDs, and the Mediator Complex (lower panel). Abbreviations: *Ac* acetylation, *EGR1* early growth response 1, *p-TEF*b positive transcription elongation factor B, *Pol II* RNA polymerase II

References

1. Simonneau G, Gatzoulis MA, Adatia I, Celermajer D, Denton C, Ghofrani A, Gomez Sanchez MA, Krishna Kumar R, Landzberg M, Machado RF, Olschewski H, Robbins IM, Souza R. Updated clinical classification of pulmonary hypertension. J Am Coll Cardiol. 2013;62(25 Suppl):D34–41.
2. Price LC, Wort SJ, Perros F, Dorfmuller P, Huertas A, Montani D, Cohen-Kaminsky S, Humbert M. Inflammation in pulmonary arterial hypertension. Chest. 2012;141(1):210–21.
3. Stenmark KR, Meyrick B, Galie N, Mooi WJ, McMurtry IF. Animal models of pulmonary arterial hypertension: the hope for etiological discovery and pharmacological cure. Am J Phys Lung Cell Mol Phys. 2009;297(6):L1013–32.
4. Das M, Burns N, Wilson SJ, Zawada WM, Stenmark KR. Hypoxia exposure induces the emergence of fibroblasts lacking replication repressor signals of PKCzeta in the pulmonary artery adventitia. Cardiovasc Res. 2008;78(3):440–8.
5. El Kasmi KC, Pugliese SC, Riddle SR, Poth JM, Anderson AL, Frid MG, Li M, Pullamsetti SS, Savai R, Nagel MA, Fini MA, Graham BB, Tuder RM, Friedman JE, Eltzschig HK, Sokol RJ, Stenmark KR. Adventitial fibroblasts induce a distinct proinflammatory/profibrotic macrophage phenotype in pulmonary hypertension. J Immunol. 2014;193(2):597–609.
6. Krick S, Hanze J, Eul B, Savai R, Seay U, Grimminger F, Lohmeyer J, Klepetko W, Seeger W, Rose F. Hypoxia-driven proliferation of human pulmonary artery fibroblasts: cross-talk between HIF-1alpha and an autocrine angiotensin system. FASEB J. 2005;19(7):857–9.
7. Li M, Riddle SR, Frid MG, El Kasmi KC, McKinsey TA, Sokol RJ, Strassheim D, Meyrick B, Yeager ME, Flockton AR, McKeon BA, Lemon DD, Horn TR, Anwar A, Barajas C, Stenmark KR. Emergence of fibroblasts with a proinflammatory epigenetically altered phenotype in severe hypoxic pulmonary hypertension. J Immunol. 2011;187(5):2711–22.
8. Panzhinskiy E, Zawada WM, Stenmark KR, Das M. Hypoxia induces unique proliferative response in adventitial fibroblasts by activating PDGFbeta receptor-JNK1 signalling. Cardiovasc Res. 2012;95(3):356–65.
9. Wang D, Zhang H, Li M, Frid MG, Flockton AR, McKeon BA, Yeager ME, Fini MA, Morrell NW, Pullamsetti SS, Velegala S, Seeger W, McKinsey TA, Sucharov CC, Stenmark KR. MicroRNA-124 controls the proliferative, migratory, and inflammatory phenotype of pulmonary vascular fibroblasts. Circ Res. 2014;114(1):67–78.
10. Molenaar JC. [From the library of the Netherlands Journal of Medicine. Rudolf Virchow: Die Cellularpathologie in ihrer Begrundung auf physiologische und pathologische Gewebelehre; 1858]. Ned Tijdschr Geneeskd. 2003;147(45):2236–44.
11. Lendahl U, Muhl L, Betsholtz C. Identification, discrimination and heterogeneity of fibroblasts. Nat Commun. 2022;13(1):3409.
12. Bloom W, Fawcett D. A textbook of histology. New York: CRC Press; 1998.
13. Movat HZ, Fernando NV. The fine structure of connective tissue. I. The fibroblast. Exp Mol Pathol. 1962;1:509–34.
14. Karsdal M. Biochemistry of collagens, laminins and elastin: structure, function and biomarkers. London: Academic; 2019.
15. Hynes RO, Naba A. Overview of the matrisome—an inventory of extracellular matrix constituents and functions. Cold Spring Harb Perspect Biol. 2012;4(1):a004903.
16. Chang HY, Chi JT, Dudoit S, Bondre C, van de Rijn M, Botstein D, Brown PO. Diversity, topographic differentiation, and positional memory in human fibroblasts. Proc Natl Acad Sci USA. 2002;99(20):12877–82.
17. Schor SL, Schor AM. Clonal heterogeneity in fibroblast phenotype: implications for the control of epithelial-mesenchymal interactions. Bioessays. 1987;7(5):200–4.
18. Gabbiani G, Ryan GB, Majne G. Presence of modified fibroblasts in granulation tissue and their possible role in wound contraction. Experientia. 1971;27(5):549–50.
19. Pakshir P, Noskovicova N, Lodyga M, Son DO, Schuster R, Goodwin A, Karvonen H, Hinz B. The myofibroblast at a glance. J Cell Sci. 2020;133(13).

20. Kalluri R. The biology and function of exosomes in cancer. J Clin Invest. 2016;126(4):1208–15.
21. Pietras K, Ostman A. Hallmarks of cancer: interactions with the tumor stroma. Exp Cell Res. 2010;316(8):1324–31.
22. Costea DE, Johannessen AC, Vintermyr OK. Fibroblast control on epithelial differentiation is gradually lost during in vitro tumor progression. Differentiation. 2005;73(4):134–41.
23. Degirmenci B, Valenta T, Dimitrieva S, Hausmann G, Basler K. GLI1-expressing mesenchymal cells form the essential Wnt-secreting niche for colon stem cells. Nature. 2018;558(7710):449–53.
24. El Ghalbzouri A, Lamme E, Ponec M. Crucial role of fibroblasts in regulating epidermal morphogenesis. Cell Tissue Res. 2002;310(2):189–99.
25. Liu Y. Cellular and molecular mechanisms of renal fibrosis. Nat Rev Nephrol. 2011;7(12):684–96.
26. Roulis M, Kaklamanos A, Schernthanner M, Bielecki P, Zhao J, Kaffe E, Frommelt LS, Qu R, Knapp MS, Henriques A, Chalkidi N, Koliaraki V, Jiao J, Brewer JR, Bacher M, Blackburn HN, Zhao X, Breyer RM, Aidinis V, Jain D, Su B, Herschman HR, Kluger Y, Kollias G, Flavell RA. Paracrine orchestration of intestinal tumorigenesis by a mesenchymal niche. Nature. 2020;580(7804):524–9.
27. Shoshkes-Carmel M, Wang YJ, Wangensteen KJ, Toth B, Kondo A, Massasa EE, Itzkovitz S, Kaestner KH. Subepithelial telocytes are an important source of Wnts that supports intestinal crypts. Nature. 2018;557(7704):242–6.
28. Heruth DP, Gibson M, Grigoryev DN, Zhang LQ, Ye SQ. RNA-seq analysis of synovial fibroblasts brings new insights into rheumatoid arthritis. Cell Biosci. 2012;2(1):43.
29. Lahiry P, Lee LJ, Frey BJ, Rupar CA, Siu VM, Blencowe BJ, Hegele RA. Transcriptional profiling of endocrine cerebro-osteodysplasia using microarray and next-generation sequencing. PLoS One. 2011;6(9):e25400.
30. Nota B, Ndika JD, van de Kamp JM, Kanhai WA, van Dooren SJ, van de Wiel MA, Pals G, Salomons GS. RNA sequencing of creatine transporter (SLC6A8) deficient fibroblasts reveals impairment of the extracellular matrix. Hum Mutat. 2014;35(9):1128–35.
31. Schaum N, et al. Tabula Muris Consortium: single-cell transcriptomics of 20 mouse organs creates a Tabula Muris. Nature. 2018;562(7727):367–72.
32. Green CD, Ma Q, Manske GL, Shami AN, Zheng X, Marini S, Moritz L, Sultan C, Gurczynski SJ, Moore BB, Tallquist MD, Li JZ, Hammoud SS. A comprehensive roadmap of murine spermatogenesis defined by single-cell RNA-Seq. Dev Cell. 2018;46(5):651–67 e610.
33. Bartoschek M, Oskolkov N, Bocci M, Lovrot J, Larsson C, Sommarin M, Madsen CD, Lindgren D, Pekar G, Karlsson G, Ringner M, Bergh J, Bjorklund A, Pietras K. Spatially and functionally distinct subclasses of breast cancer-associated fibroblasts revealed by single cell RNA sequencing. Nat Commun. 2018;9(1):5150.
34. Wei K, Korsunsky I, Marshall JL, Gao A, Watts GFM, Major T, Croft AP, Watts J, Blazar PE, Lange JK, Thornhill TS, Filer A, Raza K, Donlin LT, Accelerating Medicines Partnership Rheumatoid A, Systemic Lupus Erythematosus C, Siebel CW, Buckley CD, Raychaudhuri S, Brenner MB. Notch signalling drives synovial fibroblast identity and arthritis pathology. Nature. 2020;582(7811):259–64.
35. Chu CQ. Fibroblasts in rheumatoid arthritis. N Engl J Med. 2020;383(17):1679–81.
36. Wei K, Nguyen HN, Brenner MB. Fibroblast pathology in inflammatory diseases. J Clin Invest. 2021;131(20).
37. Wang G, Muhl L, Padberg Y, Dupont L, Peterson-Maduro J, Stehling M, le Noble F, Colige A, Betsholtz C, Schulte-Merker S, van Impel A. Specific fibroblast subpopulations and neuronal structures provide local sources of Vegfc-processing components during zebrafish lymphangiogenesis. Nat Commun. 2020;11(1):2724.
38. Muhl L, Genove G, Leptidis S, Liu J, He L, Mocci G, Sun Y, Gustafsson S, Buyandelger B, Chivukula IV, Segerstolpe A, Raschperger E, Hansson EM, Bjorkegren JLM, Peng XR, Vanlandewijck M, Lendahl U, Betsholtz C. Single-cell analysis uncovers fibroblast heterogeneity and criteria for fibroblast and mural cell identification and discrimination. Nat Commun. 2020;11(1):3953.

39. Buechler MB, Pradhan RN, Krishnamurty AT, Cox C, Calviello AK, Wang AW, Yang YA, Tam L, Caothien R, Roose-Girma M, Modrusan Z, Arron JR, Bourgon R, Muller S, Turley SJ. Cross-tissue organization of the fibroblast lineage. Nature. 2021;593(7860):575–9.
40. Di Carlo SE, Peduto L. The perivascular origin of pathological fibroblasts. J Clin Invest. 2018;128(1):54–63.
41. El Agha E, Kramann R, Schneider RK, Li X, Seeger W, Humphreys BD, Bellusci S. Mesenchymal stem cells in fibrotic disease. Cell Stem Cell. 2017;21(2):166–77.
42. Plikus MV, Wang X, Sinha S, Forte E, Thompson SM, Herzog EL, Driskell RR, Rosenthal N, Biernaskie J, Horsley V. Fibroblasts: origins, definitions, and functions in health and disease. Cell. 2021;184(15):3852–72.
43. Belknap JK, Orton EC, Ensley B, Tucker A, Stenmark KR. Hypoxia increases bromodeoxyuridine labeling indices in bovine neonatal pulmonary arteries. Am J Respir Cell Mol Biol. 1997;16(4):366–71.
44. Duffield JS, Lupher M, Thannickal VJ, Wynn TA. Host responses in tissue repair and fibrosis. Annu Rev Pathol. 2013;8:241–76.
45. Majesky MW, Dong XR, Hoglund V, Mahoney WM Jr, Daum G. The adventitia: a dynamic interface containing resident progenitor cells. Arterioscler Thromb Vasc Biol. 2011;31(7):1530–9.
46. Stenmark KR, Fagan KA, Frid MG. Hypoxia-induced pulmonary vascular remodeling: cellular and molecular mechanisms. Circ Res. 2006;99(7):675–91.
47. Stenmark KR, Yeager ME, El Kasmi KC, Nozik-Grayck E, Gerasimovskaya EV, Li M, Riddle SR, Frid MG. The adventitia: essential regulator of vascular wall structure and function. Annu Rev Physiol. 2013;75:23–47.
48. Buckley CD, Pilling D, Lord JM, Akbar AN, Scheel-Toellner D, Salmon M. Fibroblasts regulate the switch from acute resolving to chronic persistent inflammation. Trends Immunol. 2001;22(4):199–204.
49. Esquela-Kerscher A, Slack FJ. Oncomirs—microRNAs with a role in cancer. Nat Rev Cancer. 2006;6(4):259–69.
50. Li S, Ran Y, Zhang D, Chen J, Li S, Zhu D. MicroRNA-138 plays a role in hypoxic pulmonary vascular remodelling by targeting Mst1. Biochem J. 2013;452(2):281–91.
51. Small EM, Olson EN. Pervasive roles of microRNAs in cardiovascular biology. Nature. 2011;469(7330):336–42.
52. White K, Loscalzo J, Chan SY. Holding our breath: the emerging and anticipated roles of microRNA in pulmonary hypertension. Pulm Circ. 2012;2(3):278–90.
53. Adcock IM. HDAC inhibitors as anti-inflammatory agents. Br J Pharmacol. 2007;150(7):829–31.
54. Bush EW, McKinsey TA. Protein acetylation in the cardiorenal axis: the promise of histone deacetylase inhibitors. Circ Res. 2010;106(2):272–84.
55. Kawabata T, Nishida K, Takasugi K, Ogawa H, Sada K, Kadota Y, Inagaki J, Hirohata S, Ninomiya Y, Makino H. Increased activity and expression of histone deacetylase 1 in relation to tumor necrosis factor-alpha in synovial tissue of rheumatoid arthritis. Arthritis Res Ther. 2010;12(4):R133.
56. Horiuchi M, Morinobu A, Chin T, Sakai Y, Kurosaka M, Kumagai S. Expression and function of histone deacetylases in rheumatoid arthritis synovial fibroblasts. J Rheumatol. 2009;36(8):1580–9.
57. Zhang H, Laux A, Stenmark KR, Hu CJ. Mechanisms contributing to the dysregulation of miRNA-124 in pulmonary hypertension. Int J Mol Sci. 2021;22(8)
58. Cavasin MA, Demos-Davies K, Horn TR, Walker LA, Lemon DD, Birdsey N, Weiser-Evans MC, Harral J, Irwin DC, Anwar A, Yeager ME, Li M, Watson PA, Nemenoff RA, Buttrick PM, Stenmark KR, McKinsey TA. Selective class I histone deacetylase inhibition suppresses hypoxia-induced cardiopulmonary remodeling through an antiproliferative mechanism. Circ Res. 2012;110(5):739–48.

59. Zhao L, Chen CN, Hajji N, Oliver E, Cotroneo E, Wharton J, Wang D, Li M, McKinsey TA, Stenmark KR, Wilkins MR. Histone deacetylation inhibition in pulmonary hypertension: therapeutic potential of valproic acid and suberoylanilide hydroxamic acid. Circulation. 2012;126(4):455–67.
60. Zhang H, Wang D, Li M, Plecita-Hlavata L, D'Alessandro A, Tauber J, Riddle S, Kumar S, Flockton A, McKeon BA, Frid MG, Reisz JA, Caruso P, El Kasmi KC, Jezek P, Morrell NW, Hu CJ, Stenmark KR. Metabolic and proliferative state of vascular adventitial fibroblasts in pulmonary hypertension is regulated through a microRNA-124/PTBP1 (Polypyrimidine tract binding protein 1)/Pyruvate kinase muscle axis. Circulation. 2017;136(25):2468–85.
61. Dayton TL, Jacks T, Vander Heiden MG. PKM2, cancer metabolism, and the road ahead. EMBO Rep. 2016;17(12):1721–30.
62. Zhang H, D'Alessandro A, Li M, Reisz JA, Riddle S, Muralidhar A, Bull T, Zhao L, Gerasimovskaya E, Stenmark KR. Histone deacetylase inhibitors synergize with sildenafil to suppress purine metabolism and proliferation in pulmonary hypertension. Vasc Pharmacol. 2023;149:107157.
63. Plecita-Hlavata L, Tauber J, Li M, Zhang H, Flockton AR, Pullamsetti SS, Chelladurai P, D'Alessandro A, El Kasmi KC, Jezek P, Stenmark KR. Constitutive reprogramming of fibroblast mitochondrial metabolism in pulmonary hypertension. Am J Respir Cell Mol Biol. 2016;55(1):47–57.
64. Fjeld CC, Birdsong WT, Goodman RH. Differential binding of NAD+ and NADH allows the transcriptional corepressor carboxyl-terminal binding protein to serve as a metabolic sensor. Proc Natl Acad Sci USA. 2003;100(16):9202–7.
65. Zhang Q, Piston DW, Goodman RH. Regulation of corepressor function by nuclear NADH. Science. 2002;295(5561):1895–7.
66. Kim JH, Cho EJ, Kim ST, Youn HD. CtBP represses p300-mediated transcriptional activation by direct association with its bromodomain. Nat Struct Mol Biol. 2005;12(5):423–8.
67. Mirnezami AH, Campbell SJ, Darley M, Primrose JN, Johnson PW, Blaydes JP. Hdm2 recruits a hypoxia-sensitive corepressor to negatively regulate p53-dependent transcription. Curr Biol. 2003;13(14):1234–9.
68. Zhang Q, Yoshimatsu Y, Hildebrand J, Frisch SM, Goodman RH. Homeodomain interacting protein kinase 2 promotes apoptosis by downregulating the transcriptional corepressor CtBP. Cell. 2003;115(2):177–86.
69. Chinnadurai G. The transcriptional corepressor CtBP: a foe of multiple tumor suppressors. Cancer Res. 2009;69(3):731–4.
70. Li M, Riddle S, Zhang H, D'Alessandro A, Flockton A, Serkova NJ, Hansen KC, Moldovan R, McKeon BA, Frid M, Kumar S, Li H, Liu H, Caanovas A, Medrano JF, Thomas MG, Iloska D, Plecita-Hlavata L, Jezek P, Pullamsetti S, Fini MA, El Kasmi KC, Zhang Q, Stenmark KR. Metabolic reprogramming regulates the proliferative and inflammatory phenotype of adventitial fibroblasts in pulmonary hypertension through the transcriptional corepressor C-terminal binding protein-1. Circulation. 2016;134(15):1105–21.
71. Tuder RM, Archer SL, Dorfmuller P, Erzurum SC, Guignabert C, Michelakis E, Rabinovitch M, Schermuly R, Stenmark KR, Morrell NW. Relevant issues in the pathology and pathobiology of pulmonary hypertension. J Am Coll Cardiol. 2013;62(25 Suppl):D4–12.
72. Abraham NG, Levere RD, Lin JH, Beru N, Hermine O, Goldwasser E. Co-regulation of heme oxygenase and erythropoietin genes. J Cell Biochem. 1991;47(1):43–8.
73. Morita T, Mitsialis SA, Koike H, Liu Y, Kourembanas S. Carbon monoxide controls the proliferation of hypoxic vascular smooth muscle cells. J Biol Chem. 1997;272(52):32804–9.
74. Morita T, Perrella MA, Lee ME, Kourembanas S. Smooth muscle cell-derived carbon monoxide is a regulator of vascular cGMP. Proc Natl Acad Sci USA. 1995;92(5):1475–9.
75. Yet SF, Perrella MA, Layne MD, Hsieh CM, Maemura K, Kobzik L, Wiesel P, Christou H, Kourembanas S, Lee ME. Hypoxia induces severe right ventricular dilatation and infarction in heme oxygenase-1 null mice. J Clin Invest. 1999;103(8):R23–9.

76. Minamino T, Christou H, Hsieh CM, Liu Y, Dhawan V, Abraham NG, Perrella MA, Mitsialis SA, Kourembanas S. Targeted expression of heme oxygenase-1 prevents the pulmonary inflammatory and vascular responses to hypoxia. Proc Natl Acad Sci USA. 2001;98(15):8798–803.
77. Blevins MA, Kouznetsova J, Krueger AB, King R, Griner LM, Hu X, Southall N, Marugan JJ, Zhang Q, Ferrer M, Zhao R. Small molecule, NSC95397, inhibits the CtBP1-protein partner interaction and CtBP1-mediated transcriptional repression. J Biomol Screen. 2015;20(5):663–72.
78. Yang Y, Yang WS, Yu T, Yi YS, Park JG, Jeong D, Kim JH, Oh JS, Yoon K, Kim JH, Cho JY. Novel anti-inflammatory function of NSC95397 by the suppression of multiple kinases. Biochem Pharmacol. 2014;88(2):201–15.
79. Brand MD. The sites and topology of mitochondrial superoxide production. Exp Gerontol. 2010;45(7–8):466–72.
80. Roestenberg P, Manjeri GR, Valsecchi F, Smeitink JA, Willems PH, Koopman WJ. Pharmacological targeting of mitochondrial complex I deficiency: the cellular level and beyond. Mitochondrion. 2012;12(1):57–65.
81. Ryan J, Dasgupta A, Huston J, Chen KH, Archer SL. Mitochondrial dynamics in pulmonary arterial hypertension. J Mol Med (Berl). 2015;93(3):229–42.
82. Kasahara A, Scorrano L. Mitochondria: from cell death executioners to regulators of cell differentiation. Trends Cell Biol. 2014;24(12):761–70.
83. Kim JW, Tchernyshyov I, Semenza GL, Dang CV. HIF-1-mediated expression of pyruvate dehydrogenase kinase: a metabolic switch required for cellular adaptation to hypoxia. Cell Metab. 2006;3(3):177–85.
84. O'Neill LA, Hardie DG. Metabolism of inflammation limited by AMPK and pseudo-starvation. Nature. 2013;493(7432):346–55.
85. Hu CJ, Laux A, Gandjeva A, Wang L, Li M, Brown RD, Riddle S, Kheyfets VO, Tuder RM, Zhang H, Stenmark KR. The effect of hypoxia-inducible factor inhibition on the phenotype of fibroblasts in human and bovine pulmonary hypertension. Am J Respir Cell Mol Biol. 2023;69(1):73–86.
86. Huertas A, Tu L, Humbert M, Guignabert C. Chronic inflammation within the vascular wall in pulmonary arterial hypertension: more than a spectator. Cardiovasc Res. 2020;116(5):885–93.
87. Savai R, Pullamsetti SS, Kolbe J, Bieniek E, Voswinckel R, Fink L, Scheed A, Ritter C, Dahal BK, Vater A, Klussmann S, Ghofrani HA, Weissmann N, Klepetko W, Banat GA, Seeger W, Grimminger F, Schermuly RT. Immune and inflammatory cell involvement in the pathology of idiopathic pulmonary arterial hypertension. Am J Respir Crit Care Med. 2012;186(9):897–908.
88. Stenmark KR, Tuder RM, El Kasmi KC. Metabolic reprogramming and inflammation act in concert to control vascular remodeling in hypoxic pulmonary hypertension. J Appl Physiol (1985). 2015;119(10):1164–72.
89. Guilliams M, Thierry GR, Bonnardel J, Bajenoff M. Establishment and maintenance of the macrophage niche. Immunity. 2020;52(3):434–51.
90. Kelly B, O'Neill LA. Metabolic reprogramming in macrophages and dendritic cells in innate immunity. Cell Res. 2015;25(7):771–84.
91. Larionova I, Kazakova E, Patysheva M, Kzhyshkowska J. Transcriptional, epigenetic and metabolic programming of tumor-associated macrophages. Cancers (Basel). 2020;12(6).
92. O'Neill LA. A critical role for citrate metabolism in LPS signalling. Biochem J. 2011;438(3):e5–6.
93. Li M, Riddle S, Kumar S, Poczobutt J, McKeon BA, Frid MG, Ostaff M, Reisz JA, Nemkov T, Fini MA, Laux A, Hu CJ, El Kasmi KC, D'Alessandro A, Brown RD, Zhang H, Stenmark KR. Microenvironmental regulation of macrophage transcriptomic and metabolomic profiles in pulmonary hypertension. Front Immunol. 2021;12:640718.
94. Worrell JC, MacLeod MKL. Stromal-immune cell crosstalk fundamentally alters the lung microenvironment following tissue insult. Immunology. 2021;163(3):239–49.

95. Taraseviciene-Stewart L, Nicolls MR, Kraskauskas D, Scerbavicius R, Burns N, Cool C, Wood K, Parr JE, Boackle SA, Voelkel NF. Absence of T cells confers increased pulmonary arterial hypertension and vascular remodeling. Am J Respir Crit Care Med. 2007;175(12):1280–9.
96. Maston LD, Jones DT, Giermakowska W, Howard TA, Cannon JL, Wang W, Wei Y, Xuan W, Resta TC, Gonzalez Bosc LV. Central role of T helper 17 cells in chronic hypoxia-induced pulmonary hypertension. Am J Phys Lung Cell Mol Phys. 2017;312(5):L609–24.
97. Steiner MK, Syrkina OL, Kolliputi N, Mark EJ, Hales CA, Waxman AB. Interleukin-6 overexpression induces pulmonary hypertension. Circ Res. 2009;104(2):236–44. 228p following 244
98. Tian W, Jiang SY, Jiang X, Tamosiuniene R, Kim D, Guan T, Arsalane S, Pasupneti S, Voelkel NF, Tang Q, Nicolls MR. The role of regulatory T cells in pulmonary arterial hypertension. Front Immunol. 2021;12:684657.
99. Itoh M, Takahashi T, Sakaguchi N, Kuniyasu Y, Shimizu J, Otsuka F, Sakaguchi S. Thymus and autoimmunity: production of CD25+CD4+ naturally anergic and suppressive T cells as a key function of the thymus in maintaining immunologic self-tolerance. J Immunol. 1999;162(9):5317–26.
100. Gaowa S, Zhou W, Yu L, Zhou X, Liao K, Yang K, Lu Z, Jiang H, Chen X. Effect of Th17 and Treg axis disorder on outcomes of pulmonary arterial hypertension in connective tissue diseases. Mediat Inflamm. 2014;2014:247372.
101. Huertas A, Phan C, Bordenave J, Tu L, Thuillet R, Le Hiress M, Avouac J, Tamura Y, Allanore Y, Jovan R, Sitbon O, Guignabert C, Humbert M. Regulatory T cell dysfunction in idiopathic, heritable and connective tissue-associated pulmonary arterial hypertension. Chest. 2016;149(6):1482–93.
102. Plecita-Hlavata L, Brazdova A, Krivonoskova M, Hu CJ, Phang T, Tauber J, Li M, Zhang H, Hoetzenecker K, Crnkovic S, Kwapiszewska G, Stenmark KR. Microenvironmental regulation of T-cells in pulmonary hypertension. Front Immunol. 2023;14:1223122.
103. Applegate TJ, Krafsur GM, Boon JA, Zhang H, Li M, Holt TN, Ambler SK, Abrams BA, Gustafson DL, Bartels K, Garry FB, Stenmark KR, Brown RD. Brief report: case comparison of therapy with the histone deacetylase inhibitor vorinostat in a neonatal calf model of pulmonary hypertension. Front Physiol. 2021;12:712583.
104. Hu CJ, Zhang H, Laux A, Pullamsetti SS, Stenmark KR. Mechanisms contributing to persistently activated cell phenotypes in pulmonary hypertension. J Physiol. 2019;597(4):1103–19.

Chapter 4
Biology of Extracellular Matrix in Pulmonary Vascular Pathology Associated with Chronic Lung Diseases

Toyoshi Yanagihara, Kohei Otsubo, and Martin R. J. Kolb

Introduction

Vascular remodeling can occur in various chronic lung diseases, and particularly affects chronic obstructive pulmonary disease (COPD) and interstitial lung diseases (ILDs). This remodeling process involves structural changes in the pulmonary vasculature, leading to increased pulmonary vascular resistance and, ultimately, pulmonary hypertension (PH). PH is defined as elevated mean pulmonary arterial pressure (mPAP) over 20 mmHg at rest, measured by right heart catheterization [1]. According to its etiology, PH associated with chronic lung disease is classified as WHO Group 3 (group 1: pulmonary arterial hypertension, group 2: PH associated with left heart disease, group 3: PH associated with lung diseases, group 4: PH associated with pulmonary artery obstructions, group 5: PH with unclear and multifactorial mechanisms) [1]. The incidence of PH among patients with chronic lung diseases correlates with the severity of the lung condition, exceeding 30% in advanced stages of chronic lung diseases [1]. PH significantly impacts the prognosis of patients with COPD and ILD, often leading to reduced exercise tolerance, increased morbidity, and decreased survival rates [1, 2].

T. Yanagihara
Department of Respiratory Medicine, Fukuoka University Hospital, Fukuoka, Japan
e-mail: toyoshi.yana@fukuoka-u.ac.jp

K. Otsubo
Department of Respiratory Medicine, Graduate School of Medical Sciences, Kyushu University, Fukuoka, Japan

M. R. J. Kolb (✉)
Firestone Institute for Respiratory Health, Research Institute at St. Joseph's Healthcare, Department of Medicine, McMaster University, Hamilton, ON, Canada
e-mail: kolbm@mcmaster.ca

F. N. Rahaghi et al. (eds.), *The Pulmonary Vasculature in Chronic Lung Disease*, Respiratory Medicine, https://doi.org/10.1007/978-3-032-03581-3_4

The pathophysiology of vascular remodeling in chronic lung diseases is multifaceted and complex. Chronic hypoxia, inflammation, oxidative stress, and altered BMPR2 signaling play pivotal roles in initiating and perpetuating the remodeling process [3, 4]. These factors trigger endothelial dysfunction, endothelial-to-mesenchymal transition, smooth muscle cell proliferation, and fibroblast activation, collectively contributing to the thickening of the vessel walls and narrowing of the vascular lumen. Additionally, imbalances between vasoconstrictors and vasodilators, as well as pro-thrombotic and anti-thrombotic factors, further exacerbate the vascular changes observed in these diseases [5, 6].

The extracellular matrix (ECM) is intricately involved in the vascular remodeling process. The ECM, a three-dimensional network of proteins, glycoproteins, and polysaccharides, provides structural support to tissues and plays a crucial role in cell signaling, migration, and differentiation [7]. Alterations in the composition and organization of the ECM have been observed in pulmonary vasculature as well as pulmonary parenchyma in chronic lung diseases [8]. Alterations in ECM dynamics result from the modulation of matrix protein expression, degradation by metalloproteases, post-translational modifications, and topographical changes to matrix proteins. Here, we review the specific components of the ECM and their dynamics in the pathogenesis of pulmonary vascular changes. Additionally, we explore the differences in ECM composition across underlying lung diseases and potential therapeutic targets for modulating ECM in pulmonary vascular pathology.

ECM Alteration in Pulmonary Vascular Pathology

The pulmonary arterial wall, a tri-layered tapestry comprising the intima, media, and adventitia, is a dynamic structure where cellular constituents and ECM components interweave to maintain vascular integrity [9]. At the intima, endothelial cells (ECs) and the basement membrane (BM) form the first line of vascular interaction, with the BM's intricate grid of laminin and collagen type IV serving as a scaffold for cellular anchorage via integrin and dystroglycan receptors. These interactions are not merely structural; they are biologically active, mediating cellular signaling that governs vascular tone and homeostasis. The media layer, composed of vascular smooth muscle cells (VSMCs) ensconced within a matrix of elastin, fibrillin, and a diverse array of collagens, confers tensile strength and elasticity, allowing vessels to withstand and adapt to the pulsatile flow of blood. Meanwhile, the adventitia, rich in fibroblasts and a varied ECM, provides mechanical support and serves as a conduit for neurovascular and vasoactive signals.

In the context of chronic lung diseases, this harmonious architecture becomes disrupted. Pathological processes such as inflammation and aberrant repair mechanisms precipitate drastic ECM remodeling—characterized by disproportionate collagen deposition, elastin fragmentation, and dysregulated protease activity. These alterations not only stiffen the vessel walls, leading to luminal narrowing and heightened pulmonary vascular resistance but also modulate cellular behaviors, contributing to the pathology of pulmonary hypertension (PH). Understanding the molecular drivers of ECM remodeling—such as altered synthesis, post-translational modifications, and proteolytic degradation—is crucial. It opens avenues for targeted therapies that can correct the imbalances in ECM turnover and restore vascular health.

Collagens

Collagens predominantly constitute the ECM within the vascular wall. The accumulation of fibrillar collagens, such as collagen I and III, is widely acknowledged as a characteristic of vascular remodeling, which is observed in both distal and proximal pulmonary arteries [10–14]. These fibrillar collagens are mostly produced by adventitial fibroblasts and smooth muscle cells in the pulmonary vasculature [10, 15–17].

Upon synthesis, collagen fibers undergo post-translational modifications to facilitate their function in tissue reinforcement. Collagen molecules gather and form a triple-helical structure, creating procollagen molecules in the Golgi apparatus, then secreted from the Golgi to the extracellular space, where the procollagen's C-terminal and N-terminal ends are cleaved to be assembled to mature collagen molecules. Such collagen molecules begin to form fibers through self-assembly, and enzymes like lysyl oxidase (LOX), LOX-like enzymes (LOXL), and transglutaminase (TG2) crosslink the triple helices, leading to the formation of collagen fibers. LOX and LOXL catalyze the oxidative deamination of lysine and hydroxylysine residues in collagen, initiating the intermolecular crosslinking through the formation of aldehyde groups. Conversely, TG2 specifically forms isopeptide bonds between glutamine and lysine residues. In idiopathic pulmonary artery hypertension (IPAH), every isoform of the LOX is upregulated in the remodeled arteries [13]. LOXL1 and LOXL2 are also upregulated in lung tissues in idiopathic pulmonary fibrosis (IPF), the most severe form of ILD [18, 19]. These findings imply that dysregulation of collagen-modifying enzymes may be related to ECM remodeling in pulmonary hypertension, which may explain collagen maturation and vascular stiffness seen in this disease.

Collagen I and Collagen III

Collagens I and III are the most abundant collagens in the vascular wall, and they play an important role in controlling vascular homeostasis and remodeling. The multifunctional cytokine transforming growth factor-β (TGF-β) is playing an especially critical role in modulating the ECM and significantly amplifies collagen I synthesis in VSMCs, thus tying cellular responses directly to extracellular cues [20].

Collagen IV

The primary constituent of the BM is collagen IV, which binds to both integrin and nonintegrin receptors to promote cell adhesion to the basement membrane. Collagen IV is mainly synthesized by ECs. Data mining of the single-cell RNA sequencing dataset GSE136831 from healthy control, IPF, and COPD lungs revealed that collagen IV (*COL4A1* and *COL4A2*) is highly expressed in ECs from IPF lungs (Fig. 4.1). A recent study revealed venous vessel ECs (SV-ECs), localized specifically to systemically supplied vessels of the bronchial vascular plexus and of the

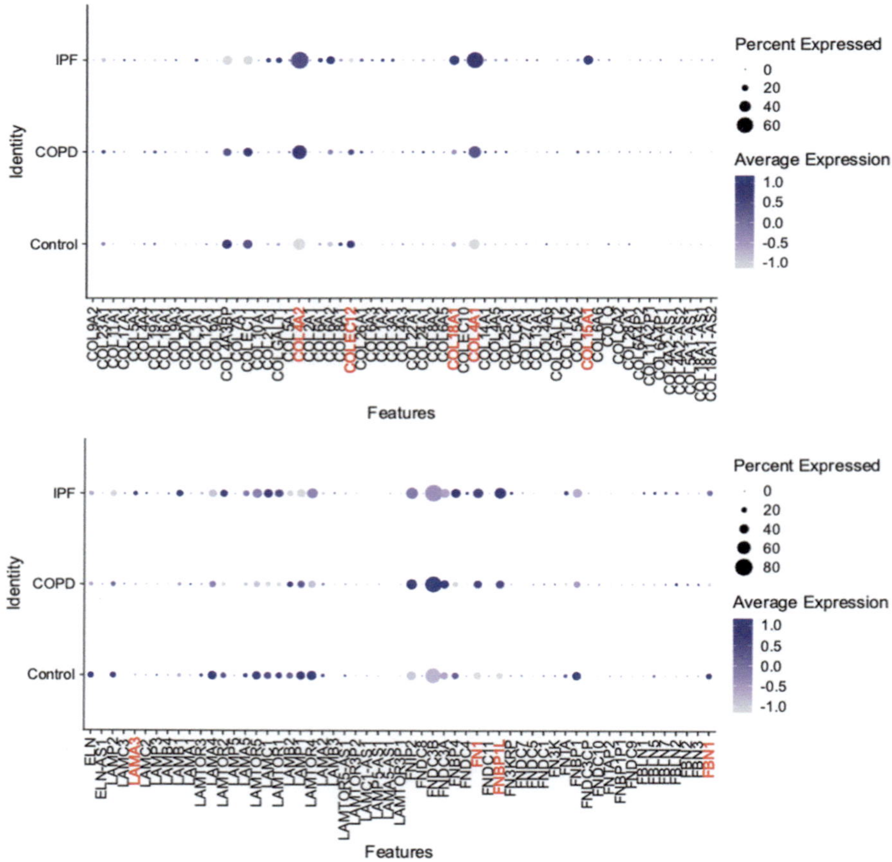

Fig. 4.1 Differential expression of collagen, elastin, laminin, fibronectin, fibrillin genes in endothelial cells from whole lung from controls, IPF, and COPDData were from the publicly available dataset GSE136831, which contains single-cell RNA sequencing data from whole lung dissociates from controls (n = 28), IPF (n = 32), and COPD (n = 18). Differential gene expression was determined using "FindMarkers," considering *p* values <0.05 as significant. Genes marked in red indicate differential expression in IPF or COPD relative to controls. [22]

visceral pleura under physiological conditions [21], are widespread in fibrotic areas of IPF lungs [22]. These SV-ECs are considered to have a central role in the endothelial regeneration process [23], and they express *COL15A1* as well as *COL4A1* and *COL4A2*, suggesting that upregulation of *COL4A1* and *COL4A2* in IPF lungs might be a consequence of regeneration of endothelial and basement membranes. The association of abnormal collagen IV with irregular angiogenesis is likely a consequence of impaired EC binding, resulting from a weakened integrin-collagen IV linkage [24]. The disrupted collagen IV-integrin axis may underlie the altered endothelial behavior, underscoring its pivotal role in the pathogenesis of IPF-linked vascular remodeling.

Collagen XV

Collagen XV is also a component of BMs. The single-cell RNA sequencing dataset GSE136831 mentioned above revealed that collagen XV (*COL15A1)* is highly expressed in ECs from IPF lungs (Fig. 4.1). As described, the composition of SV-ECs is substantially increased in IPF compared to controls and COPD [22], and these SV-ECs are characteristically expressing *COL15A1*. Thus, the upregulation of *COL15A1* in ECs from IPF might be a consequence of the increase of SV-ECs. Although the direct role of collagen XV in vascular remodeling remains unclear, its degradation product, restin, exhibits anti-angiogenic properties and hampers EC migration [25], thereby potentially modulating the vascular remodeling process.

Collagen XVIII

Collagen XVIIIα1 (*COL18A1*), another BM collagen, is reported to have increased expression in patients with pulmonary artery hypertension [26]. It is expressed in ECs as well as VSMCs. Despite similar expression levels of *COL18A1* in ECs from IPF, COPD, and healthy controls (Fig. 4.1), increased serum levels of endostatin, a functional domain of collagen XVIII within its N-terminal domain, have been reported in patients with IPF [27]. Endostatin can be cleaved from collagen XVIII by several types of proteases, including the MMPs and cathepsins. Endostatin binds integrins and glypicans on ECs, inhibiting EC proliferation and inducing EC apoptosis [28]. This indicates its engagement in the pathological remodeling of the pulmonary vasculature.

Elastin

Elastin, a resilient and fibrous protein in connective tissue, serves multiple vital functions in the lung's biomechanical properties and its vascular system. It forms the core of elastic fibers, comprised of an amorphous elastic protein and at least one microfibrillar component. These fibers impart flexibility to various parts of the lung, including alveolar walls, the interstitium of bronchioles, the arterial and venous medial layers, lymphatic vessels, and the pleura. The protein's unique hydrophobic characteristics and the extensive intermolecular crosslinks, especially desmosine, and isodesmosine, create a robust and insoluble network of polypeptide chains. This network acts as an ideal elastomer within a watery environment. Elastin is synthesized and secreted from cells, in particular, VSMCs and ECs [29]. Gaikwad et al. recently showed elastin deposition along with vascular remodeling in patients with IPF [30]. Total elastin also negatively correlated with D_{LCO} [30]. Elastin is not only a structural protein but plays a pivotal role in various physiological and pathological processes [31].

Glycoproteins

Glycoproteins are proteins that contain oligosaccharide chains covalently attached to amino acid side chains. Glycoproteins primarily influence the composition of ECM by interacting with other proteins in the surrounding microenvironment. When glycoproteins attach to cytokines or growth factors, the associated cellular signaling is often affected. Fibrillin-1, for instance, binds to TGF-β to prevent overactivation of TGF-β signaling and to preserve vascular homeostasis. Furthermore, glycoproteins function as cross-linkers, combining with elastins, collagens, proteoglycans, and glycosaminoglycans to create an ECM complex. This is exemplified by the roles played by laminin, nidogen, collagen IV, and perlecan in the production of BM.

Fibrillin

Fibrillin forms into microfibrils, which are a part of numerous connective tissues and serve as a model for the synthesis of elastic fibers. Microfibrils play a major role in tissue homeostasis by binding and sequestration of growth factors like TGF-β and through their interactions with cell surface receptors such as integrins [32, 33]. Besides, fibrillin-1 regulates endothelial sprouting during angiogenesis [34]. At the angiogenic front, fibrillin-1 functions as a dynamic signaling component to control matrix remodeling and cell specification [34]. Marfan syndrome, a rare inherited autosomal dominant connective tissue disorder involving fibrillin commonly manifests in the cardiovascular, skeletal, and ocular systems, with aortopathy being the primary concern for morbidity and mortality [35, 36]. Over 50 distinct mutations in the fibrillin-1 gene (*Fbn1*), such as Arg^{239} to Pro and Cys^{1409} to Ser, located on chromosome 15q21, are identified as causative for Marfan syndrome. These mutations disrupt the ability of fibrillin-1 to bind and regulate TGF-β, consequently leading to heightened activity of its downstream pathways. Fibrillin-2, expressed only in blood vessels in normal lungs, is specifically upregulated in IPF fibroblastic foci [37].

Fibrillin-2 changes most likely affect TGF-β availability and activation in various pulmonary compartments within the fibrotic lung.

Fibulin

Fibulins, a family of eight distinct extracellular proteins, are characterized by a conserved COOH-terminal domain, known as the "fibulin-type module," and adjacent calcium-binding EGF-like domains [38]. During fetal development, fibulin-1 is instrumental for ductus arteriosus closure by orchestrating an environment conducive to directional VSMC migration toward the subendothelial region, in synergy with EC-derived versican and its binding collaborator, hyaluronan [39]. Furthermore, fibulin-1 has been demonstrated to play major roles in the pathogenesis of airway and lung remodeling in chronic pulmonary diseases, including COPD, asthma, and pulmonary fibrosis [40]. Specifically, fibulin-1c is associated with lung fibrosis in both humans and mice, and it stabilizes collagen formation [41]. Fibulin-2 is involved in tissue development and remodeling [42]. During embryonic heart development, fibulin-2 is present in the central endometrial cushion matrix, particularly during the epithelial-mesenchymal transition [42]. Fibulin-3 and 4 play crucial roles in the assembly of elastic fibers in the lungs, and their dysregulation is associated with diseases such as emphysema and lung fibrosis [38]. Fibulin-5, indispensable for the assembly and structuring of elastic fibers, plays a paramount role in vascular remodeling and the inhibition of neointima formation. This is evidenced by the pronounced vascular remodeling and significant neointima formation observed in fbln5 null mice post-carotid artery ligation [43]. This study also unveils fibulin-5's role as a suppressor of VSMC proliferation and migration, underscoring its unexpected yet vital function in modulating the vascular response to injury. Consequently, fibulins are recognized as critical contributors to both fetal development and the pathophysiology of various diseases.

Laminin

Laminins, high molecular weight glycoproteins, are composed of three disulfide-linked polypeptide chains: alpha, beta, and gamma [44]. As a crucial element in the structural scaffolding of BM, laminins play an essential role in cell differentiation, migration, adhesion, and the maintenance of tissue structure and function. The human genome encodes 11 genetically distinct laminin chains. These chains are structurally diverse in the number, size, and configuration of several intrinsic domains, providing both shared and unique functions to the laminin family members. In the vascular ECM, the predominant laminins consist of the α4- and α5-chains that couple with laminin-β1 and γ1-chains, assembling into laminins 411 and 511 [45, 46]. Laminin 411 is crucial for vascularization by initiating Notch signaling, enhancing endothelial Dll4 expression via integrin-β binding [47]. Laminin 511 is necessary for proper shear response in ECs [48]. It engages with integrin-β1 to stabilize EC-cadherin at cellular junctions, maintaining appropriate cortical tension, which is essential as it minimizes cell surface area and results in individual cells adopting a rounded shape [48]. Among the five α isoforms, laminin-α1 is involved in BM assembly and architecture and plays a role in cell migration through interactions with integrins α3β1and α6β1 [49]. Laminin polymers create distinct networks and engage with type IV collagen networks through the proteoglycans nidogen and perlecan, contributing to increased BM stability [50]. Laminins also play a role in numerous cell-matrix interactions and functions by securing cells to the ECM, a process vital for embryonic development, maintaining tissue equilibrium, and facilitating remodeling [51].

In IPAH, laminins are expressed more abundantly, contributing to increased endothelial barrier integrity [26]. Genetically engineered mice have identified laminin α1 as a modifier influencing susceptibility to pulmonary fibrosis [52]. Notably, *Lama1* (the gene for laminin α1) mRNA expression is significantly elevated in lung tissue from patients with IPF, indicating that laminins play a critical role in both pulmonary vascular remodeling and pulmonary fibrosis. *Lama3* mRNA expression seems to be elevated in ECs from IPF compared to controls (Fig. 4.1). However, there is also literature showing reduced laminin α3 subunit in fibrotic regions of the lung from IPF [53]. Mice lacking the α3 laminin subunit specifically in the lung epithelium by crossing mice expressing Cre recombinase driven by the surfactant protein C promoter (SPC-Cre) with mice expressing floxed alleles encoding the α3 laminin gene (*Lama3*$^{fl/fl}$) exhibited increased bleomycin-induced lung fibrosis [53]. The study suggests that the laminin a3 in the lung epithelium plays a protective role in the development of fibrosis.

Periostin

Periostin is a ubiquitous and highly conserved glycoprotein first discovered in the periosteum. It facilitates cell adhesion and migration once activated during tissue damage and remodeling [54, 55]. Elevated levels of periostin are observed in conditions like asthma, IPF, and cardiac fibrosis, acting as an indicator for treatment-responsive subtypes and as a lineage marker for active fibroblasts [56–59]. Periostin levels are elevated in rodent models of hypoxia-induced experimental pulmonary hypertension and in hypoxia-treated pulmonary artery smooth muscle cells [60, 61]. Proteomic studies of lung tissues from individuals with idiopathic or heritable PAH have demonstrated a heightened presence of periostin, implying its involvement in human pulmonary vascular disease [62] (Fig. 4.2).

Nie et al. established periostin as a biomarker and contributor to pulmonary vascular remodeling in hypoxic lung diseases, with elevated levels correlating with outcomes like hospitalization and mortality in WHO group 3 PH, including IPF and COPD [63]. Reducing periostin in hypoxia-exposed mice mitigates pulmonary hypertension, through decreased cytokine release and altered PAEC dynamics,

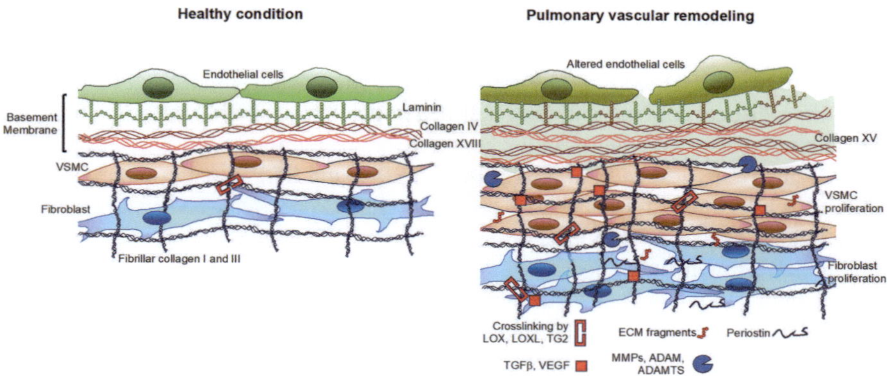

Fig. 4.2 Schematic illustration of the proposed changes in the extracellular matrix (ECM) in pulmonary vascular remodeling secondary to chronic lung diseasesIllustration of the extracellular matrix (ECM) in pulmonary vasculature under healthy conditions versus pulmonary vascular remodeling. The left panel shows a healthy condition with endothelial cells resting on a well-organized basement membrane composed of laminin, collagen IV, and collagen XVIII, and a structured arrangement of fibrillar collagen I and III, with vascular smooth muscle cells (VSMCs) and fibroblasts in their respective layers. The right panel shows pulmonary vascular remodeling, characterized by altered endothelial cells with altered laminin composition, proliferation of VSMCs and fibroblasts. Increased presence of collagen XV is noted in idiopathic pulmonary fibrosis. Additionally, it highlights the enzymatic crosslinking of collagen fibers by lysyl oxidase (LOX), LOX-like enzymes (LOXL), and transglutaminase (TG2), and the accumulation of ECM fragments and periostin. Transforming growth factor-beta (TGFβ), vascular endothelial growth factor (VEGF), matrix metalloproteinases (MMPs), A Disintegrin and Metalloproteinase (ADAM), and A Disintegrin And Metalloproteinase with ThromboSpondin motifs (ADAMTS) are indicated as contributing to the remodeling processes

making periostin attractive as a therapeutic target [63]. Furthermore, hypoxia-induced periostin secretion from PAECs stimulates proliferation and migration of VSMCs, underlining its comprehensive role in vascular pathology [63]. In PAECs, hypoxic conditions amplified the production of periostin and tropomyosin receptor kinase B (TrkB), while the synergy between periostin and hypoxia boosted the generation of TrkB's ligand, brain-derived neurotrophic factor (BDNF). Each of these elements contributes to an increase in hypoxia-inducible factor 1-alpha (HIF1α) expression, identifying it as a pivotal component in this reinforcing feedback mechanism. Additionally, this signaling pathway modulates the levels of vasoactive protein endothelin-1 and the angiogenic factor vascular endothelial growth factor. Periostin silencing reinstates the reduced BMPR2 expression and BMP-SMAD1/5/9 signaling observed in experimental PH and human ECs, while BMPR2 silencing does not affect periostin levels due to periostin's upstream position in this pathway [63]. Given periostin's regulatory role on TGF-β and BMP signaling in fibrotic remodeling [64] and the significance of BMPR2 and SMAD1/5/9 signaling in PH, these results hint at the potential of periostin-targeted therapies in PH, aligning with other experimental treatments that modulate TGF-β or bolster BMP signaling.

Thrombospondins

Thrombospondins (TSPs) are a family of secreted, calcium-binding glycoproteins that play a critical role in regulating cell-cell and cell-matrix interactions. There are five members of the protein: TSP-1 and TSP-2 are homotrimers, whereas TSP-3, TSP-4, and TSP-5 form pentamers. Both TSP-1 and TSP-2 have antiangiogenic activity, which is mostly dependent on the interaction between TSPs and CD36 on the endothelial plasma membrane [65]. Moreover, TSP-1 competes with vascular endothelial growth factor receptor 2 (VEGFR2) for interactions with CD47 [66]. TSP-1 binds to CD47 and interferes with the interaction between CD47 and VEGFR2, preventing VEGFR2 phosphorylation in ECs and nitric oxide (NO)-induced activation of cGMP-dependent protein kinase and soluble guanylate cyclase in VSMCs [67–69]. By interacting with latency-associated peptide (LAP), TSP-1 prevents LAP-TGF-β1 interactions and permits TGF-β1 to trigger downstream signaling through its receptor [70–72].

Tenascin-C

Tenascin-C belongs to a family of four glycoproteins, including tenascin-C, -R, -X, and -W. It is prevalent in the ECM during embryonic development, bone remodeling, and inflammatory processes, but is scarcely found in normal adult tissues [73]. Tenascin-C expression is upregulated in lung vessels from patients with IPF complicated with PH compared to controls [74]. Tenascin-C has several functions, including cell adhesion, angiogenesis, and promotion of the activity of growth factors, specifically, epidermal growth factor and fibroblast growth factor [75–78]. Thus, Tenascin-C might contribute to vascular remodeling in IPF.

Proteoglycans and Glycosaminoglycans

Proteoglycans are heavily glycosylated proteins. They are fundamentally composed of a "core protein" to which one or several glycosaminoglycan (GAG) chain(s) are covalently bonded. GAGs are long, unbranched polysaccharides consisting of repeating disaccharide units. Proteoglycans and GAGs usually create a gelatinous, highly hydrated "ground substance" embedded with collagens and glycoproteins. Although the content of proteoglycans and GAGs is low in the vascular tissue, these proteoglycans and GAGs within vascular walls facilitate the swift diffusion of nutrients, metabolites, and hormones between the blood and tissue cells. In the BM, perlecan and agrin are the major proteoglycans, both of them increased in patients with PH [26, 79].

The media and adventitia layers of the vessel wall are particularly rich in certain proteoglycans, such as versican, lumican, and decorin [80], and the expression of these proteoglycans can characterize distinct subsets of smooth muscle cells. Recent advancements in single-cell transcriptomic analysis have identified four unique subtypes of VSMCs in pulmonary arteries, categorized as contractile, oxygen-sensing, synthetic, and fibroblast-like/intermediate phenotypes [17]. Notably, the synthetic phenotype is markedly enriched for proteoglycans like versican and lumican. Although these four subtypes are preserved in IPAH, there's a shift in their localization and relative presence. Specifically, cells positive for versican and smooth muscle actin, typically found only in the media layer of healthy pulmonary arteries, are enriched in the neointima of remodeled arteries in patients with PAH [17]. This indicates that the proteoglycan-rich smooth muscle subtype may play a significant role in the development of vascular remodeling. Another study corroborated these results by detecting increased levels of versican and aggrecan in the pulmonary vasculature in patients with IPAH [81, 82]. Aggrecan, known as the largest and most extensively glycosylated proteoglycan, indeed exhibits a distinct distribution based on the type of vascular remodeling. In cases where vessel remodeling is characterized by media hypertrophy, aggrecan is primarily found in the media [82]. Conversely, in scenarios predominantly involving neointima formation, aggrecan is almost exclusively located in the neointima, with a notable absence in medial smooth muscle cells [82]. This indicates that VSMCs positive for aggrecan may represent a specific functional group contributing to PH pathology. Additionally, the expression of decorin, a small-leucine-rich proteoglycan, is concentrated in a particular subset of VSMCs in the pulmonary artery, specifically the intermediate/fibroblast-like subtype, marking it as a significant indicator of adventitial fibroblast.

In chronic lung diseases, altered composition of proteoglycans and GAGs is reported. Deposition of versican, the largest proteoglycan in the vessel wall, is observed in the lesions of fibroblast foci in IPF [83]. Versican expression is upregulated in VSMCs stimulated by platelet-derived growth factor (PDGF). Versican influences VSMC proliferation through epidermal growth factor sequences.

Other ECM Proteins

The ECM-associated protein, prolactin-induced protein (PIP), is highly upregulated in the parenchyma and vasculature of lungs from IPF complicated with PH compared to IPF without PH [14]. Produced by macrophages, PIP induces VSMC proliferation and thereby contributes to vascular remodeling.

Posttranslational Modifications and Matrix Degradation

Besides LOX, LOXL, and TG2 enzyme activity as mentioned above, protein function and pulmonary vascular homeostasis is affected by a variety of posttranslational modifications, including glycosylation, hydroxylation, and nitrosylation. Matrix degradation greatly alters the composition of ECM, which further impacts vascular homeostasis and remodeling. This degradation process reduces the overall matrix protein levels and generates bioactive fragments from the degraded matrix proteins. These fragments play roles in autophagy, angiogenesis, fibrosis, and wound repair, under both normal and diseased states. Herein, we discuss the post-translational modifications and ECM degradation in vascular remodeling in this section.

Posttranslational Modifications

Glycosylation

Protein glycosylation represents the most common form of posttranslational modification, affecting protein structure, folding, distribution, stability, and function. The two primary forms of glycosylation are N-linked, occurring on asparagine residues, and O-linked, which takes place on serine or threonine residues [84]. Glycation of fibrous proteins augments fiber cross-linking and increases vascular rigidity [85]. Glycated fibronectin, in comparison to its native form, has a greater impact on promoting VSMC adhesion [86].

Hydroxylation

Prolyl hydroxylase and lysyl hydroxylase enzymes catalyze hydroxylation based on the specific amino acid residues altered. Collagen chains and similar sequences often have repeated Xaa-Pro-Gly triplets, where “Xaa” represents any amino acid. Proline in these regions is hydroxylated by prolyl hydroxylases [87]. This stable and irreversible post-translational modification adds 16 Da, equivalent to an oxygen atom, to proline or lysine and is particularly prevalent in collagens. The most recognized function of hydroxylation is its contribution to the stabilization of the collagen triple helix. The hydroxylation of prolines within collagen is a critical step in the formation of collagen fibers. Lysyl hydroxylase, which specifically targets lysine, facilitates the creation of hydroxylysine within Xaa-Lys-Gly sequences found in fibrous proteins [88]. A defective mutation in the lysyl hydroxylase-1 gene (*PLOD1*) leads to Ehlers-Danlos Syndrome, with phenotypes similar to those resulting from mutations in collagen I and III, showcasing the resulting vulnerability of the skin and vascular wall [89, 90]. In a mouse model, collagen prolyl hydroxylase (*P4HA3*) was upregulated by TGF-β in fibrotic lung mesenchymal cells, while its inhibition by pyridine-2,5-dicarboxylate reduced TGF-β-stimulated collagen production in cultured fibroblasts and in bleomycin-induced mouse lung fibrosis [91].

S-Nitrosylation

S-Nitrosylation, a critical post-translational modification, involves the covalent attachment of a nitric oxide group (−NO) to a protein's cysteine thiol, forming S-nitrosothiol. In the vascular system, nitric oxide (NO) is prevalent and is key to vascular tone and other vessel functions [92]. The enzyme TG2, known for catalyzing transamidation reactions, is instrumental in matrix protein cross-linking, a process that contributes to increased vascular stiffness. Notably, endothelium-derived NO modulates this process by inducing the S-nitrosylation of TG2, thereby diminishing its cross-linking capability. Consequently, in conditions like PH where NO production is reduced [93], there's an acceleration in TG2 activity, leading to further vascular stiffening. Given the elevated levels of TG2 activity observed in IPF [94], targeting TG2 emerges as a potential therapeutic strategy in these pathologies.

Matrix Degradation

Matrix Metalloproteinases

Matrix metalloproteinases (MMPs) are a group of zinc-dependent endopeptidases, and 14 members are specifically expressed in the vasculature. MMPs degrade ECM protein substrates such as collagens, aggrecan, fibronectin, and laminin. MMPs and their degradation fragments play fundamental roles in angiogenesis, morphogenesis, and vascular remodeling. The secretion of MMP-2 and MMP-9 triggered by angiogenic factors in ECs is essential for EC proliferation, migration, and invasion into the vascular ECM associated with sprouting angiogenesis [95]. Further, several MMPs (MMP-1, -2, -7, -9, -16, and -19) mediate proteolytic cleavage of ECM to release VEGF and active TGF-β and increase their bioavailability [96]. In both human cases of PAH and experimental models of PH, there have been observations of altered expression and activity patterns of MMPs. Upregulated MMP-2 and MMP-9, while decreased levels of MMP-3 are reported [97]. Similarly, dysregulated MMP activity is reported in IPF and COPD [98, 99].

A Disintegrin and Metalloproteinases (ADAMs) and A Disintegrin and Metalloproteinase with ThromboSpondin motifs (ADAMTS)

ADAMs and ADAMTS belong to another superfamily of metallo-endopeptidases. ADAMs are known for their sheddase function, which is critical for the cleavage of membrane-bound proteins, growth factors, cytokines, as well as various ligands and receptors. ADAMTSs are crucial in embryonic development, playing significant roles in lung formation, the molecular maturation of von Willebrand factor and procollagen, as well as in the arrangement of fibrillin microfibrils within the ECM. ADAMs and ADAMTSs play numerous roles in vascular biology, including proliferation and migration, cell apoptosis of vascular cells, and angiogenesis [100]. On the contrary, as pathologic roles, ADAM10 participates in PAH [101], and ADAM10-mediated soluble ephrin-B2 is involved in pulmonary fibrosis [102]. ADAMTS8 promotes the development of PAH [103].

ECM Fragments

In recent years, it has been recognized that products cleaved by metalloproteases within the fibrotic microenvironment can contribute to disease progression. These ECM fragments, known as matrikines, possess specific bioactivities and can regulate various phenomena such as signal transduction, gene expression, angiogenesis, wound healing, and fibrosis [28]. ECM fragments interact with growth factor receptors, Toll-like receptors, integrins, and other diverse cell surface receptors, actively inducing cellular responses that differ from those caused by the parent molecules before cleavage [28].

Proline-glycine-proline (PGP), an ECM fragment derived from type I collagen, is known as a chemotactic factor for neutrophils and is involved in local inflammation within the microenvironment [104]. The C-1158/59 fragment, produced through cleavage by MMP2/9, promotes the migration of fibroblasts [105]. The non-collagenous domain at the C-terminus of type IV collagen in the basement membrane is cleaved by different enzymes, and through binding to integrins on inflammatory cells, endothelial cells, epithelial cells, and fibroblasts, and controls adhesion and migration in the microenvironment [28]. Restin (a fragment of collagen XV) and endostatin (a fragment of collagen XVIII) are already mentioned in the prior section.

Bioactive elastin fragments occur as a result of proteolytic degradation of elastin by MMPs, serine proteases, and cysteine proteases. Elastin fragments, similar to collagen fragments, promote angiogenesis, stimulate cell adhesion, EC migration, and fibrosis [106, 107]. In the lung of IPF or COPD, the activity of MMPs increases, whereby ECM fragments increase and contribute to vascular remodeling.

Conclusion

Given the significant influence of ECM dynamics on vascular remodeling, comprehending this network can help to unveil targets and therapeutic opportunities. Yet, the complexity of this regulatory system remains partially elusive, especially pulmonary remodeling secondary to chronic lung diseases. Variations in ECM composition among different etiologies of PH and distinct inflammatory environments make it challenging to the application of universal therapeutic intervention for PH. It is important to consider that the dysregulated ECM in pulmonary vascular remodeling is produced/modified by altered vascular cells and immune cells. Therefore, altered vascular cells may also be good, if not better therapeutic targets.

It is also important to consider that the candidate drugs that target ECM or ECM modulatory proteins may affect not only the vasculature but also the parenchyma. Therefore deeper understanding of ECM dynamics among vasculature and parenchyma is warranted. Recent insights into vascular-parenchymal crosstalk suggest that targeting vascular ECM remodeling may enhance treatment outcomes for underlying pulmonary conditions.

Conflict of Interest T. Yanagihara reports grants from Boehringer Ingelheim outside the submitted work. K. Otsubo reports no conflict of interest. M. Kolb reports being site PI for sponsored clinical trials for Roche and Boehringer Ingelheim, grants from Canadian Institute for Health Research, grants and personal fees for advisory board work from Boehringer Ingelheim and Roche Canada, chief editor allowance from the European Respiratory Society, personal fees for advisory board work from Horizon, Algernon, CSL Behring, DevPro, Bellerophon and BMS, personal fees for adjudication committee work from United Therapeutics, and personal fees for data monitoring committee work from LabCorp, outside the submitted work.

Appendix

Analysis of Single-Cell RNA Sequencing Data

We analyzed the publicly available dataset GSE136831, which contains single-cell RNA sequencing data from whole lung dissociates from controls ($n = 28$), IPF ($n = 32$), and COPD ($n = 18$) [22] using R package *Seurat* and *ggplot2* in RStudio (version 2023.03.0+386 with R version 4.2.3). We initiated our analysis by normalizing the filtered gene-barcode matrix using the “NormalizeData” function in Seurat version 4, applying the default settings. Subsequently, we identified the top 2000 variable genes utilizing the “vst” method available in the “FindVariableFeatures” function of Seurat. PCA and UMAP were then conducted to reduce dimensionality and visualize the data. Cell identity attached as metadata was used for cell type identification. We specifically extracted the “Endothelial” cell category to focus on endothelial cells. Collagen, elastin, laminin, fibronectin, and fibrillin genes were selected based on prefixes “^COL”, “^ELN”, “^LAM”, “^FBLN”, and “^FBN”, respectively. Differential gene expression was determined using “FindMarkers,” considering p values <0.05 as significant.

References

1. Humbert M, Kovacs G, Hoeper MM, Badagliacca R, Berger RMF, Brida M, Carlsen J, Coats AJS, Escribano-Subias P, Ferrari P, Ferreira DS, Ghofrani HA, Giannakoulas G, Kiely DG, Mayer E, Meszaros G, Nagavci B, Olsson KM, Pepke-Zaba J, Quint JK, Rådegran G, Simonneau G, Sitbon O, Tonia T, Toshner M, Vachiery J-L, Vonk Noordegraaf A, Delcroix M, Rosenkranz S. 2022 ESC/ERS Guidelines for the diagnosis and treatment of pulmonary hypertension. Eur Respir J. 2023;61:2200879.

2. Lettieri CJ, Nathan SD, Barnett SD, Ahmad S, Shorr AF. Prevalence and outcomes of pulmonary arterial hypertension in advanced idiopathic pulmonary fibrosis. Chest Am College Chest Phys. 2006;129:746–52.
3. Bousseau S, Sobrano Fais R, Gu S, Frump A, Lahm T. Pathophysiology and new advances in pulmonary hypertension. BMJ Med. 2023;2:e000137.
4. Yanagihara T, Tsubouchi K, Zhou Q, Chong M, Otsubo K, Isshiki T, Schupp JC, Sato S, Scallan C, Upagupta C, Revill S, Ayoub A, Chong SG, Dvorkin-Gheva A, Kaminski N, Tikkanen J, Keshavjee S, Paré G, Guignabert C, Ask K, Kolb MRJ. Vascular–parenchymal cross-talk promotes lung fibrosis through BMPR2 signaling. Am J Respir Crit Care Med. 2023;207:1498–514.
5. Bellaye P-S, Yanagihara T, Granton E, Sato S, Shimbori C, Upagupta C, Imani J, Hambly N, Ask K, Gauldie J, Iglarz M, Kolb M. Macitentan reduces progression of TGF-β1-induced pulmonary fibrosis and pulmonary hypertension. Eur Respir J. 2018;52:1701857.
6. Christou H, Khalil RA. Mechanisms of pulmonary vascular dysfunction in pulmonary hypertension and implications for novel therapies. Am J Physiol Heart Circ Physiol. 2022;322:H702–24.
7. Frantz C, Stewart KM, Weaver VM. The extracellular matrix at a glance. J Cell Sci. 2010;123:4195–200.
8. Burgess JK, Harmsen MC. Chronic lung diseases: entangled in extracellular matrix. Eur Respir Rev. 2022;31:210202.
9. Townsley MI. Structure and composition of pulmonary arteries, capillaries, and veins. Compr Physiol. 2012;2:675–709.
10. Mecham RP, Whitehouse LA, Wrenn DS, Parks WC, Griffin GL, Senior RM, Crouch EC, Stenmark KR, Voelkel NF. Smooth muscle-mediated connective tissue remodeling in pulmonary hypertension. Science (80-). 1987;237:423–6.
11. Jandl K, Mutgan AC, Eller K, Schaefer L, Kwapiszewska G. The basement membrane in the cross-roads between the lung and kidney. Matrix Biol Elsevier BV. 2022;105:31–52.
12. Almudéver P, Milara J, De Diego A, Serrano-Mollar A, Xaubet A, Perez-Vizcaino F, Cogolludo A, Cortijo J. Role of tetrahydrobiopterin in pulmonary vascular remodelling associated with pulmonary fibrosis. Thorax. 2013;68:938–48.
13. Nave AH, Mižíková I, Niess G, Steenbock H, Reichenberger F, Talavera ML, Veit F, Herold S, Mayer K, Vadász I, Weissmann N, Seeger W, Brinckmann J, Morty RE. Lysyl oxidases play a causal role in vascular remodeling in clinical and experimental pulmonary arterial hypertension. Arterioscler Thromb Vasc Biol. 2014;34:1446–58.
14. Ruffenach G, Umar S, Vaillancourt M, Hong J, Cao N, Sarji S, Moazeni S, Cunningham CM, Ardehali A, Reddy ST, Saggar R, Fishbein G, Eghbali M. Histological hallmarks and role of Slug/PIP axis in pulmonary hypertension secondary to pulmonary fibrosis. EMBO Mol Med. 2019;11:1–19.
15. Kong CH, Lin XY, Woo CC, Wong HC, Lee CN, Richards AM, Sorokin VA. Characteristics of aortic wall extracellular matrix in patients with acute myocardial infarction: tissue microarray detection of collagen I, collagen III and elastin levels. Interact Cardiovasc Thorac Surg. 2013;16:11–5.
16. Biasin V, Crnkovic S, Sahu-Osen A, Birnhuber A, Agha EE, Sinn K, Klepetko W, Olschewski A, Bellusci S, Marsh LM, Kwapiszewska G. PDGFRα and αSMA mark two distinct mesenchymal cell populations involved in parenchymal and vascular remodeling in pulmonary fibrosis. Am J Phys Lung Cell Mol Phys. 2020;318:L684–97.
17. Crnkovic S, Valzano F, Fließer E, Gindlhuber J, Thekkekara Puthenparampil H, Basil M, Morley MP, Katzen J, Gschwandtner E, Klepetko W, Cantu E, Wolinski H, Olschewski H, Lindenmann J, Zhao Y-Y, Morrisey EE, Marsh LM, Kwapiszewska G. Single-cell transcriptomics reveals skewed cellular communication and phenotypic shift in pulmonary artery remodeling. JCI Insight. 2022;7:e153471.
18. Yanagihara T, Sato S, Upagupta C, Kolb M. What have we learned from basic science studies on idiopathic pulmonary fibrosis? Eur Respir Rev. 2019;28:190029.

19. Tjin G, White ES, Faiz A, Sicard D, Tschumperlin DJ, Mahar A, Kable EPW, Burgess JK. Lysyl oxidases regulate fibrillar collagen remodelling in idiopathic pulmonary fibrosis. Dis Model Mech. 2017;10:1301–12.
20. Kubota K, Okazaki J, Louie O, Kent KC, Liu B. TGF-beta stimulates collagen (I) in vascular smooth muscle cells via a short element in the proximal collagen promoter. J Surg Res. 2003;109:43–50.
21. Schupp JC, Adams TS, Cosme C, Raredon MSB, Yuan Y, Omote N, Poli S, Chioccioli M, Rose KA, Manning EP, Sauler M, Deiuliis G, Ahangari F, Neumark N, Habermann AC, Gutierrez AJ, Bui LT, Lafyatis R, Pierce RW, Meyer KB, Nawijn MC, Teichmann SA, Banovich NE, Kropski JA, Niklason LE, Pe'Er D, Yan X, Homer RJ, Rosas IO, Kaminski N. Integrated single-cell atlas of endothelial cells of the human lung. Circulation. 2021;144:286–302.
22. Adams TS, Schupp JC, Poli S, Ayaub EA, Neumark N, Ahangari F, Chu SG, Raby BA, DeIuliis G, Januszyk M, Duan Q, Arnett HA, Siddiqui A, Washko GR, Homer R, Yan X, Rosas IO, Kaminski N. Single-cell RNA-seq reveals ectopic and aberrant lung-resident cell populations in idiopathic pulmonary fibrosis. Sci Adv. 2020;6:eaba1983.
23. Truchi M, Savary G, Cadis H, Lebrigand K, Baeri A, Lingampally A, Girard-Riboulleau C, Scribe C, Magnone V, Arguel M-J, Schutter C de, Gautier-isola M, Fassy J, Rezzonico R, Larrue R, Pluquet O, Perrais M, Hofman V, Marquette C, Hofman P, Günther A, Ricard N, Barbry P, Leroy S, Cauffiez C, Bellusci S, Vassaux G, Pottier N, Mari B, Arguel J, et al. Lung injury shifts pulmonary capillary endothelial cells towards regeneration-associated Lrg1+ subpopulations with delayed dynamics in aged mice. bioRxiv. 2023;2023.07.11.548522.
24. Wang H, Su Y. Collagen IV contributes to nitric oxide-induced angiogenesis of lung endothelial cells. Am J Phys Cell Physiol. 2011;300:968–9.
25. Ramchandran R, Dhanabal M, Volk R, Waterman MJF, Segal M, Lu H, Knebelmann B, Sukhatme VP. Antiangiogenic activity of restin, NC10 domain of human collagen XV: comparison to endostatin. Biochem Biophys Res Commun. 1999;255:735–9.
26. Jandl K, Marsh LM, Hoffmann J, Mutgan AC, Baum O, Bloch W, Thekkekara-Puthenparampil H, Kolb D, Sinn K, Klepetko W, Heinemann A, Olschewski A, Olschewski H, Kwapiszewska G. Basement membrane remodeling controls endothelial function in idiopathic pulmonary arterial hypertension. Am J Respir Cell Mol Biol. 2020;63:104–17.
27. Sumi M, Satoh H, Kagohashi K, Ishikawa H, Sekizawa K. Increased serum levels of endostatin in patients with idiopathic pulmonary fibrosis. J Clin Lab Anal. 2005;19:146–9.
28. Ricard-Blum S, Vallet SD. Fragments generated upon extracellular matrix remodeling: biological regulators and potential drugs. Matrix Biol Elsevier BV. 2019;75–76:170–89.
29. Halabi CM, Kozel BA. Vascular elastic fiber heterogeneity in health and disease. Curr Opin Hematol. 2020;27:190–6.
30. Gaikwad AV, Lu W, Dey S, Bhattarai P, Chia C, Larby J, Haug G, Myers S, Jaffar J, Westall G, Singhera GK, Hackett TL, Markos J, Eapen MS, Sohal SS. Vascular remodelling in idiopathic pulmonary fibrosis patients and its detrimental effect on lung physiology: potential role of endothelial-to-mesenchymal transition. ERJ Open Res. 2022;8.
31. Heinz A. Elastases and elastokines: elastin degradation and its significance in health and disease. Crit Rev Biochem Mol Biol Taylor & Francis. 2020;55:252–73.
32. Bax D V., Bernard SE, Lomas A, Morgan A, Humphries J, Shuttleworth CA, Humphries MJ, Kielty CM. Cell adhesion to fibrillin-1 molecules and microfibrils is mediated by α5β1 and αvβ3 integrins. J. Biol. Chem. Â© 2003 ASBMB. Currently published by Elsevier Inc; originally published by American Society for Biochemistry and Molecular Biology. 2003;278:34605–16.
33. Jovanovic J, Takagi J, Choulier L, Abrescia NGA, Stuart DI, Van Der Merwe PA, Mardon HJ, Handford PA. αVβ6 is a novel receptor for human fibrillin-1: Comparative studies of molecular determinants underlying integrin-RGD affinity and specificity. J Biol Chem. 2007;282:6743–51.
34. Alonso F, Dong Y, Li L, Jahjah T, Dupuy J-W, Fremaux I, Reinhardt DP, Génot E. Fibrillin-1 regulates endothelial sprouting during angiogenesis. Proc Natl Acad Sci. 2023;120.

35. Iskandar Z, Mordi I, Lang CC, Huang JTJ, Choy A-M. Biomarkers of aortopathy in Marfan syndrome. Cardiol Rev. 2020;28:92–7.
36. Pyeritz RE, McKusick VA. The Marfan syndrome: diagnosis and management. N Engl J Med. 1979;300:772–7.
37. Leppäranta O, Sens C, Salmenkivi K, Kinnula VL, Keski-Oja J, Myllärniemi M, Koli K. Regulation of TGF-β storage and activation in the human idiopathic pulmonary fibrosis lung. Cell Tissue Res. 2012;348:491–503.
38. Nakamura T. Roles of short fibulins, a family of matricellular proteins, in lung matrix assembly and disease. Matrix Biol. 2018;73:21–33.
39. Ito S, Yokoyama U, Nakakoji T, Cooley MA, Sasaki T, Hatano S, Kato Y, Saito J, Nicho N, Iwasaki S, Umemura M, Fujita T, Masuda M, Asou T, Ishikawa Y. Fibulin-1 integrates subendothelial extracellular matrices and contributes to anatomical closure of the ductus arteriosus. Arterioscler Thromb Vasc Biol. 2020;40:2212–26.
40. Liu G, Cooley MA, Jarnicki AG, Hsu AC-Y, Nair PM, Haw TJ, Fricker M, Gellatly SL, Kim RY, Inman MD, Tjin G, Wark PAB, Walker MM, Horvat JC, Oliver BG, Argraves WS, Knight DA, Burgess JK, Hansbro PM. Fibulin-1 regulates the pathogenesis of tissue remodeling in respiratory diseases. JCI Insight. 2016;1.
41. Liu G, Cooley MA, Jarnicki AG, Borghuis T, Nair PM, Tjin G, Hsu AC, Haw TJ, Fricker M, Harrison CL, Jones B, Hansbro NG, Wark PA, Horvat JC, Argraves WS, Oliver BG, Knight DA, Burgess JK, Hansbro PM. Fibulin-1c regulates transforming growth factor-β activation in pulmonary tissue fibrosis. JCI Insight. 2019;5.
42. Tsuda T, Wang H, Timpl R, Chu M. Fibulin-2 expression marks transformed mesenchymal cells in developing cardiac valves, aortic arch vessels, and coronary vessels. Dev Dyn. 2001;222:89–100.
43. Spencer JA, Hacker SL, Davis EC, Mecham RP, Knutsen RH, Li DY, Gerard RD, Richardson JA, Olson EN, Yanagisawa H. Altered vascular remodeling in fibulin-5-deficient mice reveals a role of fibulin-5 in smooth muscle cell proliferation and migration. Proc Natl Acad Sci. 2005;102:2946–51.
44. Aumailley M. The laminin family. Cell Adhes Migr. 2013;7:48–55.
45. Frieser M, Nöckel H, Pausch F, Röder C, Hahn A, Deutzmann R, Sorokin LM. Cloning of the mouse laminin alpha 4 cDNA. Expression in a subset of endothelium. Eur J Biochem. 1997;246:727–35.
46. Sorokin LM, Pausch F, Frieser M, Kröger S, Ohage E, Deutzmann R. Developmental regulation of the laminin α5 chain suggests a role in epithelial and endothelial cell maturation. Dev Biol. 1997;189:285–300.
47. Stenzel D, Franco CA, Estrach S, Mettouchi A, Sauvaget D, Rosewell I, Schertel A, Armer H, Domogatskaya A, Rodin S, Tryggvason K, Collinson L, Sorokin L, Gerhardt H. Endothelial basement membrane limits tip cell formation by inducing Dll4/Notch signalling in vivo. EMBO Rep. 2011;12:1135–43.
48. Di Russo J, Luik A, Yousif L, Budny S, Oberleithner H, Hofschröer V, Klingauf J, van Bavel E, Bakker EN, Hellstrand P, Bhattachariya A, Albinsson S, Pincet F, Hallmann R, Sorokin LM. Endothelial basement membrane laminin 511 is essential for shear stress response. EMBO J. 2017;36:183–201.
49. Tzu J, Marinkovich MP. Bridging structure with function: structural, regulatory, and developmental role of laminins. Int J Biochem Cell Biol. 2008;40:199–214.
50. Chute M, Aujla P, Jana S, Kassiri Z. The non-fibrillar side of fibrosis: contribution of the basement membrane, proteoglycans, and glycoproteins to myocardial fibrosis. J. Cardiovasc. Dev. Dis. 2019;6.
51. Farhadian F, Contard F, Sabri A, Samuel JL, Rappaport L. Fibronectin and basement membrane in cardiovascular organogenesis and disease pathogenesis. Cardiovasc Res. 1996;32:433–42.
52. Lee CM, Cho SJ, Cho WK, Park JW, Lee JH, Choi AM, Rosas IO, Zheng M, Peltz G, Lee CG, Elias JA. Laminin α1 is a genetic modifier of TGF-β1-stimulated pulmonary fibrosis. JCI Insight. 2018;3.

53. Morales-Nebreda LI, Rogel MR, Eisenberg JL, Hamill KJ, Soberanes S, Nigdelioglu R, Chi M, Cho T, Radigan KA, Ridge KM, Misharin AV, Woychek A, Hopkinson S, Perlman H, Mutlu GM, Pardo A, Selman M, Jones JCR, Budinger GRS. Lung-specific loss of α3 laminin worsens bleomycin-induced pulmonary fibrosis. Am J Respir Cell Mol Biol. 2015;52:503–12.
54. Horiuchi K, Amizuka N, Takeshita S, Takamatsu H, Katsuura M, Ozawa H, Toyama Y, Bonewald LF, Kudo A. Identification and characterization of a novel protein, periostin, with restricted expression to periosteum and periodontal ligament and increased expression by transforming growth factor β. J Bone Miner Res. 1999;14:1239–49.
55. Snider P, Standley KN, Wang J, Azhar M, Doetschman T, Conway SJ. Origin of cardiac fibroblasts and the role of periostin. Circ Res. 2009;105:934–47.
56. Naik PK, Bozyk PD, Bentley JK, Popova AP, Birch CM, Wilke CA, Fry CD, White ES, Sisson TH, Tayob N, Carnemolla B, Orecchia P, Flaherty KR, Hershenson MB, Murray S, Martinez FJ, Moore BB, COMET Investigators. Periostin promotes fibrosis and predicts progression in patients with idiopathic pulmonary fibrosis. Am J Phys Lung Cell Mol Phys. 2012;303:L1046–56.
57. Okamoto M, Fujimoto K, Johkoh T, Kawaguchi A, Mukae H, Sakamoto N, Ogura T, Ikeda S, Kondoh Y, Yamano Y, Komiya K, Umeki K, Nishikiori H, Tanino Y, Tsuda T, Arai N, Komatsu M, Sakamoto S, Yatera K, Inoue Y, Miyazaki Y, Hashimoto S, Shimizu Y, Hozumi H, Ohnishi H, Handa T, Hattori N, Kishaba T, Kato M, Inomata M, et al. A prospective cohort study of periostin as a serum biomarker in patients with idiopathic pulmonary fibrosis treated with nintedanib. Sci Rep. 2023;13:22977.
58. Woodruff PG, Boushey HA, Dolganov GM, Barker CS, Yang YH, Donnelly S, Ellwanger A, Sidhu SS, Dao-Pick TP, Pantoja C, Erle DJ, Yamamoto KR, Fahy JV. Genome-wide profiling identifies epithelial cell genes associated with asthma and with treatment response to corticosteroids. Proc Natl Acad Sci USA. 2007;104:15858–63.
59. Kaur H, Takefuji M, Ngai CY, Carvalho J, Bayer J, Wietelmann A, Poetsch A, Hoelper S, Conway SJ, Möllmann H, Looso M, Troidl C, Offermanns S, Wettschureck N. Targeted ablation of periostin-expressing activated fibroblasts prevents adverse cardiac remodeling in mice. Circ Res. 2016;118:1906–17.
60. Li P, Oparil S, Feng W, Chen Y-F. Hypoxia-responsive growth factors upregulate periostin and osteopontin expression via distinct signaling pathways in rat pulmonary arterial smooth muscle cells. J Appl Physiol. 2004;97:1550–8. discussion 1549
61. Chen Y-F, Feng J-A, Li P, Xing D, Zhang Y, Serra R, Ambalavanan N, Majid-Hassan E, Oparil S. Dominant negative mutation of the TGF-beta receptor blocks hypoxia-induced pulmonary vascular remodeling. J Appl Physiol. 2006;100:564–71.
62. Abdul-Salam VB, Wharton J, Cupitt J, Berryman M, Edwards RJ, Wilkins MR. Proteomic analysis of lung tissues from patients with pulmonary arterial hypertension. Circulation. 2010;122:2058–67.
63. Nie X, Shen C, Tan J, Wu Z, Wang W, Chen Y, Dai Y, Yang X, Ye S, Chen J, Bian J-S. Periostin: a potential therapeutic target for pulmonary hypertension? Circ Res. 2020;127:1138–52.
64. Nanri Y, Nunomura S, Terasaki Y, Yoshihara T, Hirano Y, Yokosaki Y, Yamaguchi Y, Feghali-Bostwick C, Ajito K, Murakami S, Conway SJ, Izuhara K. Cross-talk between transforming growth factor-β and periostin can be targeted for pulmonary fibrosis. Am J Respir Cell Mol Biol. 2020;62:204–16.
65. Pearce SFA, Wu J, Silverstein RL. Recombinant GST/CD36 fusion proteins define a thrombospondin binding domain. J Biol Chem. 1995;270:2981–6.
66. Kaur S, Martin-Manso G, Pendrak ML, Garfield SH, Isenberg JS, Roberts DD. Thrombospondin-1 inhibits VEGF receptor-2 signaling by disrupting its association with CD47. J Biol Chem. 2010;285:38923–32.
67. Isenberg JS, Ridnour LA, Dimitry J, Frazier WA, Wink DA, Roberts DD. CD47 is necessary for inhibition of nitric oxide-stimulated vascular cell responses by thrombospondin-1. J Biol Chem. 2006;281:26069–80.
68. Isenberg J, Wink D, Roberts D. Thrombospondin-1 antagonizes nitric oxide-stimulated vascular smooth muscle cell responses. Cardiovasc Res. 2006;71:785–93.

69. Miller TW, Isenberg JS, Roberts DD. Thrombospondin-1 is an inhibitor of pharmacological activation of soluble guanylate cyclase. Br J Pharmacol. 2010;159:1542–7.
70. Ribeiro SMF, Poczatek M, Schultz-Cherry S, Villain M, Murphy-Ullrich JE. The activation sequence of thrombospondin-1 interacts with the latency-associated peptide to regulate activation of latent transforming growth factor-β. J Biol Chem. 1999;274:13586–93.
71. Schultz-Cherry S, Chen H, Mosher DF, Misenheimer TM, Krutzsch HC, Roberts DD, Murphy-Ullrich JE. Regulation of transforming growth factor-β activation by discrete sequences of thrombospondin 1. J Biol Chem. 1995;270:7304–10.
72. Schultz-Cherry S, Lawler J, Murphy-Ullrich JE. The type 1 repeats of thrombospondin 1 activate latent transforming growth factor-beta. J Biol Chem. 1994;269:26783–8.
73. Matsumoto K, Aoki H. The roles of tenascins in cardiovascular, inflammatory, and heritable connective tissue diseases. Front Immunol. 2020;11.
74. Hoffmann J, Wilhelm J, Marsh LM, Ghanim B, Klepetko W, Kovacs G, Olschewski H, Olschewski A, Kwapiszewska G. Distinct differences in gene expression patterns in pulmonary arteries of patients with chronic obstructive pulmonary disease and idiopathic pulmonary fibrosis with pulmonary hypertension. Am J Respir Crit Care Med. 2014;190:98–111.
75. Chiquet-Ehrismann R, Tucker RP. Tenascins and the importance of adhesion modulation. Cold Spring Harb Perspect Biol. 2011;3.
76. Wang Y, Wang G, Liu H. Tenascin-C: a key regulator in angiogenesis during wound healing. Biomolecules. 2022;12.
77. Schenk S, Chiquet-Ehrismann R, Battegay EJ. The fibrinogen globe of tenascin-C promotes basic fibroblast growth factor-induced endothelial cell elongation. Matsudaira PT, editor. Mol Biol Cell. 1999;10:2933–43.
78. Jones PL, Crack J, Rabinovitch M. Regulation of tenascin-C, a vascular smooth muscle cell survival factor that interacts with the αvβ3 integrin to promote epidermal growth factor receptor phosphorylation and growth. J Cell Biol. 1997;139:279–93.
79. Hoffmann J, Marsh LM, Pieper M, Stacher E, Ghanim B, Kovacs G, König P, Wilkens H, Haitchi HM, Hoefler G, Klepetko W, Olschewski H, Olschewski A, Kwapiszewska G. Biomarkers in lung diseases: from pathogenesis to prediction to new therapiescompartment-specific expression of collagens and their processing enzymes in intrapulmonary arteries of IPAH patients. Am J Phys Lung Cell Mol Phys. 2015;308:L1002–13.
80. Wight TN. A role for proteoglycans in vascular disease. Matrix Biol. 2018;71–72:396–420.
81. Chang Y, Chan CK, Eriksson I, Johnson PY, Cao X, Westöö C, Norvik C, Andersson-Sjöland A, Westergren-Thorsson G, Johansson S, Hedin U, Kjellén L, Wight TN, Tran-Lundmark K. Versican accumulates in vascular lesions in pulmonary arterial hypertension. Pulm Circ. 2016;6:347–59.
82. van der Have O, Mead TJ, Westöö C, Peruzzi N, Mutgan AC, Norvik C, Bech M, Struglics A, Hoetzenecker K, Brunnström H, Westergren-Thorsson G, Kwapiszewska G, Apte SS, Tran-Lundmark K. Aggrecan accumulates at sites of increased pulmonary arterial pressure in idiopathic pulmonary arterial hypertension. Pulm Circ. 2023;13:e12200.
83. Bensadoun ES, Burke AK, Hogg JC, Roberts CR. Proteoglycan deposition in pulmonary fibrosis. Am J Respir Crit Care Med. 1996;154:1819–28.
84. Spiro RG. Protein glycosylation: nature, distribution, enzymatic formation, and disease implications of glycopeptide bonds. Glycobiology. 2002;12:43R–56R.
85. Slatter DA, Avery NC, Bailey AJ. Collagen in its fibrillar state is protected from glycation. Int J Biochem Cell Biol. 2008;40:2253–63.
86. Dhar S, Sun Z, Meininger GA, Hill MA. Nonenzymatic glycation interferes with fibronectin-integrin interactions in vascular smooth muscle cells. Microcirculation. 2017;24:e12347.
87. Kivirikko KI, Helaakoski T, Tasanen K, Vuori K, Myllylä R, Parkkonen T, Pihlajaniemi T. Molecular biology of prolyl 4-hydroxylase. Ann N Y Acad Sci. 1990;580:132–42.
88. Yamauchi M, Sricholpech M. Lysine post-translational modifications of collagen. Scott I, editor. Essays Biochem. 2012;52:113–33.
89. Henneton P, Legrand A, Giunta C, Frank M. Arterial fragility in kyphoscoliotic Ehlers-Danlos syndrome. BMJ Case Rep. 2018;bcr-2018-224423.

90. Malfait F. Vascular aspects of the Ehlers-Danlos Syndromes. Matrix Biol. 2018;71–72:380–95.
91. Luo Y, Xu W, Chen H, Warburton D, Dong R, Qian B, Selman M, Gauldie J, Kolb M, Shi W. A novel profibrotic mechanism mediated by *TGFβ* -stimulated collagen prolyl hydroxylase expression in fibrotic lung mesenchymal cells. J Pathol. 2015;236:384–94.
92. Naseem KM. The role of nitric oxide in cardiovascular diseases. Mol Asp Med. 2005;26:33–65.
93. Wilkins MR. Pulmonary hypertension: the science behind the disease spectrum. Eur Respir Rev. 2012;21:19–26.
94. Takeuchi T, Tatsukawa H, Shinoda Y, Kuwata K, Nishiga M, Takahashi H, Hase N, Hitomi K. Spatially resolved identification of transglutaminase substrates by proteomics in pulmonary fibrosis. Am J Respir Cell Mol Biol. 2021;65:319–30.
95. van Hinsbergh VWM, Koolwijk P. Endothelial sprouting and angiogenesis: matrix metalloproteinases in the lead. Cardiovasc Res. 2008;78:203–12.
96. Rodríguez D, Morrison CJ, Overall CM. Matrix metalloproteinases: what do they not do? New substrates and biological roles identified by murine models and proteomics. Biochim Biophys Acta. 2010;1803:39–54.
97. Chelladurai P, Seeger W, Pullamsetti SS. Series "matrix metalloproteinases in lung health and disease": matrix metalloproteinases and their inhibitors in pulmonary hypertension. Eur Respir J. 2012;40:766–82.
98. Craig VJ, Zhang L, Hagood JS, Owen CA. Matrix metalloproteinases as therapeutic targets for idiopathic pulmonary fibrosis. Am J Respir Cell Mol Biol. 2015;53:585–600.
99. Christopoulou M-E, Papakonstantinou E, Stolz D. Matrix metalloproteinases in chronic obstructive pulmonary disease. Int J Mol Sci. 2023;24.
100. Zhong S, Khalil RA. A disintegrin and metalloproteinase (ADAM) and ADAM with thrombospondin motifs (ADAMTS) family in vascular biology and disease. Biochem Pharmacol Elsevier. 2019;164:188–204.
101. Hurst LA, Dunmore BJ, Long L, Crosby A, Al-Lamki R, Deighton J, Southwood M, Yang X, Nikolic MZ, Herrera B, Inman GJ, Bradley JR, Rana AA, Upton PD, Morrell NW. TNFα drives pulmonary arterial hypertension by suppressing the BMP type-II receptor and altering NOTCH signalling. Nat Commun Nature Publishing Group. 2017;8:14079.
102. Lagares D, Ghassemi-Kakroodi P, Tremblay C, Santos A, Probst CK, Franklin A, Santos DM, Grasberger P, Ahluwalia N, Montesi SB, Shea BS, Black KE, Knipe R, Blati M, Baron M, Wu B, Fahmi H, Gandhi R, Pardo A, Selman M, Wu J, Pelletier JP, Martel-Pelletier J, Tager AM, Kapoor M. ADAM10-mediated ephrin-B2 shedding promotes myofibroblast activation and organ fibrosis. Nat Med. 2017;23:1405–15.
103. Omura J, Satoh K, Kikuchi N, Satoh T, Kurosawa R, Nogi M, Ohtsuki T, Al-Mamun ME, Siddique MAH, Yaoita N, Sunamura S, Miyata S, Hoshikawa Y, Okada Y, Shimokawa H. ADAMTS8 promotes the development of pulmonary arterial hypertension and right ventricular failure: a possible novel therapeutic target. Circ Res. 2019;125:884–906.
104. Sharma NS, Lal CV, Li J-D, Lou X-Y, Viera L, Abdallah T, King RW, Sethi J, Kanagarajah P, Restrepo-Jaramillo R, Sales-Conniff A, Wei S, Jackson PL, Blalock JE, Gaggar A, Xu X. The neutrophil chemoattractant peptide proline-glycine-proline is associated with acute respiratory distress syndrome. Am J Phys Lung Cell Mol Phys. 2018;315:L653–61.
105. Lindsey ML, Iyer RP, Zamilpa R, Yabluchanskiy A, DeLeon-Pennell KY, Hall ME, Kaplan A, Zouein FA, Bratton D, Flynn ER, Cannon PL, Tian Y, Jin Y-F, Lange RA, Tokmina-Roszyk D, Fields GB, de Castro Brás LE. A novel collagen matricryptin reduces left ventricular dilation post-myocardial infarction by promoting scar formation and angiogenesis. J Am Coll Cardiol. 2015;66:1364–74.
106. Skeie JM, Mullins RF. Elastin-mediated choroidal endothelial cell migration: possible role in age-related macular degeneration. Invest Ophthalmol Vis Sci. 2008;49:5574–80.
107. Reddel CJ, Cultrone D, Rnjak-Kovacina J, Weiss AS, Burgess JK. Tropoelastin modulates TGF-β1-induced expression of VEGF and CTGF in airway smooth muscle cells. Matrix Biol. 2013;32:407–13.

Chapter 5
Imaging in Pulmonary Hypertension Associated with Chronic Lung Disease

Andrew J. Synn and Farbod N. Rahaghi

Introduction

Imaging plays a central role in the clinical care of patients with chronic lung disease and pulmonary hypertension (PH). In particular, CT imaging is widely used to facilitate the diagnosis of various lung diseases, including emphysema, interstitial lung disease, pneumonia/pneumonitis, and lung cancer, among many others. After initial diagnosis, CT is often obtained serially during follow-up, for example, to monitor for progression of interstitial disease or for annual lung cancer screening in high-risk populations. However, CT imaging (using both traditional and more modern techniques) can also provide direct insight into abnormalities of the pulmonary circulation. Given the ubiquitous role of CT in modern clinical practice, CT may therefore be a powerful tool to enable a more effective and extensive level of screening for the development of PH among patients with lung disease who are at higher risk of pulmonary vascular disease. In patients suspected or known to have PH, imaging can also improve risk stratification by capturing the downstream hemodynamic consequences of PH, such as right ventricular dysfunction. As with other forms of PH, echocardiography continues to play a key role in screening and staging of PH associated with lung disease. Emerging methods such as dual energy CT and MRI also

A. J. Synn (✉)
Division of Pulmonary, Critical Care, and Sleep Medicine, Beth Israel Deaconess Medical Center, Harvard Medical School, Boston, MA, USA
e-mail: asynn@bidmc.harvard.edu

F. N. Rahaghi
Division of Pulmonary, Critical Care Medicine, Clinical Immunology, and Allergy, Department of Medicine, David Geffen School of Medicine at the University of California-Los Angeles, Los Angeles, CA, USA
e-mail: frahaghi@ucla.edu

F. N. Rahaghi et al. (eds.), *The Pulmonary Vasculature in Chronic Lung Disease*, Respiratory Medicine, https://doi.org/10.1007/978-3-032-03581-3_5

hold promise in assessing the parenchymal and vascular impact of perfusion and gas exchange. In this way, imaging can provide a non-invasive, quantitative, and comprehensive view into pathologies of the pulmonary parenchyma, airways, and vessels, potentially enabling better phenotyping of different subtypes of disease, improving prognostication, and enhancing our understanding of the pathophysiologic relationship between airway and parenchymal damage, vascular remodeling, and the clinical hemodynamic consequences of these abnormalities. In this chapter, we will summarize the traditional use of imaging in the context of PH and lung disease, and explore emerging frontiers that may impact clinical practice and improve outcomes for patients in the near future.

Searching for PH in Lung Disease

Pulmonary Artery Diameter

CT scans of the chest are routinely obtained for the purpose of diagnosing and monitoring of lung disease. Given that PH is a common and deadly complication of chronic lung disease (i.e., group 3 PH), there has long been interest in leveraging existing CT data to identify subgroups at higher risk for PH who would benefit for invasive testing and PH-specific treatment. The most common and traditional CT-based method of screening for PH is measurement of the diameter of the main pulmonary artery (PA) [1, 2], both as an absolute value and as a ratio of PA to aorta (PA:A), which serves to normalize the PA for body size [3]. While this metric is straightforward to calculate and has demonstrated prognostic utility [4], the data supporting its performance to screen for PH due to lung diseases such as COPD and ILD remains less consistent.

Among individuals with COPD, CT imaging is frequently obtained including as part of lung cancer screening, on which PA:A ratio can be calculated. This metric has been studied in several different cohorts, and is linked to severe disease including more frequent acute exacerbations and greater mortality [4–8]. Despite these strong clinical associations, there have been variable results in studies investigating its ability to discriminate PH as determined by gold standard right heart catheterization (RHC). For example, in a study of 92 patients with COPD who underwent RHC as part of lung transplant evaluation, a PA:A ratio >1.0 had a positive predictive value of only 63.1% and a sensitivity of only 50% (although specificity was higher at 86% for diagnosis of PH) [9]. In a similar population of 65 patients with severe COPD, Shin et al found that PA:A ratio >1.0 had good specificity at 93%, but poor sensitivity of 50% [10]. A systematic review and meta-analysis of nine studies showed an overall pooled sensitivity of 69% and specificity of 85% for a cutoff of PA:A >1 for the diagnosis of PH [11]. These results indicate that while a dilated PA on CT may suggest a more severe phenotype of COPD at higher risk of PH, a "normal" PA diameter is not sufficient to exclude the diagnosis of PH, and many vulnerable patients may be missed.

Similarly, CT imaging is standard clinical practice in the care of patients with interstitial lung disease (ILD). However, early studies in the context of pulmonary fibrosis did not show significant promise in use of PA dilation in detecting PH in IPF [12, 13]. One study showed a strong correlation between PA diameter and mPAP and PVR on RHC in a subgroup of patients without fibrosis, but no association was seen in those with fibrosis [14]. It was noted that patients with fibrosis tended to have larger PA size independent of RHC hemodynamics, raising the possibility that PA enlargement is due to traction from parenchymal fibrosis, thus rendering PA diameter as an ineffective screening tool in patients with more severe ILD who are likely at higher risk [14]. Among 28 patients with scleroderma and ILD, there was a medium-to-strong correlation between mPAP on RHC and PA diameter ($r = 0.70$), although the severity of ILD in this cohort was overall relatively mild [15]. Again, however, when examining the subset of participants with a lower FVC of ≤70% predicted, the correlation was greatly attenuated (0.42), reinforcing that PA diameter is an ineffective screening tool among patients with more severe ILD disease. As was also the case with COPD, PA dilation is consistently associated with poorer outcomes in ILD [16] despite its inconsistent performance as a screening metric for PH.

In summary, while PA dilation (as measured by absolute diameter and/or PA:A ratio) is associated with PH in lung disease, its test characteristics may limit its use as a single screening method, particularly in the context of more severe lung disease. This is likely for multifactorial reasons, including the heterogeneous nature of these diseases, the demographics and co-morbidities of people with chronic lung disease, as well as the impact of lung disease on central structures through hyperinflation and traction. An additional challenge of using imaging to screen for PH is that imaging metrics may be dynamic, as exacerbations of the underlying lung disease and hypoxemia are known to cause temporary changes in the pulmonary circulation. For example, there is an increase in the size of PA during exacerbations of both COPD and ILD [17, 18], and clinical imaging obtained during these periods of exacerbation may not accurately reflect the patient's actual PH risk in a more stable state. For these reasons, while the use of PA dilation as the sole marker for screening or ruling out PH is not recommended, it may have a role as one element of multimetric prediction rules, as discussed in the following section.

Echocardiography

Transthoracic echocardiography (TTE) is the most widely used non-invasive screening tool for all forms of PH. A finding of higher pulmonary artery systolic pressure, estimated from the peak tricuspid regurgitant jet velocity, as well as other signs of right ventricular dysfunction or dilation on echocardiography is often used to determine whether an invasive right heart catheterization is necessary. Some of the larger studies to assess the utility of TTE in the context of PH associated with lung disease have been performed in the lung transplant population, which is heavily enriched for severe lung disease and who routinely undergo RHC as part of the pre-transplant evaluation. Early studies in this population raised the potential inaccuracy of echocardiogram for determining PH status. A study in 2002 of 166 patients undergoing lung transplantation found that using a cutoff of PASP ≥45 mmHg, echocardiography had a sensitivity of 85% and a specificity of only 52% for PH as determined by RHC [19]. Similarly, in a pre-transplant population of 103 patients, the estimated correlation between PASP as measured by RHC and echocardiogram was only 0.59, with a sensitivity of 85% and specificity of 67% [20]. In a more recent and larger study of 393 subjects undergoing lung transplant evaluation, there was a similar moderate correlation of PASP on RHC and TTE of 0.61 [21]. Concerningly, TTE overestimated PASP by more than 10 mmHg in 35% of patients, while it underestimated PASP in 12%—therefore, almost half of TTE-based PASPs were inaccurate by more 10 mmHg compared to invasive measurement [21].

In the context of COPD specifically, the performance characteristics of TTE similarly appear to be limited. For example, in a study of 111 patients with severe COPD, an echocardiographic diagnosis of PH (defined as intermediate or high risk probability based on European Society of Cardiology guidelines) had a sensitivity of only 43% and TTE was consistent with RHC in ruling in/out PH in only 53% of patients [22]. Specificity was relatively higher at 83%. Of note, in a multivariable model, it was found that the diagnostic accuracy of TTE correlated inversely with lung hyperinflation, indicating that its use as a screening tool for PH is less effective in more severe disease [22]. Finally, in a subcohort of 63 participants of the National Emphysema Treatment Trial (with advanced emphysema and hyperinflation who were being evaluated for lung volume reduction surgery), there was very weak correlation between PASP on RHC and TTE, and the authors concluded that the test characteristics of echocardiographic assessments were too poor to be used as a sole method of screening for PH in the setting of COPD [23].

For ILD, the INCREASE trial demonstrated that an inhaled pulmonary vasodilator (treprostinil) improved exercise capacity (and possibly FVC) in a randomized trial of patients with ILD-PH [24, 25], which has greatly spurred the clinical need to identify noninvasive tools to screen for PH in the setting of ILD. Unfortunately, however, TTE similarly has not been shown to be sufficiently sensitive to be used as a screening tool for this purpose. In a study of 265 patients with ILD and suspected PH, 40% of patients who were classified as having "low probability of PH" based on TTE criteria were ultimately found to have PH on RHC [26]. Additionally, another limitation of PASP on TTE is that it requires the presence of tricuspid regurgitation, which is often unmeasurable or absent. For example, in one study of patients with IPF who had available TTE and RHC, PASP was unable to be assessed in almost half (50 of 110, 45%) of the entire cohort [27]. Of those 50 who could not have been screened by TTE, 16 (32%) ultimately had PH confirmed on RHC.

Magnetic Resonance Imaging

Cardiac magnetic resonance imaging (CMR) has become the standard modality to assess the structure and function of the right ventricle, and it allows for better quantification of right ventricular function compared to echocardiography [28]. Although CMR (like TTE) cannot visualize the smaller pulmonary vessels directly, it can provide accurate and reproducible assessment of the downstream hemodynamic consequences of PH, including increased RV hypertrophy (based on estimated mass), compensatory dilatation (based on end-diastolic and systolic volume indices), and reduced function (RV ejection fraction). While CMR has been widely studied in PAH as a method for initial risk stratification and for monitoring of RV function in response to therapy, its role is less clear in the setting of PH associated with chronic lung disease. A study from the ASPIRE (Assessing the Severity of Pulmonary Hypertension in a Pulmonary Hypertension Referral Center) registry analyzed 167 patients with chronic lung disease and PH who underwent both CMR and RHC [29]. The results of this study showed that an MRI-based model had high diagnostic accuracy in discriminating those with severe PH (based on mPAP $\geq$ 35 mmHg or mPAP > 25 and CI < 2 L/min/m [2]). The MRI model was also superior to a TTE-based model, especially for participants who were not positively diagnosed by a high estimated PASP on TTE—an important consideration for a screening test. Newer MRI applications, including 4D flow MRI, may allow for additional advancements including noninvasive tracking of hemodynamic parameters such as pulmonary vascular resistance [28].

Integrating Imaging into Multi-metric Screening Tools

While neither PA dilation on CT nor PASP on TTE has sufficient sensitivity to serve as a sole metric for screening of PH in lung disease [30], these metrics clearly have value as elements of a multi-metric scoring system to predict risk of PH [31]. As an example, Kovacs et al used a combination of RVSP on TTE, PA:A ratio on CT, and NT-proBNP to achieve a >0.9 NPV and PPV in detecting severe PH in patients with COPD [32]. Similarly, a study of patients with ILD found that a composite score integrating echocardiographic assessment (including measures of RV function), DLCO, and BNP could achieve great specificity in detecting PH [33]. A more recent study used an 8-variable scoring system (including PA enlargement on CT imaging) to screen for PH in ILD, again with a sensitivity and specificity of >90% [34]. Indeed, a recent expert consensus statement recommended that any initial screening for PH in ILD utilize (at minimum) a combination of biomarkers such as BNP and echocardiographic measures together, with addition of other modalities including chest CT and pulmonary function testing depending on the level of clinical suspicion [35]. This consensus statement, alongside other clinical and biological marker studies in this area [36, 37], highlight that integration of multifactorial diagnostic modalities will likely yield the most optimal screening strategies for PH in the setting of lung disease, although there are very few scoring systems that are universally accepted at present. In part, this is because the precise combination of metrics (and their cutoffs) will likely need to be tailored to each specific lung disease population, given the marked heterogeneity within and between these conditions.

Characterization of Parenchymal Lung Disease

CT imaging is the preferred method of assessing parenchymal lung abnormalities, given its high resolution and widespread availability. The degree of parenchymal tissue destruction (whether fibrosis or emphysema) has long been assumed to be a key driver of PH associated with lung disease. However, the link between parenchymal pathology in lung disease and the development of group 3 PH is very poorly understood.

In ILD, for example, histologic vascular remodeling has been observed in areas of fibrosis [38, 39], and vascular remodeling similar to that of PAH [40–42] has also been observed in areas with relatively normal parenchyma [38]. However, neither the extent of parenchymal fibrosis nor the loss of lung volume can explain the association between ILD and PH, and the degree of ILD involvement does not consistently correlate with the development or severity of the hemodynamic disturbance seen in ILD-PH [12, 43, 44]. As a result, ILD extent on imaging cannot be used clinically to screen for ILD-PH. Similarly, in COPD, there appears to be very little correlation between a CT-based emphysema score and PA pressures on RHC in participants of the NETT study mentioned previously [45]. Of note, while neither radiographic COPD nor ILD seems to be particularly strong predictors of PH, the combination of both emphysema and fibrosis seen together on imaging appears to be strongly linked to risk of PH (relative to either condition alone) [46, 47] as well as poorer gas exchange and outcomes [46]. This combination, known as CPFE, is now recognized as a unique entity [48], and this specific set of imaging features may warrant special attention for screening for PH.

In the initial work-up of pulmonary hypertension, CT imaging primarily serves to evaluate the presence and extent of lung disease to help identify the etiology of PH, as PH associated with lung disease is known as group 3 PH, and has a substantially different treatment strategy compared to group 1 PH (in which typically significant lung disease should not be present) [49, 50]. However, the mere presence of parenchymal damage may not be sufficient to answer the critical question posed to the clinician: does the extent of pulmonary parenchymal pathology on imaging sufficiently explain the presence (and severity) of the pulmonary hypertension? In clinical practice, the assessment of the "proportionality" of the pulmonary parenchymal abnormality to the hemodynamic disturbance serves as a key factor in determining whether to consider patients as group 1 or group 3, with significant implications for treatment [51]. This is of particular importance in subgroups of patients such as those with connective tissue disease (CTD) [52, 53] as these patients are at significant risk for developing both group 1 PAH and interstitial lung disease [54] with an ILD prevalence of up to 70–90% in some settings [55]. The overlap between group 1 and group 3 PH is further evident in that as many as 23% of patients classified as idiopathic PAH may have interstitial abnormalities such as centrilobular ground glass on imaging [51]. Unfortunately, despite the critical diagnostic and therapeutic importance of distinguishing between group 1 and group 3 PH, at present there remains no consensus definition of "out of proportion" PH to help guide assignment of patients with overlapping features [56], and this remains an active area of research.

Ruling Out Concurrent Thromboembolic Lung Disease

While the imaging of chronic thromboembolic pulmonary hypertension (CTEPH) is beyond the scope of this chapter, it is important to highlight that there are many shared risk factors for both CTEPH and PH associated with other traditional lung diseases [57], and also that conditions such as COPD and ILD [57–64] are themselves associated with hypercoagulable states and pulmonary thromboembolism [65–67]. This relationship is further complicated by the fact that clinical signs and symptoms, including dyspnea, hypoxemia, and right heart failure, are present in both parenchymal lung disease and CTEPH [68, 69]. As a result, imaging to rule out thromboembolic disease including CTEPH remains a key part of the work-up of patients diagnosed with PH including those with and without known chronic lung disease [50].

Emerging Imaging Approaches in PH Associated with Lung Disease

Quantitative image analysis of the intraparenchymal vasculature in PAH using clinically acquired CT imaging has demonstrated loss of vascular tree complexity [70], loss of small vessel volume [71], proximal arterial dilation [71], and increased arterial tortuosity in PAH [71, 72]. These imaging metrics can also be generated from CTs from patients with parenchymal disease to assess pulmonary vasculopathy including risk stratification for group 3 PH. However, each type of lung disease presents its own unique considerations and challenges in this regard. For example, emphysema itself can lead to loss of vascular volume due to tissue destruction, potentially obscuring the vascular signal in the remaining lung. Similarly, detection of small vessels in ILD may be impacted by the presence of perivascular fibrosis [73]. Nonetheless, associations between quantitative CT-based vascular markers and PH have been demonstrated in both COPD [74–76] and ILD [74, 77]. Given the association between vascular abnormalities and early parenchymal disease [73, 78] and parenchymal disease progression [79], it may be possible to leverage data from existing CT to better understand parenchymal/vascular interactions, detect disease earlier in its course, and identify patients with parenchymal disease who are at highest risk for PH. Additionally, CT uniquely offers the ability to simultaneously quantify both parenchymal and vascular abnormalities, which may eventually enable the use of image-based signatures to define disease sub-phenotypes and improve treatment strategy, particularly in groups for which treatment options are limited [80].

A CT-based technique that is gaining wider clinical use is that of dual-energy CT (DECT), which utilizes additional attenuation measurements along two (or more) energy spectra to create noninvasive maps of pulmonary iodine uptake as a surrogate of pulmonary perfusion [81–83]. While most research investigating DECT have focused on its ability to detect thromboembolism (including differentiating between acute pulmonary embolism from CTEPH [81]), quantification of the perfused blood volume via DECT may also be able to yield image-based signatures of PH including non-invasive surrogates of pulmonary hemodynamics [84, 85] although this has not yet been well studied for group 3 PH.

Although CT is primarily felt to reflect structural changes, prior studies have also shown that the pulmonary vascular metrics quantified using CT image analysis can also capture dynamic and/or reversible pathology, including the effect of treatment (e.g., lung volume reduction in COPD and inhaled nitric oxide in healthy controls) [86–89]. CT imaging is thus an emerging non-invasive tool to quantify longitudinal treatment response in PAH and group 3 PH, and several current and future trials (including studies of inhaled vasodilators for treatment of ILD-PH) have proposed the use of CT-based endpoints in addition to lung function testing and hemodynamic parameters [90].

Traditionally, MRI of the lung has seen limited clinical use due to complications of respiratory motion and the low proton density of lung tissue [91]. However, technological advances (to improve acquisition times), and especially the use of novel inhaled contrast agents, have significantly improved the ability of MRI to evaluate the pulmonary parenchyma and vasculature. Hyperpolarized ^{129}Xe-MRI involves inhalation of Xenon-129 gas, which diffuses from the airspaces, across the interstitial space, and into the pulmonary capillaries [92, 93]. By leveraging the distinct spectral peaks in each of these compartments, ^{129}Xe-MRI can provide information on lung ventilation, tissue diffusion, and perfusion simultaneously. In a study of 32 patients who underwent RHC and ^{129}Xe-MRI, diagnostic accuracy of MRI for pre-capillary PH was 75%, with a sensitivity of 67% and a specificity of 86%, although as we have seen with CT and TTE, the accuracy was significantly lower in mixed disease and in the presence of ILD [92]. More recently, in a small study of 10 patients with UIP on histology and/or CT, ^{129}Xe-MRI was capable of detecting alterations in both ventilation and gas exchange and may be more sensitive than pulmonary function testing or CT in detecting early UIP-related pathology [94]. Although promising, the clinical utility of ^{129}Xe-MRI in the context of group 3 PH remains to be confirmed in larger and multi-center cohorts including dedicated samples of patients with lung disease-related PH. In addition, ^{129}Xe-MRI is only available at a small number of centers, limiting its clinical use compared to TTE and CT.

Conclusion

Imaging is an essential element of modern pulmonary practice and is widely used to screen for PH among patients with chronic lung disease. While no currently available tool is well-suited to serve as a sole method of screening for PH, combinations of image-based metrics from CT, echocardiography, and MRI may help clinicians identify high-risk patients, reduce delays in definitive invasive testing, and define sub-phenotypes of lung disease-associated PH that may benefit from targeted therapeutic approaches.

References

1. Kuriyama K, Gamsu G, Stern RG, Cann CE, Herfkens RJ, Brundage BH. CT-determined pulmonary artery diameters in predicting pulmonary hypertension. Investig Radiol. 1984;19(1):16–22.
2. Schmidt HC, Kauczor HU, Schild HH, Renner C, Kirchhoff E, Lang P, et al. Pulmonary hypertension in patients with chronic pulmonary thromboembolism: chest radiograph and CT evaluation before and after surgery. Eur Radiol. 1996;6(6):817–25.
3. Ng CS, Wells AU, Padley SPG. A CT sign of chronic pulmonary arterial hypertension: the ratio of main pulmonary artery to aortic diameter. J Thorac Imaging. 1999;14(4):270–8.
4. Terzikhan N, Bos D, Lahousse L, Wolff L, Verhamme KMC, Leening MJG, et al. Pulmonary artery to aorta ratio and risk of all-cause mortality in the general population: the Rotterdam Study. Eur Respir J. 2017;49(6):1602168.
5. Wells JM, Washko GR, Han MK, Abbas N, Nath H, Mamary AJ, et al. Pulmonary arterial enlargement and acute exacerbations of COPD. N Engl J Med. 2012;367(10):913–21.
6. Cheng Y, Li L, Tu X, Pei R. The main pulmonary artery to the ascending aorta diameter ratio (PA/A) as a predictor of worse outcomes in hospitalized patients with AECOPD. Int J COPD. 2022;17:1157–65.
7. Lee JK, Kho BG, Yoon JY, Yoon CS, Na YO, Park HY, et al. The clinical characteristics associated with the ratio between the main pulmonary artery and ascending aorta diameter in patients with acute exacerbation of chronic obstructive pulmonary disease. J Thorac Dis. 2024;16(8):4924–34.
8. LaFon DC, Bhatt SP, Labaki WW, Rahaghi FN, Moll M, Bowler RP, et al. Pulmonary artery enlargement and mortality risk in moderate to severe COPD: results from COPDGene. Eur Respir J. 2020;55(2).
9. Mohamed Hoesein FA, Besselink T, Pompe E, Oudijk EJ, de Graaf EA, Kwakkel-van Erp JM, et al. Accuracy of CT pulmonary artery diameter for pulmonary hypertension in end-stage COPD. Lung. 2016;194(5):813–9.
10. Shin S, King CS, Brown AW, Albano MC, Atkins M, Sheridan MJ, et al. Pulmonary artery size as a predictor of pulmonary hypertension and outcomes in patients with chronic obstructive pulmonary disease. Respir Med. 2014;108(11):1626–32.
11. Wu X, Shi Y, Wang X, Yu X, Yang M. Diagnostic value of computed tomography-based pulmonary artery to aorta ratio measurement in chronic obstructive pulmonary disease with pulmonary hypertension: a systematic review and meta-analysis. Clin Respir J. 2022;16(4):276–83.
12. Zisman DA, Karlamangla AS, Ross DJ, Keane MP, Belperio JA, Saggar R, et al. High-resolution chest CT findings do not predict the presence of pulmonary hypertension in advanced idiopathic pulmonary fibrosis. Chest. 2007;132(3):773–9.

13. Condliffe R, Radon M, Hurdman J, Davies C, Hill C, Akil M, et al. CT pulmonary angiography combined with echocardiography in suspected systemic sclerosis-associated pulmonary arterial hypertension. Rheumatology. 2011;50(8):1480–6.
14. Devaraj A, Wells AU, Meister MG, Corte TJ, Hansell DM. The effect of diffuse pulmonary fibrosis on the reliability of CT signs of pulmonary hypertension. Radiology. 2008;249(3):1042–9.
15. Mccall RK, Ravenel JG, Nietert PJ, Granath A, Silver RM. Relationship of main pulmonary artery diameter to pulmonary arterial pressure in scleroderma patients with and without interstitial fibrosis. J Comput Assist Tomogr. 2014;38(2):163–8.
16. Shin S, King CS, Puri N, Shlobin OA, Brown AW, Ahmad S, et al. Pulmonary artery size as a predictor of outcomes in idiopathic pulmonary fibrosis. Eur Respir J. 2016;47(5):1445–51.
17. Matsushita S, Matsuoka S, Yamashiro T, Fujikawa A, Yagihashi K, Kurihara Y, et al. Pulmonary arterial enlargement in patients with acute exacerbation of interstitial pneumonia. Clin Imaging. 2014;38(4):454–7.
18. Michael Wells J, Morrison JB, Bhatt SP, Nath H, Dransfield MT. Pulmonary artery enlargement is associated with cardiac injury during severe exacerbations of COPD. Chest. 2016;149(5):1197–204.
19. Arcasoy SM, Christie JD, Ferrari VA, Sutton MSJ, Zisman DA, Blumenthal NP, et al. Echocardiographic assessment of pulmonary hypertension in patients with advanced lung disease. Am J Respir Crit Care Med. 2003;167(5):735–40.
20. Balcı MK, Arı E, Vayvada M, Salturk C, Aşıcıoğlu E, Kahveci G, et al. Assessment of pulmonary hypertension in lung transplantation candidates: correlation of doppler echocardiography with right heart catheterization. Transplant Proc. 2016;48(8):2797–802.
21. Abu T, Levi A, Hasdai D, Kramer MR, Bental T, Bdolah-Abram T, et al. Preoperative evaluation of pulmonary hypertension in lung transplant candidates: echocardiography versus right heart catheterization. BMC Cardiovasc Disord. 2022;22(1):53.
22. Younis M, Al-Antary N, Dalbah R, Qarajeh A, Khanfar AN, Kar AA, et al. Echocardiography and pulmonary hypertension in patients with chronic obstructive pulmonary disease undergoing lung transplantation evaluation. Am J Med Sci. 2024;367(2):95–104.
23. Fisher MR, Criner GJ, Fishman AP, Hassoun PM, Minai OA, Scharf SM, et al. Estimating pulmonary artery pressures by echocardiography in patients with emphysema. Eur Respir J. 2007;30(5):914–21.
24. Waxman A, Restrepo-Jaramillo R, Thenappan T, Ravichandran A, Engel P, Bajwa A, et al. Inhaled treprostinil in pulmonary hypertension due to interstitial lung disease. N Engl J Med. 2021;384(4):325–34.
25. Nathan SD, Waxman A, Rajagopal S, Case A, Johri S, DuBrock H, et al. Inhaled treprostinil and forced vital capacity in patients with interstitial lung disease and associated pulmonary hypertension: a post-hoc analysis of the INCREASE study. Lancet Respir Med. 2021;9(11):1266–74.
26. Keir GJ, Wort SJ, Kokosi M, George PM, Walsh SLF, Jacob J, et al. Pulmonary hypertension in interstitial lung disease: limitations of echocardiography compared to cardiac catheterization. Respirology. 2018;23(7):687–94.
27. Nathan SD, Shlobin OA, Barnett SD, Saggar R, Belperio JA, Ross DJ, et al. Right ventricular systolic pressure by echocardiography as a predictor of pulmonary hypertension in idiopathic pulmonary fibrosis. Respir Med. 2008;102(9):1305–10.
28. Zhou Y, Panda A, Jokerst CE. Editorial for "Evaluation of pulmonary hypertension using 4D flow MRI" J Magn Reson Imaging 2022;56(1):246-247.
29. Alkhanfar D, Dwivedi K, Alandejani F, Shahin Y, Alabed S, Johns C, et al. Non-invasive detection of severe PH in lung disease using magnetic resonance imaging. Front Cardiovasc Med. 2023;10:1016994.
30. Alkukhun L, Wang XF, Ahmed MK, Baumgartner M, Budev MM, Dweik RA, et al. Non-invasive screening for pulmonary hypertension in idiopathic pulmonary fibrosis. Respir Med. 2016;117:65–72.

31. Parikh R, Konstantinidis I, O'Sullivan DM, Farber HW. Pulmonary hypertension in patients with interstitial lung disease: a tool for early detection. Pulm Circ. 2022;12(4):e12141.
32. Kovacs G, Avian A, Bachmaier G, Troester N, Tornyos A, Douschan P, et al. Severe pulmonary hypertension in COPD: impact on survival and diagnostic approach. Chest. 2022;162(1):202–12.
33. Ruocco G, Cekorja B, Rottoli P, Refini RM, Pellegrini M, Di Tommaso C, et al. Role of BNP and echo measurement for pulmonary hypertension recognition in patients with interstitial lung disease: an algorithm application model. Respir Med. 2015;109(3):406–15.
34. Parikh R, O'Sullivan DM, Farber HW. The PH-ILD Detection tool: external validation and use in patients with ILD. Pulm Circ. 2023;13(3):e12273.
35. Rahaghi FF, Kolaitis NA, Adegunsoye A, de Andrade JA, Flaherty KR, Lancaster LH, et al. Screening strategies for pulmonary hypertension in patients with interstitial lung disease: a multidisciplinary Delphi study. Chest. 2022;162(1):145–55.
36. Furukawa T, Kondoh Y, Taniguchi H, Yagi M, Matsuda T, Kimura T, et al. A scoring system to predict the elevation of mean pulmonary arterial pressure in idiopathic pulmonary fibrosis. Eur Respir J. 2018;51(1).
37. Sonti R, Gersten RA, Barnett S, Brown AW, Nathan SD. Multimodal noninvasive prediction of pulmonary hypertension in IPF. Clin Respir J. 2019;13(9):567–73.
38. Colombat M, Mal H, Groussard O, Capron F, Thabut G, Jebrak G, et al. Pulmonary vascular lesions in end-stage idiopathic pulmonary fibrosis: histopathologic study on lung explant specimens and correlations with pulmonary hemodynamics. Hum Pathol. 2007;38(1):60–5.
39. Parra ER, David YR, Da Costa LRS, Ab'Saber A, Sousa R, Kairalla RA, et al. Heterogeneous remodeling of lung vessels in idiopathic pulmonary fibrosis. Lung. 2005;183(4):291–300.
40. King CS, Shlobin OA. The trouble with group 3 pulmonary hypertension in interstitial lung disease: dilemmas in diagnosis and the conundrum of treatment. Chest. 2020;158(4):1651–64.
41. Klinger Jr. Group III Pulmonary hypertension: pulmonary hypertension associated with lung disease: epidemiology, pathophysiology, and treatments. Cardiol Clin. 2016;34(3):413-33.
42. Dotan Y, Stewart J, Gangemi A, Wang H, Aneja A, Chakraborty B, et al. Pulmonary vasculopathy in explanted lungs from patients with interstitial lung disease undergoing lung transplantation. BMJ Open Respir Res. 2020;7(1).
43. Nathan SD, Shlobin OA, Ahmad S, Urbanek S, Barnett SD. Pulmonary hypertension and pulmonary function testing in idiopathic pulmonary fibrosis. Chest. 2007;131(3):657–63.
44. Ruffenach G, Hong J, Vaillancourt M, Medzikovic L, Eghbali M. Pulmonary hypertension secondary to pulmonary fibrosis: clinical data, histopathology and molecular insights. Respir Res. 2020;21(1):303.
45. Scharf SM, Iqbal M, Keller C, Criner G, Lee S, Fessler HE. Hemodynamic characterization of patients with severe emphysema. 2012;166(3):314–22. https://doi.org/10.1164/rccm2107027.
46. Caceres JD, Venkata A. Combined pulmonary fibrosis and emphysema. Curr Opin Pulm Med. 2024;30(2):167–73.
47. Ni H, Wei Y, Yang L, Wang Q. An increased risk of pulmonary hypertension in patients with combined pulmonary fibrosis and emphysema: a meta-analysis. BMC Pulm Med. 2023;23(1):221.
48. Cottin V, Inoue Y, Selman M, Ryerson CJ, Wells AU, Agusti A, et al. Syndrome of combined pulmonary fibrosis and emphysema an official ATS/ERS/JRS/ALAT research statement. Am J Respir Crit Care Med. 2022;206(4):E7–E41.
49. Remy-Jardin M, Ryerson CJ, Schiebler ML, Leung ANC, Wild JM, Hoeper MM, et al. Imaging of pulmonary hypertension in adults: a position paper from the Fleischner Society. Eur Respir J. 2021;57(1).
50. Kiely DG, Levin DL, Hassoun PM, Ivy D, Jone PN, Bwika J, et al. Statement on imaging and pulmonary hypertension from the Pulmonary Vascular Research Institute (PVRI). Pulm Circ. 2019;9(3):2045894019841990.

51. Dwivedi K, Condliffe R, Sharkey M, Lewis R, Alabed S, Rajaram S, et al. Computed tomography lung parenchymal descriptions in routine radiological reporting have diagnostic and prognostic utility in patients with idiopathic pulmonary arterial hypertension and pulmonary hypertension associated with lung disease. ERJ Open Res. 2022;8(1).
52. Rodolfi S, Ong VH, Denton CP. Recent developments in connective tissue disease associated pulmonary arterial hypertension. Int J Cardiol Congenit Hear Dis. 2024;16:100513.
53. Vonk MC, Vandecasteele E, van Dijk AP. Pulmonary hypertension in connective tissue diseases, new evidence and challenges. Eur J Clin Investig. 2021;51(4):e13453.
54. Joy GM, Arbiv OA, Wong CK, Lok SD, Adderley NA, Dobosz KM, et al. Prevalence, imaging patterns and risk factors of interstitial lung disease in connective tissue disease: a systematic review and meta-analysis. Eur Respir Rev. 2023;32(167).
55. Solomon JJ, Olson AL, Fischer A, Bull T, Brown KK, Raghu G. Scleroderma lung disease. Eur Respir Rev. 2013;22(127):6–19.
56. Zanatta E, Polito P, Famoso G, Larosa M, De Zorzi E, Scarpieri E, et al. Pulmonary arterial hypertension in connective tissue disorders: pathophysiology and treatment. Exp Biol Med. 2019;244(2):120–31.
57. Shimoda M, Nunokawa H, Tanaka Y, Morimoto K, Moue I, Yoshimori K, et al. Predictive factors of the presence of pulmonary embolism in patients with interstitial lung disease: observational study. Medicine (Baltimore). 2024;103(1):e36828.
58. Park SH. Pulmonary embolism is more prevalent than deep vein thrombosis in cases of chronic obstructive pulmonary disease and interstitial lung diseases. Springerplus. 2016;5(1):1777.
59. Alsilmi R. The prevalence of pulmonary embolism in patients with interstitial lung disease: a cross-sectional retrospective study. Cureus. 2022;14(3):e23063.
60. Sode BF, Dahl M, Nielsen SF, Nordestgaard BG. Venous thromboembolism and risk of idiopathic interstitial pneumonia: a nationwide study. Am J Respir Crit Care Med. 2010;181(10):1085–92.
61. Hubbard RB, Smith C, Le Jeune I, Gribbin J, Fogarty AW. The association between idiopathic pulmonary fibrosis and vascular disease: a population-based study. Am J Respir Crit Care Med. 2008;178(12):1257–61.
62. Navaratnam V, Fogarty AW, McKeever T, Thompson N, Jenkins G, Johnson SR, et al. Presence of a prothrombotic state in people with idiopathic pulmonary fibrosis: a population-based case-control study. Thorax. 2014;69(3):207–15.
63. Sprunger DB, Olson AL, Huie TJ, Fernandez-Perez ER, Fischer A, Solomon JJ, et al. Pulmonary fibrosis is associated with an elevated risk of thromboembolic disease. Eur Respir J. 2012;39(1):125–32.
64. Sobiecka M, Szturmowicz M, Lewandowska K, Kowalik A, Łyżwa E, Zimna K, et al. Chronic hypersensitivity pneumonitis is associated with an increased risk of venous thromboembolism: a retrospective cohort study. BMC Pulm Med. 2021;21(1):416.
65. Kyriakopoulos C, Chronis C, Papapetrou E, Tatsioni A, Gartzonika K, Tsaousi C, et al. Prothrombotic state in patients with stable copd: an observational study. ERJ Open Res. 2021;7(4)
66. Ashitani JI, Mukae H, Arimura Y, Matsukura S. Elevated plasma procoagulant and fibrinolytic markers in patients with chronic obstructive pulmonary disease. Intern Med. 2002;41(3):181–5.
67. Rahaghi FN, Pistenmaa CL. Hypercoagulation in COPD: the clot thickens. ERJ Open Res. 2021;7(4).
68. Aleva FE, Voets LWLM, Simons SO, de Mast Q, van der Ven AJAM, Heijdra YF. Prevalence and localization of pulmonary embolism in unexplained acute exacerbations of COPD: a systematic review and meta-analysis. Chest. 2017;151(3):544–54.
69. Couturaud F, Bertoletti L, Pastre J, Roy PM, Le Mao R, Gagnadoux F, et al. Prevalence of pulmonary embolism among patients with COPD hospitalized with acutely worsening respiratory symptoms. J Am Med Assoc. 2021;325(1):59–68.

70. Moledina S, De Bruyn A, Schievano S, Owens CM, Young C, Haworth SG, et al. Fractal branching quantifies vascular changes and predicts survival in pulmonary hypertension: a proof of principle study. Heart. 2011;97(15):1245–9.
71. Rahaghi FN, Nardelli P, Harder E, Singh I, Sánchez-Ferrero GV, Ross JC, et al. Quantification of arterial and venous morphologic markers in pulmonary arterial hypertension using CT imaging. Chest. 2021;160(6):2220–31.
72. Helmberger M, Pienn M, Urschler M, Kullnig P, Stollberger R, Kovacs G, et al. Quantification of tortuosity and fractal dimension of the lung vessels in pulmonary hypertension patients. PLoS One. 2014;9(1):e87515.
73. Synn AJ, Li W, Hunninghake GM, Washko GR, San José Estépar R, O'Connor GT, et al. Vascular pruning on CT and interstitial lung abnormalities in the Framingham Heart Study. Chest. 2021;159(2):663–72.
74. Alkhanfar D, Shahin Y, Alandejani F, Dwivedi K, Alabed S, Johns C, et al. Severe pulmonary hypertension associated with lung disease is characterised by a loss of small pulmonary vessels on quantitative computed tomography. ERJ Open Res. 2022;8(2).
75. Matsuoka S, Washko GR, Yamashiro T, Estepar RSJ, Diaz A, Silverman EK, et al. Pulmonary hypertension and computed tomography measurement of small pulmonary vessels in severe emphysema. Am J Respir Crit Care Med. 2010;181(3):218–25.
76. Rahaghi FN, Wells JM, Come CE, De La Bruere IA, Bhatt SP, Ross JC, et al. Arterial and venous pulmonary vascular morphology and their relationship to findings in cardiac magnetic resonance imaging in smokers. J Comput Assist Tomogr. 2016;40(6):948–52.
77. Harder EM, Abtin F, Nardelli P, Brownstein A, Channick RN, Washko GR, et al. Pulmonary hypertension in idiopathic interstitial pneumonia is associated with small vessel pruning. Am J Respir Crit Care Med. 2024;209(9):1170–3.
78. Harder EM, Nardelli P, Pistenmaa CL, Ash SY, Balasubramanian A, Bowler RP, et al. Preacinar arterial dilation mediates outcomes of quantitative interstitial abnormalities in COPDGene. Am J Respir Crit Care Med. 2024;210(9):1132–42.
79. Pistenmaa CL, Nardelli P, Ash SY, Come CE, Diaz AA, Rahaghi FN, et al. Pulmonary arterial pruning and longitudinal change in percent emphysema and lung function: the genetic epidemiology of COPD study. Chest. 2021;160(2):470–80.
80. Johnson SW, Wan ES, San Jose Estépar R, Nardelli P, Pistenmaa C, Piccari L, et al. Chest computed tomography to improve phenotyping in pulmonary hypertension associated with chronic obstructive pulmonary disease. Ann Am Thorac Soc. 2025;22(2):175–80.
81. Gertz RJ, Gerhardt F, Pienn M, Lennartz S, Kröger JR, Caldeira L, et al. Dual-layer dual-energy CT-derived pulmonary perfusion for the differentiation of acute pulmonary embolism and chronic thromboembolic pulmonary hypertension. Eur Radiol. 2024;34(5):2944–56.
82. McCollough CH, Leng S, Yu L, Fletcher JG. Dual- and multi-energy CT: principles, technical approaches, and clinical applications. Radiology. 2015;276(3):637–53.
83. Miwa K, Taniguchi Y, Fujii H, Matsuoka Y, Onishi H, Yanaka K, et al. Microvasculopathy evaluated by dual-energy computed tomography in patients with chronic thromboembolic pulmonary hypertension and pulmonary arterial hypertension. Life. 2022;12(8):1232.
84. Ugawa S, Akagi S, Ejiri K, Nakamura K, Ito H. Quantification of lung perfusion blood volume in dual-energy computed tomography in patients with pulmonary hypertension. Life. 2022;12(5):684.
85. Ameli-Renani S, Rahman F, Nair A, Ramsay L, Bacon JL, Weller A, et al. Dual-energy CT for imaging of pulmonary hypertension: challenges and opportunities. Radiographics. 2014;34(7):1769–90.
86. Rahaghi FN, Winkler T, Kohli P, Nardelli P, Martí-Fuster B, Ross JC, et al. Quantification of the pulmonary vascular response to inhaled nitric oxide using noncontrast computed tomography imaging. Circ Cardiovasc Imaging. 2019;12(1):8338.
87. Rahaghi F, Come C, Ross J, Harmouche R, Diaz A, Estépar RSJ, et al. Morphologic response of the pulmonary vasculature to endoscopic lung volume reduction. Chronic Obstr Pulm Dis. 2015;2(3):214–22.

88. Iyer KS, Newell JD, Jin D, Fuld MK, Saha PK, Hansdottir S, et al. Quantitative dual-energy computed tomography supports a vascular etiology of smoking-induced inflammatory lung disease. Am J Respir Crit Care Med. 2016;193(6):652–61.
89. Ando K, Kuraishi H, Nagaoka T, Tsutsumi T, Hoshika Y, Kimura T, et al. Potential role of CT metrics in chronic obstructive pulmonary disease with pulmonary hypertension. Lung. 2015;193(6):911–8.
90. Newman JH, Rich S, Abman SH, Alexander JH, Barnard J, Beck GJ, et al. Enhancing insights into pulmonary vascular disease through a precision medicine approach: a joint nhlbi-cardiovascular medical research and education fund workshop report. Am J Respir Crit Care Med. 2017;195(12):1661–70.
91. Kumar S, Liney G, Rai R, Holloway L, Moses D, Vinod SK. Magnetic resonance imaging in lung: a review of its potential for radiotherapy. Br J Radiol. 2016;89(1060):20150431.
92. Bier EA, Alenezi F, Lu J, Wang Z, Mammarappallil JG, O'sullivan-Murphy B, et al. Noninvasive diagnosis of pulmonary hypertension with hyperpolarised129Xe magnetic resonance imaging and spectroscopy. ERJ Open Res. 2022;8(2).
93. Alenezi F, Covington TA, Mukherjee M, Mathai SC, Yu PB, Rajagopal S. Novel approaches to imaging the pulmonary vasculature and right heart. Circ Res. 2022;130(9):1445–65.
94. Qing K, Altes TA, Mugler JP, Mata JF, Tustison NJ, Ruppert K, et al. Hyperpolarized xenon-129: a new tool to assess pulmonary physiology in patients with pulmonary fibrosis. Biomedicine. 2023;11(6):1533.

Chapter 6
Omics and Precision Medicine Approaches in Pulmonary Vascular Diseases Associated with Chronic Lung Disease

Kevin Schwalbach and Anna R. Hemnes

Introduction

Precision medicine is an approach to healthcare that uses an individual's unique genetic, environmental, and lifestyle factors to inform healthcare recommendations and decisions [1]. While nearly universally agreed that this approach should improve patient-centered care, the details of its implementation remain elusive in many fields, including lung disease. That said, bedside clinicians can readily recount how some patients with significant parenchymal lung disease develop severe pulmonary vascular disease while others, who may appear in a cursory look to be indistinguishable, do not develop this dreaded comorbidity. This unexplained yet common clinical observation provides ample rationale for the study of precision medicine approaches to pulmonary vascular disease in chronic lung disease, as features other than parenchymal lung disease drivers may be mediating the development of pulmonary vascular disease, e.g., genetic risk or specific environmental exposures. Improved understanding of an individual's risk for pulmonary vascular disease or a specific patient's likelihood to respond to a particular intervention through precision medicine approaches would be a major advance in the field. This chapter will discuss what is known and not known in precision medicine approaches to pulmonary vascular disease in chronic lung disease and provide a roadmap for future studies to move the field forward through lessons learned in other similar disease states.

K. Schwalbach · A. R. Hemnes (✉)
Division of Allergy, Pulmonary and Critical Care Medicine, Vanderbilt University Medical Center, Nashville, TN, USA
e-mail: kevin.t.schwalbach@vumc.org; anna.r.hemnes@vumc.org

F. N. Rahaghi et al. (eds.), *The Pulmonary Vasculature in Chronic Lung Disease*, Respiratory Medicine, https://doi.org/10.1007/978-3-032-03581-3_6

"Omics" and Lung Disease

Omics comes from the Greek word "ome" meaning whole of class. The field of biological sciences has applied this term to many biologic processes or molecules to mean the study of the whole class. For instance, genomics is the study of an organism's entire genome and transcriptomics is the study of an organism's entire RNA transcripts. Other Omics that are commonly used include metabolomics and proteomics, but many other molecules that have many permutations can be studied. Further, we can expand our Omics to include factors external to the individual, for instance, the entirety of a person's exposures in the exposome.

In the field of lung disease, there are many nuances to consider in the discussion of Omics. First is the source of the Omic. There are benefits to studying the tissue of interest, for instance, the lungs from explants at the time of lung transplant may inform on the state of Omics in end-stage disease. Now with advanced single cell or special transcriptomics, we often are able to further differentiate the cell of interest so that Omics that are specifically relevant to the pulmonary vasculature can be identified even when changes are small in the entire lung. Second is the timing of the Omic study. In the aforementioned explanted lungs, the observations in Omics may be limited to end-stage disease and one may prefer to study early Omic initiators of disease, which may be particularly relevant in the exposome. Third is the availability of Omics to clinicians treating patients. While we understand lung tissue and cells to be the most informative of disease drivers and state, these studies are generally not relevant to clinicians in their day-to-day practice where access to lung tissue is limited, if present at all. This practicality is often provided as a rationale to study blood-based Omics, given their ready availability to clinicians via simple venipuncture. While these Omics may be biomarkers, they may be actually participating in pulmonary vascular disease promotion or resolution, as there is an intimate relationship between the pulmonary vasculature and circulating factors as the entire cardiac output must pass through the pulmonary vasculature. With confirmation in human tissue, experimental models, and translational approaches, these circulating Omic biomarkers may be demonstrated to participate in disease processes. As the field of precision medicine in pulmonary vascular disease in chronic lung disease is in its infancy, all of these Omics may be informative to disease risk, progression, and therapeutic response.

What We Can Learn from Precision Medicine Approaches in Pulmonary Hypertension Due to Other Causes

In the field of pulmonary vascular disease which is intimately linked to pulmonary hypertension (PH), precision medicine approaches have been most frequently been applied to pulmonary arterial hypertension (PAH) or Group 1 PH. While PAH is not entirely homogeneous, the subtypes do generally share similar pathology and response to therapy [2], which makes this condition amenable to the use of Omics to advance precision medicine ideals. Some examples of this include differentiation of PAH from healthy controls with a focus on underlying disease mechanisms using plasma Omics [3–5] and using Omics to identify PAH patients at high risk of disease progression [6–8]. Further, Omics have been used to develop prediction models of therapeutic response in PAH [9, 10] and even to identify Omic markers of target activation in novel therapies of PAH [4, 11]. And more recently, the integration of multiple Omics, so-called multiomics, has been applied, harnessing the power of these multiple, varied molecules, to understand PAH pathogenesis [12]. Thus, while a major challenge to using Omics to study a rare disease like PAH includes the potential for false discovery with thousands of Omics applied in few patients, this limitation has been largely mitigated through international consortiums raising the number of included individuals, advanced analytic techniques, and confirmation using translational approaches.

The PVDOMICS cohort (Redefining Pulmonary Hypertension through Pulmonary Vascular Disease Phenomics [13]) has taken a more expansive approach to Omics in pulmonary vascular disease of all types, including chronic lung disease. The goals of the project are to enhance or refine the current clinical classification of pulmonary hypertension using precision medicine approaches to uncover endophenotypes of pulmonary vascular disease. This US-based study enrolled a total of 1195 individuals including 172 subjects with chronic lung disease-associated PH and 119 with chronic lung disease and no PH or mild PH in addition to 96 healthy controls and other forms of PH and disease comparators [14]. While Omic data is presently limited to metabolomics, there will be in the future genomic, transcriptomic, and other Omics available for analysis. Key approaches used by this consortium include unbiased analyses to uncover novel phenotypes of pulmonary vascular disease. Early work has shown a key role for the kynurenine pathway in the development of scleroderma-associated PAH [15], suggesting that metabolomics may be useful in early identification of subjects at risk for pulmonary vascular disease. The impact of similar Omic analyses to chronic lung disease-associated pulmonary vascular disease will be enhanced by the deep clinical phenotyping in the cohort including imaging (chest CT and ventilation/perfusion scans) and pulmonary function testing in addition to traditional pulmonary vascular disease testing including echocardiography and right heart catheterization.

The State of Precision Medicine Approaches in Chronic Lung Disease

PH can occur in nearly any form of chronic lung disease. While hypoxia is undoubtedly a common driver of PH in all of these, whether regional or global, there are likely myriad other contributors dependent on the type of chronic lung disease. As such, it would appear to be a risk to scientific advancement to include all forms of chronic-lung disease-associated PH into a single analysis. In accordance with this approach, the 2024 World Symposium on Pulmonary Hypertension's working group on Group 3 PH suggested that deep phenotyping of the nature of lung disease is critical to understanding pathogenesis and potential therapy of PH in this context [16]. Here, we will discuss several key forms of chronic lung disease-associated PH separately.

One of the most remarkable applications of precision medicine in recent years has been in the development of medications targeting gene mutations in cystic fibrosis (CF). The causative mutations in CF transmembrane conductance regulator (*CFTR*) gene lead to impairment in CFTR mRNA expression, stability, processing, and/or function. The consequent malfunctioning CFTR protein results in the inability of cells to appropriately move chloride ions across cell membranes. Within the lung, this leads to viscous secretions, poor clearance of bacteria, and repeated cycles of infection and inflammation that destroy the architecture of the airways. A new class of medications known as CFTR modulators target various gene mutations and has drastically changed CF care and management. Agents are classified into five main groups depending on their effects on CFTR protein: potentiators, correctors, stabilizers, read-through agents, and amplifiers [17]. It is now standard practice to sequence a patient's *CFTR* gene at diagnosis [18]. This allows modulators to be precisely applied to treat an individual's specific protein defect. At present, more than 180 gene mutations have been approved for treatment with modulator therapy [17]. Efficacy of this approach has been shown in several RCTs to date, but one needs only look at a lung transplant list before and after modulators were approved for market use to truly see the effect these have had on the outcomes of CF patients [19–22].

The success of CFTR modulators has become a model for other chronic lung diseases such as idiopathic pulmonary fibrosis (IPF) and chronic obstructive lung disease (COPD). One major challenge that separates these later diseases from CF is the reality that the resultant phenotypes and endotypes are not the product of single gene mutations but rather heterogenous conditions resulting from a complicated interplay of many genotypes, proteins, and environmental factors [23, 24].

At present, there is limited data that we can use an individual's genetic profile in clinical application of those with COPD. A notable exception to this is in those who have COPD related to alpha-1 antitrypsin deficiency. Guidelines now suggest early screening of patients with COPD for mutations in the *SERPINA1* gene [25]. Those carrying mutations in this gene and resultant A1AT deficiency have been shown to benefit from replacement with plasma-purified alpha-1 antitrypsin (AAT) [26]. However, more useful clinical applications of precision medicine in COPD have included use of phenotypes, biomarkers, and imaging to navigate care. Current recommendations from the Global Obstructive Lung Disease Initiative (GOLD) suggest using the patient's exacerbation history and symptom severity to decide on inhaler therapy [25]. In those with high burden of symptoms based on scoring on Modified Medical Research Council or Chronic obstructive pulmonary disease assessment test, or exacerbation history ≥2 per year or ≥1 leading to hospitalization, consideration should be given to adding an inhaled corticosteroid. If exacerbations continue despite high-dose inhaled corticosteroid, then medications such as roflumilast or azithromycin are often added to inhaler therapy. One biomarker gaining traction for clinical use in COPD is blood eosinophil level. It has been suggested that serum eosinophil level may help predict patient response to ICS therapy [27, 28]. Although debate remains about the exact thresholds that predict response, GOLD currently uses >300 eosinophils/uL and <100 eosinophils/uL to identify individuals with higher and lower probability, respectively, of experiencing treatment benefit. Recently, the use of biologic therapy has shown promising results in those with serum eosinophils >300. Believed to be an indicator of patients with high levels of type 2 inflammation, it was shown that treatment with Dupilumab, a monoclonal antibody blocking interleukin-4 and interleukin-13 receptor, results in lower rates of exacerbation, improved lung function and less severe respiratory symptoms [29]. Lastly, several surgical and bronchoscopy techniques including lung volume reduction surgery (LVRS) and endobronchial valves have been applied on an individual level. Suitable candidates are assessed based on specific radiographic features identifying the pattern of emphysema combined with extent of hyperinflation and interlobar collateral ventilation [25, 30]. Omic predictors of drug response are thus beginning to gain traction in COPD, but the use of Omics in the context of PH associated with COPD is not yet studied.

Advances in the understanding of IPF pathogenesis, susceptibility, and disease progression have led to improved recognition and the advent of two anti-fibrotic medications that slow morbidity. However, precision medicine as a clinical application in IPF remains stubbornly within the realm of research. Genome-wide association studies have identified several polymorphisms in genes that increase susceptibility or severity in IPF [31]. Most well described are those with genetic variation in the *MUC5B* gene, known to increase risk of disease 6-fold [32]. Whom to perform genetic testing for is not an easy decision, but recent publication by the Pulmonary Fibrosis Foundation Genetic Testing Work Group attempts to address this question with clinical guidance for high-yield scenarios [33]. A growing number of biomarkers have been suggested for the diagnosis of IPF, but clinical applicability remains limited [34–36]. A notable exception to this is the Envisia Genomic Classifier, a commercially available biomarker that analyzes transbronchial biopsies and can identify histopathologic features of usual interstitial pneumonia (UIP) with high accuracy [37, 38]. Its main limitation is the inability to decipher UIP due to IPF from UIP due to other interstitial lung diseases (ILD). IPF has a variable clinical course, where some experience rapid progression and others experience gradual decline accompanied by acute respiratory deteriorations. Which category patients will fall into, and best ways to treat each subset remains unknown. Gene variations, micro-RNAs and telomere shortening have all been shown to predict IPF mortality. For example, one study identified signature endotypes in peripheral blood able to predict high and low risk of disease progression based on transcriptomic and proteomic data, although not yet available to clinicians [39]. It has also been recognized that up to one-third of individuals with familial IPF and 1 in 10 with sporadic IPF have telomere-related shortening [40]. Regardless of cause, individuals with short telomeres have a more rapid disease course and worse survival. Two anti-fibrotic drugs, nintedanib and pirfenidone, have been shown to slow decline in lung function [41, 42]. These therapies are now applied broadly across all subsets of patients. Research into prediction of treatment response is ongoing, but more work is needed in order to translate this research into actionable information. Overall, several outstanding questions remain despite a plethora of primary research into the area and which of the above Omic markers will ultimately prove useful in clinical practice is yet to be determined [43].

Group 3 PH unites several disparate diseases under one heading, despite a wide variety of different phenotypes, endotypes, and genetics. Although a number of animal models have helped discover some of the molecular mechanisms underlying pulmonary vascular remodeling in chronic hypoxia – including HIF-1α and TBF-β signaling pathways – none have yet been moved to the bedside clinician [44]. PAH-specific therapies have been tested in trials for Group 3 PH with mixed results [45–47]. The INCREASE trial recently evaluated inhaled treprostinil in patients with ILD-PH and showed it may increase 6MWD and delay time to clinical worsening [46]. However, other trials including endothelin receptor antagonists, riociguat, and PDE-5 inhibitors have actually signaled some harm when applied to Group 3 PH broadly [48]. The success of the INCREASE trial can, at least in part, be ascribed to enrollment of a specific form of Group 3 PH (ILD-associated PH) rather than all forms, the stringent phenotyping required for enrollment, and the potential efficacy of the drug. This has now opened the door to precision-based approaches to Group 3 PH in which a distinct clinical phenotype with a specific drug response may allow investigators to understand how these patients differ from other forms of Group 3 PH using an Omics-based approach.

Specific Challenges to Precision Medicine Approaches Using Omics in Chronic Lung Disease-Associated Pulmonary Hypertension

The primary challenge to precision medicine in Group 3 PH is the heterogeneous diseases that can lead to pulmonary vascular disease. While they all incorporate some measure of hypoxia either regionally localized to specific alveoli or diffusely across the parenchyma, there is little evidence that the pulmonary vascular histopathology they elicit is identical or even quite similar as is the case in PAH [49]. Further, there is clear heterogeneity in treatment response, as thus far ILD-associated PH is the only disease with an approved therapy (inhaled Treprostinil [46]) and the same drug showed no efficacy in COPD-associated PH [45]. Thus, the field has moved to studies of specific disease phenotypes in this heterogeneous condition.

A second major challenge is clinical detection of early or sub-clinical disease. A major goal of precision medicine approaches is often to identify subjects at risk for disease development. In the case of Group 3 PH, this would be identification of patients with parenchymal lung disease and no PH who are at high risk to develop mild PH, at a time when therapy may be most effective. However, detection of early pulmonary vascular disease is difficult as PH in early forms is often associated with fatigue and dyspnea, which are seminal symptoms of all parenchymal lung disease including those without PH. Echocardiography and DLCO may be useful in detection of PH [16, 50], however they are not 100% sensitive and the gold standard for diagnosis, right heart catheterization, may be infeasible for many patients. Thus, ensuring that people without PH on non-invasive screening are in fact true negatives is a major challenge. Consequently, detection of early disease and application of Omics to detect risk for early PH is a major challenge.

A third challenge is identification of predictors of drug responses in Group 3 PH. While this is possible in the context of a well-conducted Phase II or III clinical trial, samples need to be collected, and Omics analyses planned for prior to enrollment of subjects in the trial. Moreover, the discovery that there are Omic predictors of response may limit drug use in patients without these predictors, which gives both prescribers and pharma pause about limited access to drugs that meet FDA-approved endpoints for approval in the general disease population. That said, this is a potential application of precision medicine using omics in chronic lung disease-associated PH, which could mimic the tremendous success outlined above in cystic fibrosis.

Future Directions for Precision Medicine and Omics in Chronic Lung Disease-Associated Pulmonary Vascular Disease

Despite these challenges, there are some features of chronic lung disease-associated PH that make them amenable to precision medicine-based approaches using Omics. In contrast to PAH, very few of the diseases that lead to group 3 PH are rare improving confidence in findings through stronger statistical approaches. There is ever-advancing knowledge on the genetics of ILD, in particular, that may be used to identify endophenotypes including potentially those at high risk of PH. The more common event of lung transplant in Group 3 PH allows for comparison of Omics in the peripheral blood with Omics identified specifically in the pulmonary vasculature. This feature will improve confidence in blood-based Omic findings and potentially point to Omics that participate in disease pathogenesis in comparison with biomarkers of disease that are not participating in disease initiation or progression.

There are existing cohorts that could be used to identify Omic differences between chronic lung disease with and without PH. As mentioned above, the PVDOMICS cohort includes rich phenotyping and extensive Omics that can be used to compare subjects with and without PH. Other cohorts of ILD or COPD have extensive Omic data but frequently do not have a comprehensive phenotyping of pulmonary vascular disease, which would be a limitation.

To move the field forward, a longitudinal cohort including multiple forms of chronic lung disease with deep phenotyping of the pulmonary vasculature at baseline and over time would be a worthy investment. Studying subjects at risk for PH over time would be a major advance in the field and allow for Omic analyses of predictors of PH development. Further, collection of peripheral blood (and explant lung tissue where available) in the context of placebo-controlled trials of interventions in chronic lung disease-associated PH therapeutics will allow investigators to understand both predictors of drug response at entry and, potentially, early detection of regression of pulmonary vascular disease with therapy.

Lastly, to develop one day highly impactful therapies, better disease models are needed. In particular, validation of human discoveries in animal models that faithfully recapitulate human disease or cell culture models using human cells where possible would allow Omics discoveries to be studied in a dynamic fashion using Koch's postulates. While the field is improving, further opportunities to validate large-scale Omic data in a hypothesis-driven approach would move the field forward.

References

1. Shah SH, Arnett D, Houser SR, et al. Opportunities for the cardiovascular community in the precision medicine initiative. Circulation. 2016;133(2):226–31. https://doi.org/10.1161/CIRCULATIONAHA.115.019475.
2. Kovacs G, Bartolome S, Denton CP, et al. Definition, classification and diagnosis of pulmonary hypertension. Eur Respir J. 2024;64(4). https://doi.org/10.1183/13993003.01324-2024.
3. Ulrich A, Wu Y, Draisma H, et al. Blood DNA methylation profiling identifies cathepsin Z dysregulation in pulmonary arterial hypertension. Nat Commun. 2024;15(1):330. https://doi.org/10.1038/s41467-023-44683-0.
4. Guignabert C, Savale L, Boucly A, et al. Serum and pulmonary expression profiles of the activin signaling system in pulmonary arterial hypertension. Circulation. 2023;147(24):1809–22. https://doi.org/10.1161/CIRCULATIONAHA.122.061501.
5. Harbaum L, Rhodes CJ, Wharton J, et al. Mining the plasma proteome for insights into the molecular pathology of pulmonary arterial hypertension. Am J Respir Crit Care Med. 2022;205(12):1449–60. https://doi.org/10.1164/rccm.202109-2106OC.
6. Rhodes CJ, Wharton J, Swietlik EM, et al. Using the plasma proteome for risk stratifying patients with pulmonary arterial hypertension. Am J Respir Crit Care Med. 2022;205(9):1102–11. https://doi.org/10.1164/rccm.202105-1118OC.
7. Rhodes CJ, Batai K, Bleda M, et al. Genetic determinants of risk in pulmonary arterial hypertension: international genome-wide association studies and meta-analysis. Lancet Respir Med. 2019;7(3):227–38. https://doi.org/10.1016/S2213-2600(18)30409-0.
8. Rhodes CJ, Otero-Nunez P, Wharton J, et al. Whole-blood RNA profiles associated with pulmonary arterial hypertension and clinical outcome. Am J Respir Crit Care Med. 2020;202(4):586–94. https://doi.org/10.1164/rccm.202003-0510OC.
9. Hemnes AR, Trammell AW, Archer SL, et al. Peripheral blood signature of vasodilator-responsive pulmonary arterial hypertension. Circulation. 2015;131(4):401–9; discussion 409. https://doi.org/10.1161/circulationaha.114.013317.

10. Benza RL, Gomberg-Maitland M, Demarco T, et al. Endothelin-1 pathway polymorphisms and outcomes in pulmonary arterial hypertension. Am J Respir Crit Care Med. 2015;192(11):1345–54. https://doi.org/10.1164/rccm.201501-0196OC.
11. Hemnes AR, Rathinasabapathy A, Austin EA, et al. A potential therapeutic role for angiotensin-converting enzyme 2 in human pulmonary arterial hypertension. Eur Respir J. 2018;51(6). https://doi.org/10.1183/13993003.02638-2017.
12. Hong J, Medzikovic L, Sun W, et al. Integrative multiomics in the lung reveals a protective role of asporin in pulmonary arterial hypertension. Circulation. 2024;150(16):1268–87. https://doi.org/10.1161/CIRCULATIONAHA.124.069864.
13. Hemnes AR, Beck GJ, Newman JH, et al. PVDOMICS: a multi-center study to improve understanding of pulmonary vascular disease through phenomics. Circ Res. 2017;121(10):1136–9. https://doi.org/10.1161/CIRCRESAHA.117.311737.
14. Hemnes AR, Leopold JA, Radeva MK, et al. Clinical characteristics and transplant-free survival across the spectrum of pulmonary vascular disease. J Am Coll Cardiol. 2022;80(7):697–718. https://doi.org/10.1016/j.jacc.2022.05.038.
15. Simpson CE, Ambade AS, Harlan R, et al. Kynurenine pathway metabolism evolves with development of preclinical and scleroderma-associated pulmonary arterial hypertension. Am J Phys Lung Cell Mol Phys. 2023;325(5):L617–27. https://doi.org/10.1152/ajplung.00177.2023.
16. Shlobin OA, Adir Y, Barbera JA, et al. Pulmonary hypertension associated with lung diseases. Eur Respir J. 2024;64(4). https://doi.org/10.1183/13993003.01200-2024.
17. Lopes-Pacheco M. CFTR modulators: the changing face of cystic fibrosis in the era of precision medicine. Front Pharmacol. 2019;10:1662. https://doi.org/10.3389/fphar.2019.01662.
18. Southern KW, Castellani C, Lammertyn E, et al. Standards of care for CFTR variant-specific therapy (including modulators) for people with cystic fibrosis. J Cyst Fibros. 2023;22(1):17–30. https://doi.org/10.1016/j.jcf.2022.10.002.
19. Middleton PG, Mall MA, Drevinek P, et al. Elexacaftor-tezacaftor-ivacaftor for cystic fibrosis with a single Phe508del allele. N Engl J Med. 2019;381(19):1809–19. https://doi.org/10.1056/NEJMoa1908639.
20. Nichols DP, Paynter AC, Heltshe SL, et al. Clinical effectiveness of elexacaftor/tezacaftor/ivacaftor in people with cystic fibrosis: a clinical trial. Am J Respir Crit Care Med. 2022;205(5):529–39. https://doi.org/10.1164/rccm.202108-1986OC.
21. Flume PA, Biner RF, Downey DG, et al. Long-term safety and efficacy of tezacaftor-ivacaftor in individuals with cystic fibrosis aged 12 years or older who are homozygous or heterozygous for Phe508del CFTR (EXTEND): an open-label extension study. Lancet Respir Med. 2021;9(7):733–46. https://doi.org/10.1016/S2213-2600(20)30510-5.
22. Shteinberg M, Taylor-Cousar JL. Impact of CFTR modulator use on outcomes in people with severe cystic fibrosis lung disease. Eur Resp Rev. 2020;29(155). https://doi.org/10.1183/16000617.0112-2019.
23. Leung JM, Obeidat M, Sadatsafavi M, Sin DD. Introduction to precision medicine in COPD. Eur Respir J. 2019;53(4). https://doi.org/10.1183/13993003.02460-2018.
24. Rennard SI, Vestbo J. The many “small COPDs”: COPD should be an orphan disease. Chest. 2008;134(3):623–7. https://doi.org/10.1378/chest.07-3059.
25. Agusti A, Celli BR, Criner GJ, et al. Global initiative for chronic obstructive lung disease 2023 report: GOLD executive summary. Am J Respir Crit Care Med. 2023;207(7):819–37. https://doi.org/10.1164/rccm.202301-0106PP.
26. McElvaney NG, Burdon J, Holmes M, et al. Long-term efficacy and safety of alpha1 proteinase inhibitor treatment for emphysema caused by severe alpha1 antitrypsin deficiency: an open-label extension trial (RAPID-OLE). Lancet Respir Med. 2017;5(1):51–60. https://doi.org/10.1016/S2213-2600(16)30430-1.
27. Pascoe S, Barnes N, Brusselle G, et al. Blood eosinophils and treatment response with triple and dual combination therapy in chronic obstructive pulmonary disease: analysis of the IMPACT trial. Lancet Respir Med. 2019;7(9):745–56. https://doi.org/10.1016/S2213-2600(19)30190-0.

28. Singh D. Blood eosinophil counts in chronic obstructive pulmonary disease: a biomarker of inhaled corticosteroid effects. Tuberc Respir Dis (Seoul). 2020;83(3):185–94. https://doi.org/10.4046/trd.2020.0026.
29. Bhatt SP, Rabe KF, Hanania NA, et al. Dupilumab for COPD with type 2 inflammation indicated by eosinophil counts. N Engl J Med. 2023;389(3):205–14. https://doi.org/10.1056/NEJMoa2303951.
30. Marchetti N, Criner GJ. Surgical approaches to treating emphysema: lung volume reduction surgery, bullectomy, and lung transplantation. Semin Respir Crit Care Med. 2015;36(4):592–608. https://doi.org/10.1055/s-0035-1556064.
31. Partanen JJ, Happola P, Zhou W, et al. Leveraging global multi-ancestry meta-analysis in the study of idiopathic pulmonary fibrosis genetics. Cell Genom. 2022;2(10):100181. https://doi.org/10.1016/j.xgen.2022.100181.
32. Peljto AL, Zhang Y, Fingerlin TE, et al. Association between the MUC5B promoter polymorphism and survival in patients with idiopathic pulmonary fibrosis. JAMA. 2013;309(21):2232–9. https://doi.org/10.1001/jama.2013.5827.
33. Newton CA, Oldham JM, Applegate C, et al. The role of genetic testing in pulmonary fibrosis: a perspective from the pulmonary fibrosis foundation genetic testing work group. Chest. 2022;162(2):394–405. https://doi.org/10.1016/j.chest.2022.03.023.
34. White ES, Xia M, Murray S, et al. Plasma surfactant protein-D, matrix metalloproteinase-7, and osteopontin index distinguishes idiopathic pulmonary fibrosis from other idiopathic interstitial pneumonias. Am J Respir Crit Care Med. 2016;194(10):1242–51. https://doi.org/10.1164/rccm.201505-0862OC.
35. Stainer A, Faverio P, Busnelli S, et al. Molecular biomarkers in idiopathic pulmonary fibrosis: state of the art and future directions. Int J Mol Sci. 2021;22(12). https://doi.org/10.3390/ijms22126255.
36. Todd JL, Neely ML, Overton R, et al. Peripheral blood proteomic profiling of idiopathic pulmonary fibrosis biomarkers in the multicentre IPF-PRO Registry. Respir Res. 2019;20(1):227. https://doi.org/10.1186/s12931-019-1190-z.
37. Raghu G, Flaherty KR, Lederer DJ, et al. Use of a molecular classifier to identify usual interstitial pneumonia in conventional transbronchial lung biopsy samples: a prospective validation study. Lancet Respir Med. 2019;7(6):487–96. https://doi.org/10.1016/S2213-2600(19)30059-1.
38. Richeldi L, Scholand MB, Lynch DA, et al. Utility of a molecular classifier as a complement to high-resolution computed tomography to identify usual interstitial pneumonia. Am J Respir Crit Care Med. 2021;203(2):211–20. https://doi.org/10.1164/rccm.202003-0877OC.
39. Ruan P, Todd JL, Zhao H, et al. Integrative multi-omics analysis reveals novel idiopathic pulmonary fibrosis endotypes associated with disease progression. Respir Res. 2023;24(1):141. https://doi.org/10.1186/s12931-023-02435-0.
40. Courtwright AM, El-Chemaly S. Telomeres in interstitial lung disease: the short and the long of it. Ann Am Thorac Soc. 2019;16(2):175–81. https://doi.org/10.1513/AnnalsATS.201808-508CME.
41. Efficacy and safety of nintedanib in idiopathic pulmonary fibrosis. N Engl J Med. 2015;373(8):782. https://doi.org/10.1056/NEJMx150012.
42. King TE Jr, Bradford WZ, Castro-Bernardini S, et al. A phase 3 trial of pirfenidone in patients with idiopathic pulmonary fibrosis. N Engl J Med. 2014;370(22):2083–92. https://doi.org/10.1056/NEJMoa1402582.
43. Karampitsakos T, Juan-Guardela BM, Tzouvelekis A, Herazo-Maya JD. Precision medicine advances in idiopathic pulmonary fibrosis. EBioMedicine. 2023;95:104766. https://doi.org/10.1016/j.ebiom.2023.104766.
44. Singh N, Dorfmuller P, Shlobin OA, Ventetuolo CE. Group 3 pulmonary hypertension: from bench to bedside. Circ Res. 2022;130(9):1404–22. https://doi.org/10.1161/CIRCRESAHA.121.319970.

45. Nathan SD, Argula R, Trivieri MG, et al. Inhaled treprostinil in pulmonary hypertension associated with COPD: PERFECT study results. Eur Respir J. 2024;63(6). https://doi.org/10.1183/13993003.00172-2024.
46. Waxman A, Restrepo-Jaramillo R, Thenappan T, et al. Inhaled treprostinil in pulmonary hypertension due to interstitial lung disease. N Engl J Med. 2021;384(4):325–34. https://doi.org/10.1056/NEJMoa2008470.
47. Nathan SD, Behr J, Collard HR, et al. Riociguat for idiopathic interstitial pneumonia-associated pulmonary hypertension (RISE-IIP): a randomised, placebo-controlled phase 2b study. Lancet Respir Med. 2019;7(9):780–90. https://doi.org/10.1016/S2213-2600(19)30250-4.
48. King CS, Shlobin OA. The trouble with group 3 pulmonary hypertension in interstitial lung disease: dilemmas in diagnosis and the conundrum of treatment. Chest. 2020;158(4):1651–64. https://doi.org/10.1016/j.chest.2020.04.046.
49. Guignabert C, Aman J, Bonnet S, et al. Pathology and pathobiology of pulmonary hypertension: current insights and future directions. Eur Respir J. 2024;64(4). https://doi.org/10.1183/13993003.01095-2024.
50. Vitulo P, Piccari L, Wort SJ, et al. Screening and diagnosis of pulmonary hypertension associated with chronic lung disease (PH-CLD): a consensus statement from the pulmonary vascular research institute's innovative drug development initiative-group 3 pulmonary hypertension. Pulm Circ. 2024;14(4):e70005. https://doi.org/10.1002/pul2.70005.

Chapter 7
RV/PA Coupling in Pulmonary Hypertension Secondary to Chronic Lung Disease

Fatima Zeba, Paul M. Heerdt, and Inderjit Singh

Introduction

Pulmonary hypertension (PH) secondary to pulmonary arterial remodeling is associated with a variety of chronic lung diseases (CLD), most commonly chronic obstructive pulmonary disease (COPD), interstitial lung disease (ILD), and hypoventilation syndromes. Proposed mechanisms include hypoxia, endothelial dysfunction, mechanical factors, and genetic predisposition leading to precapillary vascular remodeling. In contrast, granulomatous infiltration with resultant pulmonary vaso- and veno-occlusion plays a role in PH secondary to sarcoidosis, while in obesity hypoventilation syndrome (OHS) or in patients with overlap syndrome (obstructive sleep apnea and COPD), alveolar hypoventilation and subsequent alveolar hypoxia is the major driver for PH development [1, 2].

The exact prevalence of PH in CLD is unclear due to variations in the diagnostic method, the definition of PH used, the patient population studied and the severity of CLD at time of evaluation [3–7]. More recently, these data are further complicated by studies utilizing different definitions for PH, following a change in guideline recommendations from a mPAP $\geq$ 25 to mPAP > 20 in 2022 [8].

The presence of PH in patients with chronic lung disease portends a poor prognosis [9–11] and some data suggest a worse prognosis than in patients with idiopathic pulmonary arterial hypertension (PAH). Hemnes et al reported that among

F. Zeba (✉) · I. Singh
Division of Pulmonary, Critical Care, and Sleep Medicine, Department of Internal Medicine, Yale School of Medicine, New Haven, CT, USA
e-mail: fatima.zeba@yale.edu; inderjit.singh@yale.edu

P. M. Heerdt
Department of Anesthesiology, Yale School of Medicine, New Haven, CT, USA

F. N. Rahaghi et al. (eds.), *The Pulmonary Vasculature in Chronic Lung Disease*, Respiratory Medicine, https://doi.org/10.1007/978-3-032-03581-3_7

750 patients with PH, transplant-free survival was poorest in group 3 PH. Using group 1 PH as the reference group, the hazard ratio for death or relevant transplant was 3.1 in group 3 PH vs. 1.47 in group 2 PH. This effect was also seen among comparators (enrollees with similar underlying diseases but with milder or no pulmonary vascular phenotype), where group 3 subjects had a >5-fold increased risk of death or heart/lung transplant over the follow-up period compared to group 1 patients [12].

Among patients with CLD who develop PH, prognostication and selection of patients for treatment presents a unique challenge. Understanding the impact of RV dysfunction on exercise tolerance, over and above limitations from gas exchange, can help inform these clinical questions. RV-PA coupling is emerging as a valuable measurement that provides insight into this relationship.

Right Ventricular (RV) Pulmonary Artery (PA) Coupling

Methods of RV-PA Coupling Assessment: Invasive Hemodynamic Assessment

RV-PA coupling describes the mechanical interaction between the RV and the pulmonary artery (PA), and its most objective metric is the ratio between ventricular elastance (Ees), a load-independent measure of contractility, and arterial elastance (Ea), a lump sum measure of total arterial afterload. The normal Ees/Ea ratio for the RV has been reported to be between 1.5 and 2.0, which corresponds to an optimal balance between RV mechanical work and oxygen consumption [13, 14].

The ability of the RV to adapt to the increasing afterload has been shown to confer important prognostic significance in patients with PH. The compensatory response of the RV to increasing afterload is first to dilate to preserve stroke volume (heterometric autoregulation). With a continued increase in afterload, the RV transitions to homeometric adaptation and increases contractility (the Anrep effect) to maintain stroke volume. Ultimately, with sustained pressure overload, RV-PA uncoupling ensues with a resultant mismatch between RV contractility and its afterload. Eventually, these changes cause RV failure, LV underfilling, and hemodynamic instability [15].

The reference standard measurement for Ees and Ea is derived by plotting the continuous relationship between pressure and volume (PV loops) over a range of preload (Fig. 7.1). Data acquisition for RV PV loops typically involves the use of a micromanometer and conductance catheter [16]. However, in routine clinical practice, this technique is impractical for several reasons. These include cost, complexity, and the need for application of controlled maneuvers that acutely alter the RV preload (valsalva, external abdominal compression, balloon occlusion of the inferior vena cava). As an alternative, single-beat (SB) methods for deriving Ees and Ea have been described that do not require preload variation and combine analysis of

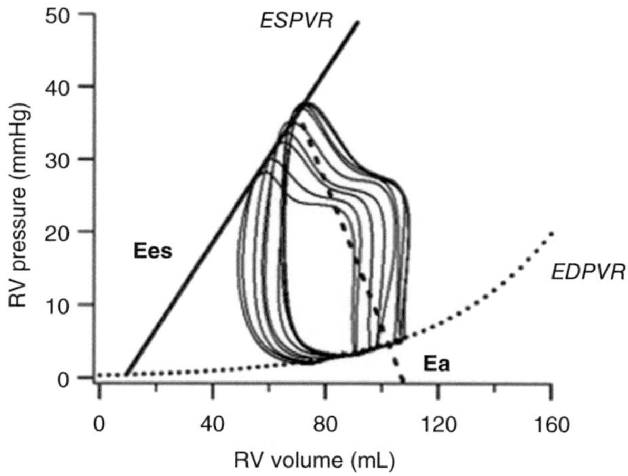

Fig. 7.1 Representative multi-beat right ventricular (RV) pressure-volume analysis. Data were acquired during occlusion of the inferior vena cava in a swine model. Regression of the point of end-systolic pressure for each loop during decreasing preload was used to define the end-systolic pressure-volume relationship (ESPVR, solid line). The ESPVR slope represents end-systolic elastance (Ees, expressed in mmHg/mL), a load-independent measure of contractility. Regression of the point of end-diastolic pressure was used to define the end-diastolic pressure-volume relationship (EDPVR, dotted line) with the equation for this non-linear relationship then used to derive a stiffness constant. From the first loop of the sequence, the end-systolic pressure/(end-diastolic volume—end-systolic volume) was used to summarize afterload as arterial elastance (Ea, hatched line, expressed in mmHg)

the RV pressure waveform with SV alone or maximal and minimal RV volume measured by imaging [17, 18].

The most common SB method for estimating RV-PA coupling is centered on two factors: (1) Pmax, the predicted maximum RV pressure generated during an isovolumic contraction; and (2) RV end-systolic pressure (ESP). Pmax is determined by extrapolation of early and late isovolumic portions of the RV pressure curve [19]. With these data, Ees is calculated as (Pmax-ESP)/SV, and Ea is calculated as ESP/SV [16]. However, variation in how Pmax is predicted and, more importantly how ESP is defined, can affect the derived values for Ees and Ea, potentially complicating comparison of absolute values reported for different studies. For example, RV ESP has been estimated using mPAP, peak RV systolic pressure, a correction equation for mPAP (ESP = 1.65 × mPAP − 7.79), or the second derivative square method [20, 21]. The comparison of the different ESP permutations as well as whether pulmonary artery wedge pressure should be considered is beyond the scope of the current chapter and is described in detail elsewhere [20]. A representative figure describing the SB method of RV-PA coupling using the ESP correction equation in two patients with scleroderma PAH with and without associated interstitial lung disease is depicted in Fig. 7.2. A limitation of the Pmax SB method is that it does not account for changes in the end-systolic pressure-volume relationship (ESPVR) volume intercept (Vo), the theoretical volume remaining at a ventricular pressure of

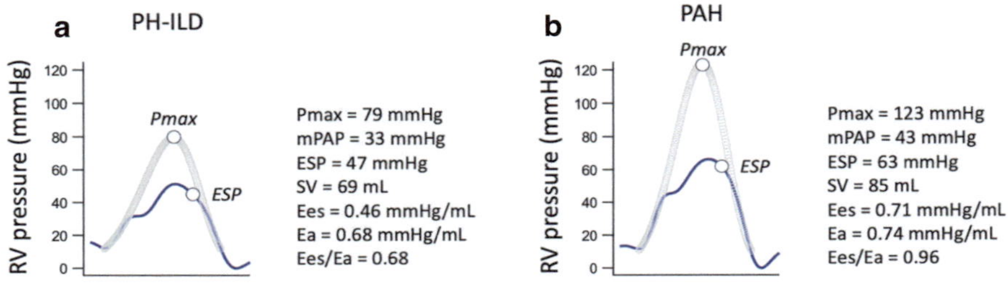

Fig. 7.2 Representative Pmax single beat method of right ventricular-pulmonary artery (RV-PA) coupling estimation in scleroderma patients with PH-ILD (**a**) and PAH (**b**). The blue waveform represents the native RV pressure waveform while the superimposed hatched grey waveform is the theoretical isovolumic contraction beat. ESP was estimated using the previously validated correction equation (ESP = 1.65 × mPAP − 7.79). Both patients exhibited reduced RV-PA coupling (Ees/Ea) with the PH-ILD patients demonstrating more significantly reduced Ees/Ea compared to the PAH patient*PH* pulmonary hypertension, *ILD* interstitial lung disease, *RV* right ventricle, *PA* pulmonary artery, *Pmax* maximum RV pressure generated during an isovolumic contraction, *PA mPAP* mean pulmonary artery pressure, *SV* stroke volume, *Ee* end-systolic elastance, *Ea* pulmonary arterial elastance, *PAH* pulmonary arterial hypertension

0 mmHg. Instead, the model assumes that Vo ~ 0 mmHg potentially affecting the accuracy of the Ees given that in a hypertensive RV, Vo does not typically equal 0 mmHg. As an alternative, recent data have demonstrated the potential clinical utility of applying a SB model that does not require Pmax prediction and integrates measurement of maximal and minimal RV volume to calculate Vo and improve accuracy of the derived Ees [22].

Methods of RV-PA Coupling Assessment: Non-invasive RV-PA Coupling Assessment

The ratio of TAPSE/PASP measured by 2D Echo has been used as a non-invasive surrogate for RV-PA coupling. This measurement has been validated by comparison to conductance catheter measurements, and a cutoff of 0.31 mm/mmHg is found to detect RV-arterial uncoupling (with a sensitivity 87.5% and a specificity 75.9%) [23, 24]. Ghio et al. non-invasively examined measures of RV function during dobutamine stress testing in patients with PAH versus controls. They noted a decline in the TAPSE/PASP ratio in patients with PAH, indicating uncoupling, and decreased contractile reserve in agreement with findings from invasive cardiopulmonary stress testing (CPET) [25]. However, the measurement of the tricuspid regurgitant (TR) jet (which is used to estimate PASP in practice) is often unreliable, especially in chronic lung disease [26]. Echo parameters are also dependent on the scale of RV dysfunction. It is important to note that severe TR may lead to an underestimation of PASP and an overestimation of TAPSE [27, 28].

Other echocardiographic-derived parameters such as RV FAC/mPAP and RV FAC/RV ESA (end-systolic area) have also been found to correlate with reference standard conductance catheter-measured Ees/Ea in patients with PAH and CTEPH [23]. Cardiac magnetic resonance imaging (MRI)-derived ratio of stroke volume to end-systolic volume (SV/ESV) was shown to independently predict survival as a measure of RV-PA coupling in 50 patients evaluated for suspected PH [29]. This ratio has prognostic relevance in patients with PAH with a cutoff of 0.5 [30]. However, the inherent limitation of this "volumetric method" of estimating RV-PA coupling is the assumption, like that of the Pmax SB model, that Vo = 0 mmHg, which, as mentioned earlier, is not the case in a hypertensive RV [18].

It is important to highlight here that echocardiographic estimations of PA pressure have limited accuracy in detecting PH in lung disease, with an accuracy rate of 40–48% reported when compared to RHC in two separate studies [3, 4]. In a study of 265 patients with ILD and suspected PH, RHC confirmed PH in 86% of subjects with a peak tricuspid regurgitation (TR) velocity >3.4 m/s and in 40% of ILD subjects with a TR velocity <2.8 m/s, highlighting the limitation of using the latter threshold to exclude PH in this patient population [5].

Exercise Pulmonary Hypertension in Chronic Lung Disease

With exercise, cardiac output increases, initially accompanied by decreased PVR due to pulmonary vessel distension and subsequent recruitment. With continued increase in RV SV and PA pressure, RV afterload increases, and PA compliance decreases [31]. In a normal RV-PA unit, this is followed by a commensurate increase in RV contractility to maintain RV-PA coupling.

COPD-PH

Even under moderate exercise conditions, COPD patients may show a rapid rise in mPAP, indicating loss of lung vasculature, vascular distensibility, or loss of vessel recruitment ability. Hilde et al. reported a comparable abnormal pulmonary vascular response in COPD patients with and without PH suggesting that factors other than fixed pulmonary vascular remodeling (e.g., dynamic air trapping) also contribute to abnormal exercise pulmonary vascular response in COPD [32]. Exercise PH in COPD patients may also be due to other factors including comorbid left heart disease with resultant pulmonary venous hypertension and deconditioning.

ILD-PH

Exercise PH defined as mPAP/cardiac output >3 has a prevalence of 28% in patients with ILD [33]. Oliveira et al conducted an invasive CPET study to examine the relative contributions of pulmonary vascular burden and RV work in patients with established resting ILD-PH and ILD patients with exercise PH (ILD-ePH). They found that patients with ILD-PH and ILD-ePH had a greater pulmonary vascular disease burden, reflected by an increase in pulmonary vascular resistance and a reduction in PA compliance. Patients with ILD-PH also demonstrated greater exercise RV work (measured by RV stroke work index) compared to ILD-ePH patients with similarly reduced peak exercise aerobic capacity compared to ILD patients without resting or exercise PH. The findings from this study highlight the significant role of increased pulmonary vascular and RV burden on exercise capacity in ILD patients with PH [34].

An abnormal pulmonary vascular response in ILD can also be elicited using non-invasive CPET where exercise results in ventilation-perfusion mismatch represented by inefficient ventilation, abnormalities in gas exchange, and increased dead space [33, 35, 36]. Sub-maximal CPET confers several advantages over conventional non-invasive CPET. In submaximal CPET, unlike conventional CPET, a maximal exercise effort is not required, making it an attractive option for PH and/or ILD patients with baseline cardiopulmonary limitation or patients with preexisting musculoskeletal disorders (e.g., those with connective tissue disease) and elderly patients who often are unable to undergo maximum exercise testing [37, 38].

In a small single-center study examining the utility of submaximal CPET in distinguishing between ILD-PH and ILD patients without PH [37], a gas exchange-derived estimate of pulmonary vascular capacitance (GXcap) measurement ≤416 ml*mmHg offered a high probability of ILD-PH (82%). When the GXcap value was combined with estimated RVSP (>43 mmHg) and FVC/DLCO ratio (<1.7), the predictive ability for PH-ILD improved. These variables taken together had an AUC of 0.94 (sensitivity 86% and specificity 93%). Submaximal exercise testing may therefore serve as an important adjunct to screen ILD patients for PH.

Prognostic Significance of RV PA Coupling in Group 3 PH

The ability of the RV to adapt to the increased afterload (coupling) is an important prognostic factor in PH. Ees and Ees/Eea are lower in systemic sclerosis (SSc)-PAH compared with IPAH at a similar afterload, potentially due to worse or inherent RV systolic dysfunction in patients with SSc [39, 40]. Multi-beat Ees/Ea < 0.65 can predict a shorter time to clinical worsening in pre-capillary pulmonary hypertension [40, 41] and PH secondary to left heart disease [42]. As discussed earlier, when uncoupling occurs (indicated by Ees/Ea decreasing below a critical value), RVEF decreases, end-diastolic volume increases, and RV failure can ultimately ensue.

While there have been several studies examining the prognostic significance of RV-PA coupling in PAH and group 2 PH, clinical outcomes studies on RV-PA coupling in PH-ILD are lacking. Prinz et al examined 122 patients with group 3 PH and 155 patients with group 1 PAH to assess RV function in PH. Patients with group 3 PH in this study had lower mPAP and PVR, higher pulmonary vascular compliance, and cardiac output compared to group 1 patients. Despite this, the group 3 cohort had worse RV function (lower RV fractional area change values for any given mPAP), reduced exercise capacity, and worse survival than the group 1 cohort [43]. The mechanisms underlying this finding are unclear, and one possible explanation is the mechanical effect of COPD on the RV [44, 45]. Another explanation may be the increased burden of pulmonary vascular disease imposed by the underlying lung disease on the RV, especially during exercise.

Conclusion

Mortality from group 3 PH remains unacceptably high despite our improved understanding of CLD-PH patho-mechanism and advances in PAH treatment. Recent studies have demonstrated that treatment with inhaled treprostinil can delay time to clinical worsening [46] and perhaps even improve lung function [47, 48].

While RV-PA coupling has been shown to confer prognostic significance in PH without CLD, outcome data pertaining to RV-PA coupling in CLD-PH is lacking. In CLD patients with normal resting right heart catheterization, hemodynamic perturbations can often be unmasked with exercise testing (e.g., inability to recruit and distend the small pulmonary vasculature to accommodate antecedent increase in stroke volume). Accordingly, future studies should investigate resting and dynamic RV-PA coupling measurements and their prognostic significance in CLD-PH vs CLD without PH and examine the mechanism of action of approved targeted therapies in PAH (e.g., decrease in Ea with or without a concomitant increase in Ees) to help inform a precision medicine approach for this patient population.

References

1. Singh I, Ma KC, Berlin DA. Pathophysiology of pulmonary hypertension in chronic parenchymal lung disease. Am J Med. 2016;129(4):366–71.
2. Adir Y, Humbert M, Chaouat A. Sleep-related breathing disorders and pulmonary hypertension. Eur Respir J. 2021;57(1).
3. Nathan SD, Shlobin OA, Barnett SD, Saggar R, Belperio JA, Ross DJ, Ahmad S, Saggar R, Libre E, Lynch JP 3rd, Zisman DA. Right ventricular systolic pressure by echocardiography as a predictor of pulmonary hypertension in idiopathic pulmonary fibrosis. Respir Med. 2008;102(9):1305–10.

4. Arcasoy SM, Christie JD, Ferrari VA, Sutton MS, Zisman DA, Blumenthal NP, Pochettino A, Kotloff RM. Echocardiographic assessment of pulmonary hypertension in patients with advanced lung disease. Am J Respir Crit Care Med. 2003;167(5):735–40.
5. Keir GJ, Wort SJ, Kokosi M, George PM, Walsh SLF, Jacob J, Price L, Bax S, Renzoni EA, Maher TM, MacDonald P, Hansell DM, Wells AU. Pulmonary hypertension in interstitial lung disease: limitations of echocardiography compared to cardiac catheterization. Respirology. 2018;23(7):687–94.
6. Nathan SD, Barbera JA, Gaine SP, Harari S, Martinez FJ, Olschewski H, Olsson KM, Peacock AJ, Pepke-Zaba J, Provencher S, Weissmann N, Seeger W. Pulmonary hypertension in chronic lung disease and hypoxia. Eur Respir J. 2019;53(1).
7. Hoeper MM, Humbert M, Souza R, Idrees M, Kawut SM, Sliwa-Hahnle K, Jing ZC, Gibbs JS. A global view of pulmonary hypertension. Lancet Respir Med. 2016;4(4):306–22.
8. Humbert M, Kovacs G, Hoeper MM, Badagliacca R, Berger RMF, Brida M, Carlsen J, Coats AJS, Escribano-Subias P, Ferrari P, Ferreira DS, Ghofrani HA, Giannakoulas G, Kiely DG, Mayer E, Meszaros G, Nagavci B, Olsson KM, Pepke-Zaba J, Quint JK, Radegran G, Simonneau G, Sitbon O, Tonia T, Toshner M, Vachiery JL, Vonk Noordegraaf A, Delcroix M, Rosenkranz S, Group EESD. 2022 ESC/ERS Guidelines for the diagnosis and treatment of pulmonary hypertension. Eur Respir J. 2022.
9. Nunes H, Humbert M, Capron F, Brauner M, Sitbon O, Battesti JP, Simonneau G, Valeyre D. Pulmonary hypertension associated with sarcoidosis: mechanisms, haemodynamics and prognosis. Thorax. 2006;61(1):68–74.
10. Piccari L, Wort SJ, Meloni F, Rizzo M, Price LC, Martino L, Salvaterra E, Scelsi L, Lopez Meseguer M, Blanco I, Callari A, Perez Gonzalez V, Tuzzolino F, McCabe C, Rodriguez Chiaradia DA, Vitulo P, Investigators RR. The effect of borderline pulmonary hypertension on survival in chronic lung disease. Respiration. 2022;101(8):717–27.
11. Shorr AF, Wainright JL, Cors CS, Lettieri CJ, Nathan SD. Pulmonary hypertension in patients with pulmonary fibrosis awaiting lung transplant. Eur Respir J. 2007;30(4):715–21.
12. Hemnes AR, Leopold JA, Radeva MK, Beck GJ, Abidov A, Aldred MA, Barnard J, Rosenzweig EB, Borlaug BA, Chung WK, Comhair SAA, Desai AA, Dubrock HM, Erzurum SC, Finet JE, Frantz RP, Garcia JGN, Geraci MW, Gray MP, Grunig G, Hassoun PM, Highland KB, Hill NS, Hu B, Kwon DH, Jacob MS, Jellis CL, Larive AB, Lempel JK, Maron BA, Mathai SC, McCarthy K, Mehra R, Nawabit R, Newman JH, Olman MA, Park MM, Ramos JA, Renapurkar RD, Rischard FP, Sherer SG, Tang WHW, Thomas JD, Vanderpool RR, Waxman AB, Wilcox JD, Yuan JX, Horn EM, Group PS. Clinical characteristics and transplant-free survival across the spectrum of pulmonary vascular disease. J Am Coll Cardiol. 2022;80(7):697–718.
13. Vonk-Noordegraaf A, Haddad F, Chin KM, Forfia PR, Kawut SM, Lumens J, Naeije R, Newman J, Oudiz RJ, Provencher S, Torbicki A, Voelkel NF, Hassoun PM. Right heart adaptation to pulmonary arterial hypertension: physiology and pathobiology. J Am Coll Cardiol. 2013;62(25 Suppl):D22–33.
14. Tello K, Dalmer A, Axmann J, Vanderpool R, Ghofrani HA, Naeije R, Roller F, Seeger W, Sommer N, Wilhelm J, Gall H, Richter MJ. Reserve of right ventricular-arterial coupling in the setting of chronic overload. Circ Heart Fail. 2019;12(1):e005512.
15. Tarras E, Khosla A, Heerdt PM, Singh I. Right heart failure in the intensive care unit: etiology, pathogenesis, diagnosis, and treatment. J Intensive Care Med. 2023:8850666231216889.
16. Brener MI, Masoumi A, Ng VG, Tello K, Bastos MB, Cornwell WK 3rd, Hsu S, Tedford RJ, Lurz P, Rommel KP, Kresoja KP, Nagueh SF, Kanwar MK, Kapur NK, Hiremath G, Sarraf M, Van Den Enden AJM, Van Mieghem NM, Heerdt PM, Hahn RT, Kodali SK, Sayer GT, Uriel N, Burkhoff D. Invasive right ventricular pressure-volume analysis: basic principles, clinical applications, and practical recommendations. Circ Heart Fail. 2022;15(1):e009101.
17. Heerdt PM, Kheyfets V, Charania S, Elassal A, Singh I. A pressure-based single beat method for estimation of right ventricular ejection fraction: proof of concept. Eur Respir J. 2020;55(3).
18. Trip P, Kind T, van de Veerdonk MC, Marcus JT, de Man FS, Westerhof N, Vonk-Noordegraaf A. Accurate assessment of load-independent right ventricular systolic function in patients with pulmonary hypertension. J Heart Lung Transplant. 2013;32(1):50–5.

19. Inuzuka R, Hsu S, Tedford RJ, Senzaki H. Single-beat estimation of right ventricular contractility and its coupling to pulmonary arterial load in patients with pulmonary hypertension. J Am Heart Assoc. 2018;7(10).
20. Singh I, Oakland H, Elassal A, Heerdt PM. Defining end-systolic pressure for single-beat estimation of right ventricle-pulmonary artery coupling: simple... but not really. ERJ Open Res. 2021;7(3).
21. Tello K, Richter MJ, Axmann J, Buhmann M, Seeger W, Naeije R, Ghofrani HA, Gall H. More on single-beat estimation of right ventriculo-arterial coupling in pulmonary arterial hypertension. Am J Respir Crit Care Med. 2018.
22. Heerdt PM, Martin-Flores M, Oakland HT, Joseph P, Singh I. Integrating right ventricular pressure waveform analysis with two-point volume measurement for quantification of systolic and diastolic function: experimental validation and clinical application. J Cardiothorac Vasc Anesth. 2023.
23. Tello K, Wan J, Dalmer A, Vanderpool R, Ghofrani HA, Naeije R, Roller F, Mohajerani E, Seeger W, Herberg U, Sommer N, Gall H, Richter MJ. Validation of the tricuspid annular plane systolic excursion/systolic pulmonary artery pressure ratio for the assessment of right ventricular-arterial coupling in severe pulmonary hypertension. Circ Cardiovasc Imaging. 2019;12(9):e009047.
24. Richter MJ, Peters D, Ghofrani HA, Naeije R, Roller F, Sommer N, Gall H, Grimminger F, Seeger W, Tello K. Evaluation and prognostic relevance of right ventricular-arterial coupling in pulmonary hypertension. Am J Respir Crit Care Med. 2019.
25. Ghio S, Fortuni F, Greco A, Turco A, Lombardi C, Scelsi L, Raineri C, Matrone B, Vullo E, Guida S, Badagliacca R, Oltrona Visconti L. Dobutamine stress echocardiography in pulmonary arterial hypertension. Int J Cardiol. 2018;270:331–5.
26. Fisher MR, Criner GJ, Fishman AP, Hassoun PM, Minai OA, Scharf SM, Fessler HE, Group NR. Estimating pulmonary artery pressures by echocardiography in patients with emphysema. Eur Respir J. 2007;30(5):914–21.
27. Galie N, Humbert M, Vachiery JL, Gibbs S, Lang I, Torbicki A, Simonneau G, Peacock A, Vonk Noordegraaf A, Beghetti M, Ghofrani A, Gomez Sanchez MA, Hansmann G, Klepetko W, Lancellotti P, Matucci M, McDonagh T, Pierard LA, Trindade PT, Zompatori M, Hoeper M, Group ESCSD. 2015 ESC/ERS Guidelines for the diagnosis and treatment of pulmonary hypertension: The Joint Task Force for the Diagnosis and Treatment of Pulmonary Hypertension of the European Society of Cardiology (ESC) and the European Respiratory Society (ERS): Endorsed by: Association for European Paediatric and Congenital Cardiology (AEPC), International Society for Heart and Lung Transplantation (ISHLT). Eur Heart J. 2016;37(1):67–119.
28. Li Y, Guo D, Gong J, Wang J, Huang Q, Yang S, Zhang X, Hu H, Jiang Z, Yang Y, Lu X. Right ventricular function and its coupling with pulmonary circulation in precapillary pulmonary hypertension: a three-dimensional echocardiographic study. Front Cardiovasc Med. 2021;8:690606.
29. Vanderpool RR, Pinsky MR, Naeije R, Deible C, Kosaraju V, Bunner C, Mathier MA, Lacomis J, Champion HC, Simon MA. RV-pulmonary arterial coupling predicts outcome in patients referred for pulmonary hypertension. Heart. 2015;101(1):37–43.
30. Brewis MJ, Bellofiore A, Vanderpool RR, Chesler NC, Johnson MK, Naeije R, Peacock AJ. Imaging right ventricular function to predict outcome in pulmonary arterial hypertension. Int J Cardiol. 2016;218:206–11.
31. Singh I, Rahaghi FN, Naeije R, Oliveira RKF, Vanderpool RR, Waxman AB, Systrom DM. Dynamic right ventricular-pulmonary arterial uncoupling during maximum incremental exercise in exercise pulmonary hypertension and pulmonary arterial hypertension. Pulm Circ. 2019;9(3):2045894019862435.
32. Hilde JM, Skjorten I, Hansteen V, Melsom MN, Hisdal J, Humerfelt S, Steine K. Haemodynamic responses to exercise in patients with COPD. Eur Respir J. 2013;41(5):1031–41.

33. Degani-Costa LH, Levarge B, Digumarthy SR, Eisman AS, Harris RS, Lewis GD. Pulmonary vascular response patterns during exercise in interstitial lung disease. Eur Respir J. 2015;46(3):738–49.
34. Oliveira RKF, Waxman AB, Hoover PJ, Dellaripa PF, Systrom DM. Pulmonary vascular and right ventricular burden during exercise in interstitial lung disease. Chest. 2020;158(1):350–8.
35. Armstrong HF, Thirapatarapong W, Dussault NE, Bartels MN. Distinguishing pulmonary hypertension in interstitial lung disease by ventilation and perfusion defects measured by cardiopulmonary exercise testing. Respiration. 2013;86(5):407–13.
36. Glaser S, Noga O, Koch B, Opitz CF, Schmidt B, Temmesfeld B, Dorr M, Ewert R, Schaper C. Impact of pulmonary hypertension on gas exchange and exercise capacity in patients with pulmonary fibrosis. Respir Med. 2009;103(2):317–24.
37. Joseph P, Savarimuthu S, Zhao J, Yan X, Oakland HT, Cullinan M, Heerdt PM, Singh I. Noninvasive determinants of pulmonary hypertension in interstitial lung disease. Pulm Circ. 2023;13(1):e12197.
38. Oakland HT, Joseph P, Elassal A, Cullinan M, Heerdt PM, Singh I. Diagnostic utility of submaximum cardiopulmonary exercise testing in the ambulatory setting for heart failure with preserved ejection fraction. Pulm Circ. 2020;10(4):2045894020972273.
39. Tedford RJ, Mudd JO, Girgis RE, Mathai SC, Zaiman AL, Housten-Harris T, Boyce D, Kelemen BW, Bacher AC, Shah AA, Hummers LK, Wigley FM, Russell SD, Saggar R, Saggar R, Maughan WL, Hassoun PM, Kass DA. Right ventricular dysfunction in systemic sclerosis-associated pulmonary arterial hypertension. Circ Heart Fail. 2013;6(5):953–63.
40. Hsu S, Houston BA, Tampakakis E, Bacher AC, Rhodes PS, Mathai SC, Damico RL, Kolb TM, Hummers LK, Shah AA, McMahan Z, Corona-Villalobos CP, Zimmerman SL, Wigley FM, Hassoun PM, Kass DA, Tedford RJ. Right ventricular functional reserve in pulmonary arterial hypertension. Circulation. 2016;133(24):2413–22.
41. Hsu S, Simpson CE, Houston BA, Wand A, Sato T, Kolb TM, Mathai SC, Kass DA, Hassoun PM, Damico RL, Tedford RJ. Multi-beat right ventricular-arterial coupling predicts clinical worsening in pulmonary arterial hypertension. J Am Heart Assoc. 2020;9(10):e016031.
42. Schmeisser A, Rauwolf T, Groscheck T, Fischbach K, Kropf S, Luani B, Tanev I, Hansen M, Meissler S, Schafer K, Steendijk P, Braun-Dullaeus RC. Predictors and prognosis of right ventricular function in pulmonary hypertension due to heart failure with reduced ejection fraction. ESC Heart Fail. 2021;8(4):2968–81.
43. Prins KW, Rose L, Archer SL, Pritzker M, Weir EK, Kazmirczak F, Misialek JR, Thenappan T. Disproportionate right ventricular dysfunction and poor survival in group 3 pulmonary hypertension. Am J Respir Crit Care Med. 2018;197(11):1496–9.
44. Visca D, Aiello M, Chetta A. Cardiovascular function in pulmonary emphysema. Biomed Res Int. 2013;2013:184678.
45. Fessler HE. Heart-lung interactions: applications in the critically ill. Eur Respir J. 1997;10(1):226–37.
46. Nathan SD, Tapson VF, Elwing J, Rischard F, Mehta J, Shapiro S, Shen E, Deng C, Smith P, Waxman A. Efficacy of inhaled treprostinil on multiple disease progression events in patients with pulmonary hypertension due to parenchymal lung disease in the INCREASE trial. Am J Respir Crit Care Med. 2022;205(2):198–207.
47. Waxman A, Restrepo-Jaramillo R, Thenappan T, Ravichandran A, Engel P, Bajwa A, Allen R, Feldman J, Argula R, Smith P, Rollins K, Deng C, Peterson L, Bell H, Tapson V, Nathan SD. Inhaled treprostinil in pulmonary hypertension due to interstitial lung disease. N Engl J Med. 2021;384(4):325–34.
48. Nathan SD, Waxman A, Rajagopal S, Case A, Johri S, DuBrock H, De La Zerda DJ, Sahay S, King C, Melendres-Groves L, Smith P, Shen E, Edwards LD, Nelsen A, Tapson VF. Inhaled treprostinil and forced vital capacity in patients with interstitial lung disease and associated pulmonary hypertension: a post-hoc analysis of the INCREASE study. Lancet Respir Med. 2021;9(11):1266–74.

Chapter 8
The Pathophysiology, Diagnosis, and Clinical Impact of Pulmonary Hypertension in Emphysema, COPD, and Smoking-Related Lung Disease

Lucilla Piccari, Aparna Balasubramanian, Karys Khilzi, Mona Lichtblau, and Diego A. Rodríguez Chiaradía

Pathophysiology of Pulmonary Hypertension in Chronic Obstructive Pulmonary Disease

Chronic obstructive pulmonary disease (COPD) is a highly prevalent and heterogenous disease, characterized by airflow obstruction and chronic respiratory symptoms [1]. While the presence of pulmonary vascular abnormalities and development

L. Piccari (✉) · K. Khilzi
Department of Pulmonology, Hospital del Mar, Barcelona, Spain

Hospital del Mar Research Institute, Barcelona, Spain
e-mail: lpiccari@researchmar.net; kkhilzi@psmar.cat

A. Balasubramanian
Division of Pulmonary and Critical Care Medicine, Department of Medicine, Johns Hopkins University School of Medicine, Baltimore, MD, USA
e-mail: abalasu2@jhmi.edu

M. Lichtblau
Department of Pulmonology, University Hospital Zürich, Zürich, Switzerland

University of Zürich, Zürich, Switzerland
e-mail: mona.lichtblau@usz.ch

D. A. Rodríguez Chiaradía
Department of Pulmonology, Hospital del Mar, Barcelona, Spain

Hospital del Mar Research Institute, Barcelona, Spain

Department of Medicine and Life Sciences (MELIS), Universitat Pompeu Fabra (UPF), Barcelona, Spain

Centro de Investigación en Red de Enfermedades Respiratorias (CIBERES), Instituto de Salud Carlos III (ISCIII), Madrid, Spain
e-mail: darodriguez@psmar.cat

F. N. Rahaghi et al. (eds.), *The Pulmonary Vasculature in Chronic Lung Disease*, Respiratory Medicine, https://doi.org/10.1007/978-3-032-03581-3_8

of pulmonary hypertension (PH) among individuals with COPD is well-known, the pathophysiology of COPD-PH is poorly understood and likely to be multifactorial. Understanding the pathophysiology of PH in COPD first requires defining the factors that may predispose individuals to also develop pulmonary hypertension.

Etiopathogenesis of Pulmonary Hypertension in COPD

Commonly cited etiopathogenesis mechanisms for COPD involve a susceptible host subjected to environmental toxin exposures. For example, there are numerous genetic loci thought to predispose individuals to an exaggerated lung response to cigarette smoking exposure. The same concept likely applies to the development of PH in COPD as well, with individuals carrying a genetic predisposition for abnormal vascular responses to environmental exposures that ultimately trigger pulmonary vascular injury. Genetic abnormalities in COPD with PH have been seldom studied, but there is some evidence related to genes regulating smooth muscle cell proliferation being associated with the presence [2] and severity [3] of PH in COPD patients, regardless of the severity of the airflow obstruction. Additionally, genetic analysis has evidenced how COPD patients with PH might share gene expression profiles with pulmonary arterial hypertension [4], where genetic abnormalities are well-known to be associated with disease. Among environmental exposures, the use of tobacco products is the most studied in the context of COPD and PH, with evidence of endothelial dysfunction [5] and apoptosis [6]. Beyond cigarette smoking, air pollution is directly linked to development, severity and exacerbation of COPD [7, 8], and the Global Initiative for Chronic Obstructive Lung Disease has recently issued a comprehensive report on its effect on COPD [8]. To date, there are no studies demonstrating the direct influence of air pollution on the development of PH in COPD, however if the prevalence and severity of COPD is increasing with air pollution, an increase in PH-COPD may reasonably be expected.

The etiopathogenesis of COPD-PH also raises the question of temporal associations between COPD and PH development: pulmonary vascular disease may precede or develop concurrently with lung parenchymal injury, versus mechanisms for PH development that may be pathophysiologic responses to the COPD disease manifestations. It is likely that both pathways occur across the heterogeneity of COPD-PH, and this remains an area of active research, focusing on phenotypes defined by hemodynamic patterns. The 6th World Symposium on Pulmonary Hypertension (6WSPH) notes that Group 3 disease, including COPD-PH, classically has a pre-capillary hemodynamic profile characterized by an elevated pulmonary vascular resistance (PVR) without elevation in pulmonary capillary wedge pressure (PCWP) [9]. However, in registry studies of COPD patients who undergo right heart catheterization [10–12], pre-capillary, isolated post-capillary, and combined pre- and post-capillary pulmonary hypertension have all been observed. The pathophysiologic mechanisms that lead to these various hemodynamic patterns can be viewed as mechanisms that increase pulmonary vascular resistance, or those that increase left atrial pressure.

Pathophysiology of Increased Pulmonary Vascular Resistance in COPD

Hypoxia

The most commonly cited pathophysiologic mechanism for pulmonary hypertension in lung disease is hypoxia. Alveolar hypoxia is known to precipitate hypoxic vasoconstriction leading to increases in pulmonary vascular resistance. Further, hypoxia is thought to induce vascular remodeling, with intimal thickening and smooth muscle cell proliferation of small pulmonary arterioles, as has been demonstrated in animal models and among individuals at high altitude who develop hypoxia-related pulmonary hypertension [13]. Chronic hypoxia is also associated with polycythemia, and with resultant increases in blood viscosity has been theorized as contributing to increased pulmonary vascular resistance.

Although widely accepted as a driver of pulmonary hypertension in COPD, hypoxia may not be the primary pathophysiologic mechanism for developing COPD-PH. Studies of COPD have noted development of pulmonary hypertension without evidence of hypoxia [14]. In severe PH associated with COPD, there is evidence for more prominent pulmonary vascular remodeling, with hypoxic pulmonary vasoconstriction potentially being less prominent; in this context, reduced cardiac output may also be implicated in the very profound hypoxemia observed in these patients [15]. Additionally, partial pressures of arterial oxygen have not been found to be associated with pulmonary pressures [16, 17]. The response of oxygen administration on pulmonary pressures has been variable [18], and associations between polycythemia and pulmonary hemodynamics are similarly inconsistent [19, 20]. Thus, these findings suggest that while hypoxia is a contributor to pulmonary vasoconstriction and vascular remodeling, it is unlikely to be a sufficient pathophysiologic explanation to fully explain the development of PH in COPD.

Hyperinflation

Gas-trapping, related to airflow obstruction in small to medium airways, and associated hyperinflation has been postulated to be associated with increases in pulmonary vascular resistance related to direct compression of the pulmonary vasculature and larger swings in intrathoracic pressures during the respiratory cycle [16, 21, 22]. There is limited evidence supporting this pathophysiologic mechanism, with some studies noting no association between residual lung volumes and pulmonary pressures [12, 22], while other small studies suggesting improvement in pulmonary pressures with bronchoscopic or surgical lung volume reduction [23, 24]. In acute settings of exacerbations, hyperventilation, or exercise, dynamic hyperinflation has been associated with an increase in pulmonary pressures [25–27], suggesting hyperinflation may be a contributory factor to increases in pulmonary vascular resistance particularly when there is increased flow.

Pulmonary Vascular Disease

The pulmonary vasculature has been demonstrated to have significant remodeling in cigarette smokers with and without COPD. Notably, intimal thickening, smooth muscle proliferation, and elastin and collagen deposition have been consistently observed across autopsy and explanted lung histopathologic studies [28–30]. Wall thickness has been associated with reduced distensibility in response to exercise, offering an explanation for how vascular remodeling may precipitate increased pulmonary vascular resistance [31]. While many studies have noted these structural alterations in the pulmonary vasculature, there are inconsistent associations with pulmonary pressures [32–34]. The prevailing hypothesis is that early vascular alterations in response to cigarette smoking may not have a sustained impact on distensibility responses to increased flow, but prolonged injury can eventually alter vessel compliance increasing resistance to flow. This hypothesis has yet to be thoroughly assessed, but prolonged smoke exposure has shown changes in pulmonary artery compliance [33].

A trigger for vascular remodeling in response to cigarette smoking may be endothelial dysfunction. Endothelial dysfunction is a primary pathophysiologic mechanism in other forms of pulmonary hypertension, and it refers broadly to morphologic abnormalities and injury to the endothelium with alterations in mediator production or response to endothelial mediators such as endothelial nitric oxide, endothelin, and vascular endothelial growth factor [34]. Cigarette smoking has been observed in animal models to upregulate endothelin and vascular endothelial growth factor [35, 36], and chronic exposure altered gene expression of those mediators as well as endothelial nitric oxide synthase with effects persisting for months [37]. Supporting these findings, in humans with mild COPD, pulmonary arteries demonstrate impaired relaxation in response to nitric oxide-dependent vasodilators [14]. Further, immunohistochemical studies in populations of smokers with and without COPD have noted reductions in endothelial nitric oxide synthase, increased endothelin, and increased vascular endothelial growth factor [30, 35, 38, 39]. Together, these findings begin to illuminate pathways of the direct effects of cigarette smoking on endothelial dysfunction which may trigger vascular remodeling and hemodynamic abnormalities.

In addition to endothelial dysfunction as a stimulus for vascular remodeling, imbalances in protease and anti-protease activity have been posited to play a role. Serine elastases and metalloproteases have been associated with vascular remodeling in hypoxia or monocrotaline animal models of pulmonary hypertension [40–42], and are implicated in development and progression of emphysema [43, 44], but there is very limited data on the impact of proteases on vascular remodeling in individuals with COPD or in models of cigarette smoking. One study of cigarette smoke-exposed rats has demonstrated that administration of an elastase inhibitor decreases small vessel muscularization [45].

Finally, there may be genetic factors that predispose individuals to vascular remodeling and increased pulmonary pressures in COPD. Genetic polymorphisms in endothelial nitric oxide synthase and 5-hydroxytryptamine, a serotonin transporter associated with pulmonary vascular smooth muscle hyperplasia and vascular remodeling in hypoxic models and non-COPD pulmonary hypertension, have been associated with endothelial dysfunction, vascular remodeling, and pulmonary pressures in COPD [2, 46]. Additionally, interleukin-6 has been clinically associated with pulmonary pressures, and the interleukin-6 GG genotype has been associated with development of COPD-PH [47]. Further study of genetic predisposition to both COPD and COPD-PH is still needed, with promising inflammatory and endothelial targets identified thus far.

Other COPD-Specific Mechanisms

Emphysema, and associated destruction of the pulmonary vasculature, has been purported as a major pathophysiologic mechanism for COPD-PH, however, there is limited literature to support this hypothesis. Degree of radiographic emphysema has not been associated with pulmonary pressures in registry studies [16, 48], and preclinical studies of smoking exposure demonstrate increases in pulmonary arterial pressures preceding development of emphysema [49, 50]. However, peripheral vascular pruning by imaging has been observed in patients with severe emphysema and associated with mean pulmonary artery pressure (mPAP) [51]. Similarly, computed tomography vascular pruning has been observed in COPD patients with severe hemodynamics, suggesting that pulmonary vascular loss in the periphery of the lung may contribute to elevated pulmonary pressures [52]. However, studies in severe emphysematous patients of lung volume reduction surgery, where pulmonary vasculature is resected alongside distended airspaces thereby reducing available pulmonary vasculature even further, are conflicting and do not consistently demonstrate increases in subsequent pulmonary pressures [23, 53–55]. These paradoxical findings may be related to the contributions of the degree of resection across patients, the beneficial effect of relief of hyperinflation, or the presence of recruitable capillaries. However, together these findings suggest that destruction of the vasculature is not the only contributor to increases in pulmonary vascular resistance or the development of COPD-PH, though likely plays a role alongside other pathophysiologic mechanisms.

Early physiologic studies of hypercapnia in COPD demonstrated increases in cardiac output which led to increased pulmonary pressures, and some evidence of acidosis-mediated increases in pulmonary vascular resistance [56–58]. However, hypercapnia also recruits additional capillaries, which frequently will offset the vasoconstrictive effects on pulmonary hemodynamics. In the setting of emphysema, this balance is disrupted allowing for a greater impact of hypercapnia on pulmonary vascular resistance. In epidemiologic studies however, degree of hypercapnia has not been associated with pulmonary pressures.

COPD is also a known risk factor for the development of thromboembolic disease and increases the odds of chronic thromboembolic pulmonary hypertension after thromboembolism [59, 60]. Nearly a quarter of those diagnosed with chronic thromboembolic pulmonary hypertension also have concurrent COPD [60]. Increased pulmonary vascular resistance from chronic pulmonary thromboembolism is therefore also an important consideration in COPD.

In summary, increases in pulmonary vascular resistance in COPD are likely a combination of factors related to hypoxic vasoconstriction, hyperinflation, vascular remodeling related to inhalational exposures and/or genetics, vessel loss or pruning both within and outside the context of emphysema, hypercapnia, and/or thromboembolic disease. The relative contributions of each of these mechanisms likely define the observed phenotypes of COPD-PH.

Pathophysiology of Elevated Left Atrial Pressures in COPD

Elevated left atrial pressures in COPD may be related to a variety of cardiovascular system abnormalities, including LV systolic dysfunction, LV diastolic dysfunction, or valvular disease. Evidence of elevated wedge pressure is common in COPD-PH with 11–60% of patients having an elevated wedge pressure [10–12, 16]. Cigarette smoking is a common risk factor for both COPD as well as cardiovascular disease, being implicated in creating a state of low-level chronic inflammation and accelerated aging [61–63]. There is an estimated 50% increase in the risk of developing heart failure with smoking [64]. In studies of general COPD populations, prevalence of clinically diagnosed heart failure is approximately 20%, however this is likely to be an underestimate, in particular as the prevalence of diastolic dysfunction or heart failure with preserved ejection fraction is thought to be highly underappreciated in COPD patients [65, 66].

Systolic heart failure or heart failure with reduced ejection fraction is believed to primarily be related to coronary artery disease, with the frequency of ischemic adverse cardiovascular events associated with levels of inflammation and FEV_1, independent of other cardiovascular risk factors [67, 68]. Inflammation is also implicated in both systolic and diastolic heart failure independent of myocardial ischemia [69]. Further, emphysema and hyperinflation have been associated with impaired left ventricular filling and diastolic heart failure, and overall smaller cardiac chamber sizes have been observed in epidemiologic imaging studies of COPD [70, 71]. Thus, COPD and heart failure are closely linked with common underlying triggers and inflammatory pathways in both disease states, as well as additional direct effects of airflow obstruction and airspace destruction on cardiac filling, morphology, and function which can lead to increases in left atrial pressures.

Diagnosis of Pulmonary Hypertension in COPD

Diagnosis of PH in COPD, as in other forms of pulmonary hypertension, hinges on invasive hemodynamics. There are currently no agreed-upon criteria to select which individuals with COPD should undergo right heart catheterization or who should be considered as highly likely to have pulmonary hypertension. As such, both non-invasive and invasive assessment remains crucial in diagnosing COPD-related pulmonary hypertension and defining phenotypes of disease (Fig. 8.1).

Comprehensive Non-invasive Approach to Diagnosis of Pulmonary Hypertension in Patients with COPD

Clinical Features

Evaluating risk of pulmonary hypertension in a patient with COPD begins with thorough characterization of symptoms such as shortness of breath, fatigue, cough, and exercise intolerance. In particular, rapid trajectory for symptom progression without a justifiable cause and/or pronounced symptoms that do not seem to match the extent of airflow obstruction should raise suspicion for possible pulmonary hypertension [72]. On physical examination, some common findings like a loud second heart sound, pansystolic murmur, and right ventricular enlargement could suggest pulmonary hypertension; lower limb oedema, however, is nonspecific in COPD patients [73] due to an imbalance in the renin-angiotensin-aldosterone system and other incompletely understood pathophysiological mechanisms [74]. An important component of initial evaluation in COPD includes identifying signs and symptoms that suggest risk for either PAH or CTEPH, since the diagnostic and prognostic considerations for those diseases are different. These conditions also have a much clearer potential for treatment with pulmonary vasodilators or, in the case of CTEPH, with pulmonary endarterectomy or balloon pulmonary angioplasty [75]. Further, given the ubiquity of COPD and relative rarity of PAH or CTEPH, not assessing for these diseases may result in delays in diagnosis as symptoms are attributed to COPD.

Beyond history and physical examination, other non-invasive objective testing may inform the probability of diagnosing PH. For example, the electrocardiogram can be a useful tool to provide some information for the potential presence of pulmonary hypertension; rightward deviation of the axial axis or signs of right heart overload are suggestive of PH [76]. Increased levels of NT-pro BNP can also indicate the presence of pulmonary hypertension in patients with COPD. However, it is important to note that its elevation is not solely linked to pulmonary hypertension and should be assessed within the patient's clinical context [77].

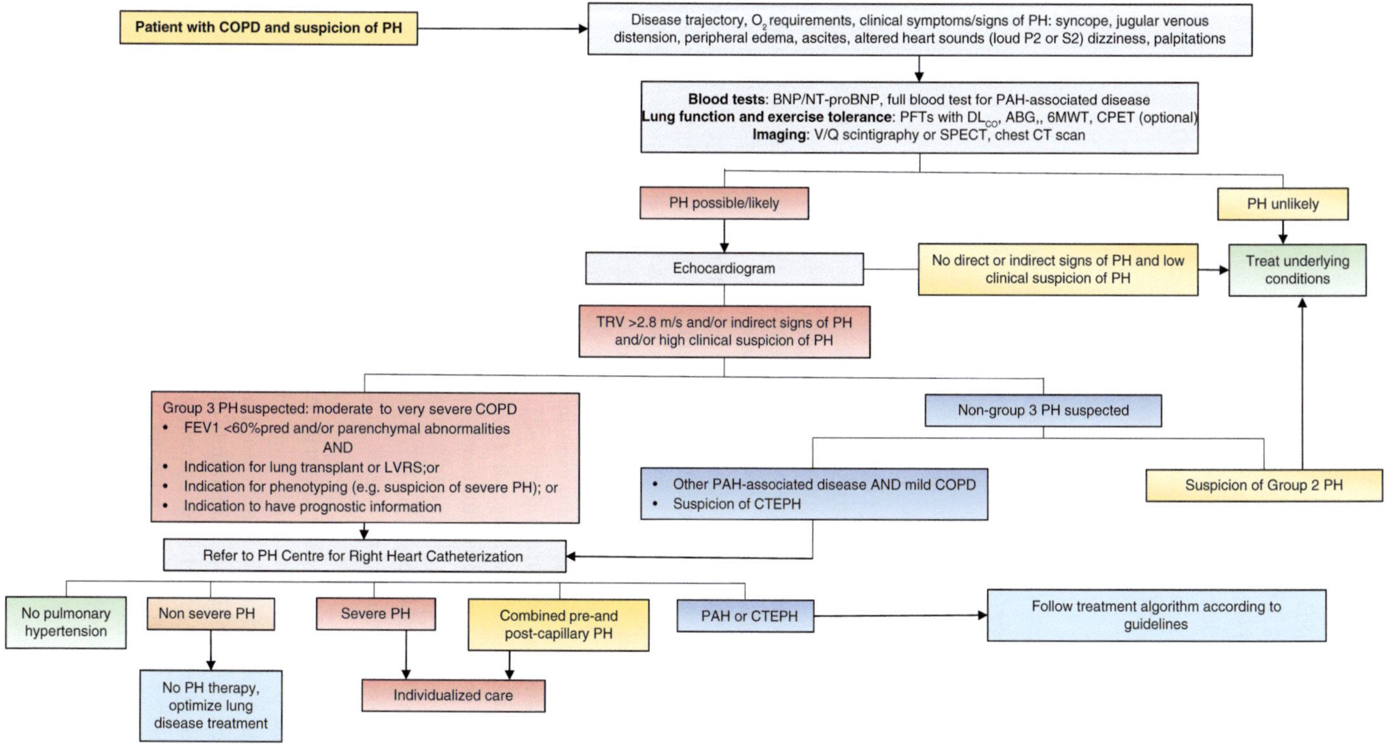

Fig. 8.1 Diagnostic algorithm in COPD-PH. Definition of abbreviations: *6MWT* 6-minute walking test, *ABG* arterial blood gas, *BNP* brain natriuretic peptide, *CPET* cardio-pulmonary exercise test, *CT* computer tomography, *CTEPH* chronic thromboembolic pulmonary hypertension, DL_{CO} diffusing capacity of the lung for carbon monoxide, FEV_1 forced expiratory volume in 1 s, *LVRS* lung volume reduction surgery, *NT-proBNP* N-terminal proB type natriuretic peptide, *PFTs* pulmonary function test, *PH* pulmonary hypertension, *V/Q* ventilation-perfusion lung scan, *SPECT* single-photon emission CT

Pulmonary Function

In general, patients with PH associated with COPD exhibit impaired gas exchange at rest or during exercise, and this impairment may manifest more severely than expected based on ventilatory impairments [78]. A clear deterioration in PaO_2 levels, sometimes also accompanied by a reduction in $PaCO_2$, in patients with no obvious progression of the underlying lung disease, warrants suspicion of PH.

Exercise Capacity

The presence of PH independently affects exercise tolerance in COPD [79]. The 6-minute walking test (6MWT) is an easy, standardized, and useful assessment to screen for PH in patients with COPD: in fact, low SaO_2 during the 6MWT has been found useful in predicting PH in COPD patients [80]. Furthermore, a recent meta-analysis found that in COPD patients the presence of PH was associated with lower peak oxygen consumption, workload, and oxygen pulse compared to COPD patients without PH during cardiopulmonary exercise test [81]. Further, a PaO_2 below 61 mmHg (8.1 kPa) during unloaded pedaling was observed to predict PH with a sensitivity of 86% and a specificity of 78% [82].

Echocardiogram

In the context of COPD, the echocardiogram remains the most commonly used non-invasive test for the evaluation of a patient who may have developed PH. The likelihood of PH by echocardiography (high, intermediate, or low) is determined by measuring the speed of the tricuspid regurgitant jet along with the presence of signs suggesting increased right ventricular size or dysfunction [75]. However, the accuracy of echocardiography in these patients may be markedly low, especially in those with severe emphysema [83]. There is evidence that in up to 50% of patients suspected of having PH associated with respiratory disease, tricuspid regurgitation cannot be measured and, if detected, its value is overestimated [84]. These findings may lead to misclassification of patients, which is particularly important for those who may have severe PH; for these reasons, other echocardiographic data can be useful in identifying these patients, such as the RA area, the RV/LV ratio, or the eccentricity index. A pilot study [85] suggested a role for exercise Doppler echocardiography in identifying exercise PH; however, its clinical utility remains uncertain due to the lack of validated criteria and prospective confirmatory data.

Imaging

Chest radiography may also suggest PH: cardiomegaly and features suggestive of right atrial enlargement may be observed in the context of COPD. Over the last two decades, there have been major advances in imaging techniques such as nuclear medicine, computed tomography (CT) scanning, and magnetic resonance imaging (MRI). There is growing evidence to support the value of imaging in screening for PH and in some cases these techniques may be extremely valuable to understand the pathophysiologic mechanisms involved. When the patient is clinically stable, a pulmonary artery diameter of 30 mm or greater, right ventricular outflow hypertrophy of 6 mm or more, a septal angle of 140° or higher, or a right ventricle to left ventricle ratio of 1 or higher on CT pulmonary angiography indicate the possible presence of pulmonary hypertension [86]; the combination between echocardiography with a contrast-enhanced CT may also aid diagnostic assessment and disease classification [87].

The application of techniques of artificial Intelligence is a growing field of research, as these techniques could improve the accuracy of CT imaging in predicting pulmonary hypertension. In this line, the evaluation of small vessels and the application of artificial intelligence may help to obtain more detailed phenotypes [52, 88]. Cardiac MRI could also assist in identifying patients with severe PH in the context of COPD [89]. The utility of these techniques still needs confirmation in large, prospective clinical trials.

The different non-invasive modalities of screening for PH in COPD may be more useful in combination to predict the likelihood of PH. One study identified the combination of systolic pulmonary artery pressure ≥56 mmHg measured at echocardiography, an NT-proBNP ≥650 pg/mL, and PA/Ao ratio ≥0.93 is able to predict severe PH with high sensitivity and specificity [78]; however, more research is needed to develop validated tools that can be applied to different phenotypes of PH in COPD and that can be used in clinical practice .

Approach to Right Heart Catheterization in Patients with COPD

As in any form of PH, right heart catheterization (RHC) is the gold standard procedure for confirming the diagnosis [75]. While in patients with COPD or smoking-related lung disease, this test is widely indicated before surgical treatment (lung transplantation or volume reduction surgery) or in case of suspected PAH or CTEPH, its performance is also very relevant when obtaining hemodynamic information and will aid in evaluating the patient's phenotype. However, shifting hemodynamic definitions of PH and lack of data on optimal timing to perform RHC in patients with lung disease make it difficult to compare accumulated evidence on phenotypes.

Hemodynamic Definition of PH and of PH Severity in Lung Disease

A majority of studies on the epidemiology of COPD-PH have used the ESC/ERS 2015 definition of PH, which included mPAP ≥25 mmHg, and which for lung diseases garnered a diagnosis of severe PH at mPAP ≥35 mmHg or cardiac index (CI) <2.5 L/min/m^2 (not explained by other causes) [90]. The 6WSPH [91] changed the diagnostic criteria of Group 3 PH to mPAP ≥21 mmHg with PAWP ≤15 mmHg (the criterion for elevated PVR >3 WU only being included in the proceedings relating to PAH) [9]. In 2022, the hemodynamic thresholds were again lowered by the ESC/ERS guidelines to mPAP >20 mmHg and PVR > 2 WU [75]. Thus, in the space of only 4 years, the definition of PH has changed multiple times, and this has made the results of observational studies and randomized-controlled trials a jigsaw puzzle of changing definitions.

Based on two recently published studies focusing on PH in lung disease, the ESC/ERS 2022 guideline also revised the definition of severe Group 3 PH, establishing for the first time in all groups of PH a cutoff point based on PVR, with severe hemodynamic involvement at PVR >5 WU [92, 93]. Both these studies included patients using the previous threshold for PH (mPAP ≥25 mmHg with PAWP ≤15 mmHg), excluded transplanted patients and both found that in this group a threshold of PVR >5 WU conferred worse survival (although in the study by Olsson et al. for ILD, the highest statistical significance was reached for a PVR >8 WU). A subsequent multicenter study [94] enrolling COPD and ILD patients with RHC data and excluding lung transplant recipients, stratified them using the definitions of the 6WSPH for PH in lung disease as: no PH (mPAP <21 mmHg), "borderline" PH (mPAP 21–24 with PVR >3 WU), mild-moderate PH (mPAP 25–35 mmHg) and severe PH (mPAP ≥35 mmHg or CI <2 L/min/m^2). This analysis found that while in COPD only severe PH was associated with worse survival, in ILD any degree of hemodynamic impairment, compared to patients without PH, conferred worse survival. Furthermore, it confirmed the significance of PVR >5 WU for COPD patients but not for ILD patients (possibly because it enrolled them according to a broader definition of PH). Thus, there is at least some indication that COPD might behave differently than ILD with regard to hemodynamic severity and prognosis. Confirming the importance of PH severity in COPD, another work using the 6WSPH definitions found that those with a combination of mild GOLD stage (1–2) and mild-moderate PH (mPAP 21–24 with PVR >3 WU or mPAP 25–35 mmHg) had the best prognosis, while those with more severe GOLD stage (3–4) and severe PH (mPAP ≥35 mmHg or CI <2 L/min/m^2) had the worst prognosis; the other two combinations of COPD and PH severity were grouped together and featured an intermediate mortality risk [78].

Hemodynamic assessment is also helpful in assessing whether patients have other factors that may contribute to increased pulmonary pressure. As previously mentioned, numerous patients with respiratory diseases have common risk factors for cardiovascular diseases [95], so it is not uncommon to detect a post-capillary component explaining the increase in pulmonary pressure in some cases. Indeed, the discovery of PH of cardiac origin (or Group 2 in the current classification) or combined PH introduces a new element of complexity, with implications for therapeutic management [75] and possibly a different prognosis [96] compared to patients with exclusively pre-capillary PH associated with COPD.

In contrast, there are situations in which RHC is not advisable: typically, in patients where the procedure's outcome will not change the therapeutic approach, patients with advanced disease and end-of-life situations, or in the setting of acute-on-chronic critical illness [75].

Several technical considerations should be taken into account to perform RHC in COPD patients [97]. The ideal scenario in which a patient should undergo RHC is always during a period of clinical stability and with optimized medical therapy, oxygen supplementation and no intervening acute infection because an exacerbation of the underlying disease might lead to an overestimation of pulmonary pressures [75]. Furthermore, pressure measurements should be obtained from the average value of several respiratory cycles, especially in the case of pulmonary artery wedge pressure, in contrast to the recommendation to measure pulmonary pressures at the end of expiration in case of suspected PAH or CTEPH. This is to minimize the effects of thoracic pressure during the respiratory cycle, especially in patients with air trapping and dynamic hyperinflation [97], where the end-expiration pressure in the airways may not be the lowest point of pressure. Unlike in other group of PH, vasodilator testing is not recommended in these patients, as there is no data on its meaning in clinical practice.

Phenotypes of COPD-PH

Just as there are numerous mechanisms for hemodynamic abnormalities in COPD, the pathophysiology of COPD-PH in any given patient is a combined effect encompassing airflow obstruction, lung parenchymal injury, pulmonary vascular alterations, and cardiovascular disease. Given the heterogeneity and multifactorial nature of each of these individual components in a COPD population, there is an observed wide range of manifestations and burden of disease. Epidemiologic studies from registries of individuals, often who have been referred clinically for RHC, have helped identify potential phenotypes of COPD-PH.

Most individuals with COPD-PH are found to have mild elevations in pulmonary arterial pressures. Furthermore, these individuals tend to have fairly slow progression of pulmonary pressures [98, 99], allowing time for the right ventricle to adequately compensate. As a result, often these individuals have preserved cardiac outputs and RV contractility measures on echocardiography or cardiac magnetic resonance imaging. Their airflow obstruction can range from mild to severe, but the prevalence of COPD-PH has been associated with lower FEV_1 values [12, 17, 48, 100].

By contrast, approximately 5–20% of individuals are observed to have severe elevations in pulmonary pressures [22, 48, 101]. The presence of severe pulmonary hypertension may be related to severe airflow obstruction and emphysematous destruction, which is considered a pathophysiologic progression of severe COPD into severe PH. Additionally, severe hemodynamics can be observed alongside severe left ventricular dysfunction and elevations in left atrial pressures, chronic thromboembolic disease, or pulmonary vasculopathy. Individuals who tend to have severe pre-capillary hemodynamics with mild to moderate lung parenchymal injury have been deemed a "pulmonary vascular phenotype" and are noted to have significantly worse prognosis than those with mild-moderate PH in multiple different registry studies [48, 101, 102]. However, in one registry study, patients with severe PH and severe COPD presented the worst prognosis of all the combinations of airflow obstruction and hemodynamic severity [78].

Finally, there has been evidence of abnormal pulmonary pressures in specific settings for COPD patients. Hemodynamic responses to exercise in COPD have noted significant elevations in pulmonary pressures regardless of whether or not individuals have resting pulmonary hypertension [103], suggesting that morbidity in the form of exercise limitation may be related to circulatory limitations from pulmonary pressures during exertion. During sleep, nocturnal hypoxemia increases pulmonary pressures and these increases are mitigated by oxygen administration, but there is conflicting evidence over whether nocturnal desaturation alone is sufficient for resting pulmonary hypertension while awake [29, 104, 105]. Finally, during acute exacerbations of COPD, where hypoxia, hypercapnia, potential dynamic hyperinflation, LV dysfunction, and volume overload may all be present, patients with increased pulmonary artery diameters on chest imaging, and those with elevations in serum biomarkers of heart failure, even in the absence of left ventricular disease, have worse prognosis [106, 107]. There are numerous manifestations and phenotypes defined by the various pathophysiologic mechanisms for COPD-PH and encompassing various hemodynamic profiles.

Clinical Impact of Pulmonary Hypertension in COPD

Prevalence

The current global prevalence of COPD is estimated to be around 10.3% (GOLD Report 2023), with projections indicating a further increase in the coming decades. In the context of COPD, the prevalence of PH has been reported at 39% based on a comprehensive meta-analysis including 38 studies with a total of 16,345 patients with COPD from 16 different countries [100]. However, it is important to note that there is considerable variability in estimated prevalence due to a lack of consistency and standardization in definitions, diagnostic modalities, and studied populations (Table 8.1). The studies pooled in the meta-analysis used different definitions of PH and of severe PH, which as previously explained varied in the years from guideline to guideline. Furthermore, 61% (23/38) of the studies included in the meta-analysis used data from articles estimating prevalence of PH through echocardiography,

Table 8.1 Prevalence of pulmonary hypertension in COPD

1st Author	Year	Country	N	PH criteria	Population	FEV_1 in PH group, % mean (SD)	mPAP in PH group, mmHg mean (SD)	Prevalence	Study design
Andersen et al. [142]	2012	Denmark	409	mPAP ≥25 mmHg PCP ≤15 mmHg	Pre-transplant	22 (6)	29 (5)	36% (+13% post-capillary PH)	Retrospective
Cuttica et al. [143]	2010	USA	4930	mPAP ≥25 mmHg PCP ≤15 mmHg	Pre-transplant	22 (10)	–	30% (+17% post-capillary PH)	Retrospective
Thabut et al. [144]	2005	France	215	mPAP ≥25 mmHg PCP ≤15 mmHg	Pre-transplant LVRS	29 (7)	32 (7)	50%	Retrospective
Hilde et al. [145]	2013	Norway	98	mPAP ≥25 mmHg PCP ≤15 mmHg	Outpatient clinic	32 (12)	29 (4)	27%	Prospective
Portillo et al. [146]	2015	Spain	139	mPAP ≥25 mmHg PCP ≤15 mmHg	–	–	–	18%	Retrospective
Nathan et al. [147]	2021	USA	6572	mPAP >20 mmHg PVR >3 WU PCP <15 mmHg	Pre-transplant			28% (+18% post-capillary PH)	Retrospective
Zhang et al. [148]	2022	Various	16345	Including both echocardiography and right heart catheterization studies	Meta-analysis	–	–	39%	Retrospective

FEV1 forced expiratory volume in 1 second, *LVRS* lung volume reduction surgery, *mPAP* mean pulmonary artery pressure, *PCP* pulmonary capillary pressure, *PH* pulmonary hypertension, *PVR* pulmonary vascular resistance, *SD* standard deviation

which is only considered a detection tool and not a diagnostic tool in COPD, due to the many pitfalls it entails especially in patients with significant emphysema [83].

Estimates of the prevalence of PH associated with COPD have exhibited a wide range, spanning from 11% [108] to exceeding 80% [109]. Notably, among individuals with COPD listed for lung transplantation, a substantial 80% have been documented to exhibit pulmonary hypertension as confirmed by RHC. This wide variability is at least somewhat related to severity of airflow obstruction [110], although mPAP elevation does not correlate with the severity of emphysema [111]. Additionally, hemodynamic severity and varying COPD-PH phenotypes display varying prevalence; in fact, in the meta-analysis by Zhang mild PH was found in the majority of cases (30.2%) whereas severe PH was only reported in 7.2% [100]. Other studies report even lower numbers for severe PH in COPD with 1–5% of the cases [101, 110, 112].

Increased awareness and improved diagnostic techniques have led to more frequent diagnosis of PH in COPD and independent of the limitations mentioned above, the global burden of PH in COPD is likely substantial and still increasing due to increasing prevalence of COPD [113].

Morbidity and Mortality

Survival for PH secondary to lung disease is worse when compared to the other forms of PH [48, 114, 115]. Especially in light of the new treatment era where vast improvements for patients with PAH and CTEPH have been achieved, the survival for PH secondary to lung disease has not improved significantly in the last 10 years [115]. Several studies have illuminated the correlation between severity of PH in COPD and mortality. An mPAP of $\geq$40 mmHg [77], or mPAP $\geq$35 mmHg and/or cardiac index < 2 l/min/m^2 [94], and recently a PVR >5 WU [92] have been identified as relevant cut-offs for prognostication.

Morbidity can be highly determined by co-morbidities and especially in patients with COPD the risk of cardiovascular co-morbidities is important. The risk of ischemic heart disease, arrhythmias, chronic heart failure, pulmonary vascular diseases, and diseases of the peripheral arteries is increased two to five-fold in COPD patients compared to those without COPD. Additionally, hypertension, diabetes, and smoking were reported more often in patients with COPD, thus increasing their cardiovascular risk profile [95]. Therefore, suspicion of post-capillary PH should be high in COPD patients and the workup of PH should include careful assessment of cardiovascular diseases; furthermore, preventive strategies for cardiovascular risk factors such as cholesterol and hypertension should be part of medical care of COPD patients with PH.

Quality of Life and Exercise Capacity

COPD patients with PH perform poorer compared to COPD patients without PH during maximal as well as endurance exercise tests (incremental exercise testing, constant workload endurance time, 6MWT) [79]. Even without manifest PH at rest, patients with COPD that develop PH with exercise have a reduced peak oxygen uptake and 6-minute walk distance when compared to matched controls [116].

A correlation between severity of the pulmonary pressure in COPD-PH and St. George's Respiratory Questionnaire has been described by several groups [117]. Interestingly, PH-targeted therapy does not seem to improve the symptomatic burden, dyspnea, or quality of life (as measured by the St. George's Questionnaire) when compared to placebo or standard of care [118].

Altitude Travel

Non-hypercapnic patients with moderate to severe COPD living at low altitude (lowlanders) experience dyspnea, exercise limitation, and sleep disturbances when traveling to moderate to high altitude. Hypoxic pulmonary vasoconstriction causes a rise in pulmonary artery pressure. Patients might become severely hypoxemic, even at moderate altitudes (2500–3000 m). While hypoxemia may be asymptomatic but poses an increased risk for systemic and pulmonary hypertension, cardiac arrhythmias, myocardial infarction, and cerebral ischemia [119]. Randomized, placebo-controlled trials have shown that preventive treatment with acetazolamide reduces the risk of altitude-related health effects, such as severe hypoxemia or acute mountain sickness, and lowers the altitude-induced increase in pulmonary pressure [120]. Preventive dexamethasone treatment improves oxygenation and altitude-induced excessive sleep apnea, and lowers systemic and pulmonary artery pressure [121, 122].

Therapy

Effective treatment of COPD-PH is still not available, so standard of care is mainly focused on treating the underlying lung disease. There have been several trials including oxygen therapy and targeted PH-therapy with moderate success, and which will be discussed in more detail below (Table 8.2).

While pulmonary vasodilator therapy might improve pulmonary hemodynamics, no clear efficacy was found for clinically relevant outcomes such as exercise capacity or quality of life in the treatment of cohorts of COPD patients with PH of any severity. Indeed, many trials have not considered the severity of the PH or airway disease as inclusion/exclusion criteria and therefore the results are uncertain. Retrospective studies have shown longer survival in patients with respiratory diseases and severe PH treated with PH therapy, mostly including PDE-5 inhibitors

Table 8.2 Randomised clinical trials with pulmonary vasodilators in COPD

1st Author	Year	n	Drug	Design	Follow-up	PH status	Main endpoint	Results
Stolz D	2008	30	Bosentan	RCT	12 weeks	No	6MWD	NS
Rao RV	2011	33	Sildenafil	RCT	12 weeks	TTE with sPAP >40 mmHg	6MWD	Positive
Lederer DJ	2012	10	Sildenafil	RCT	4 weeks	PH patients excluded	6MWD VO2 max	Negative
Blanco I	2013	60	Sildenafil + respiratory rehabilitation	RCT	3 months	RHC or TTE with TRV >2.7 m/s	Endurance time	NS
Goudie AR	2014	120	Tadalafil	RCT	12 weeks	TTE with PAT <120 m/s o RVSP >30 mmHg	6MWD	NS
Vitulo P	2017	28	Sildenafil	RCT	16 weeks	RHC	PVR, BODE DL_{CO}, QoL	Positive

6MWD 6-minute walking distance, *BODE* body mass index, airflow obstruction, dyspnea, and exercise capacity score, *DL_{CO}* carbon monoxide diffusion capacity, *n* number of patients enrolled in the study, *NS* not significant, *PAT* pulmonary acceleration time, *PH* pulmonary hypertension, *PVR* pulmonary vascular resistance, *QoL* quality of life, *RCT* randomised-controlled trial, *RHC* right heart catheterization, *RVSP* right ventricle systolic pressure, *sPAP* systolic pulmonary artery pressure, *TRV* tricuspid regurgitation velocity, *TTE* trans-thoracic echocardiography, *VO_2* max peak oxygen consumption

[123, 124]. Furthermore, a double-blind, randomized controlled trial focusing on patients with significant pulmonary vasculopathy (mPAP ≥35 mmHg if FEV_1 <30% and mPAP ≥30 mmHg if FEV_1 > 30%) in which sildenafil was compared to placebo during 16 weeks found that patients on sildenafil not only presented with improved hemodynamics (PVR and CI) but also had improved DL_{CO}, BODE index (body mass index, airflow obstruction, dyspnea, and exercise) and quality of life (according to the Short Form Health Survey 36 Questionnaire) [125]. Thus, COPD patients with severe PH, especially those with the so-called "pulmonary vascular phenotype" might benefit from pulmonary vasodilator therapy, although larger studies are needed to confirm these results.

Oxygen Therapy

Decades ago, the famous studies "Medical Research Council Trial" [99] and "Nocturnal Oxygen Therapy Trial" [126] showed that long-term oxygen therapy (15 h/day) prevented the progression of mPAP increase in patients with COPD-PH and severe hypoxemia. Studies with longer duration of oxygen therapy (more than 18 h/day) showed a decrease of mPAP [98, 127, 128]. Acute oxygen application improves pulmonary hemodynamics [18] at the cost of increased VA/Q mismatch [129].

The above-mentioned trials are famous for their results on survival benefit of oxygen therapy which however does not translate into long-term effects on pulmonary hemodynamics [99, 126]. Furthermore, the positive results on survival have not been found in patients with moderate resting or exercise-induced desaturation [130].

Targeted PH Therapy

Multiple attempts have been made with PH targeted therapy in patients with COPD PH including several randomized controlled trials as well as meta-analyses [131–133]. While PH therapy, especially sildenafil [125] and bosentan [134], improved pulmonary hemodynamics in patients with COPD-PH in some small studies, others failed to show any effect of sildenafil on RV stroke volume at rest and during exercise measured with MRI [135]. Results on exercise capacity in patients with COPD-PH treated with targeted PH therapy are inconclusive: while two meta-analyses did not show improvement in 6MWD [132, 133], another showed the contrary but only included two RCTs [131]. The effect of a pulmonary rehabilitation program can furthermore not be improved by adding sildenafil in COPD patients with moderate PH [136]. Neither can PH-targeted therapy in COPD-PH improve patient-relevant outcomes such as dyspnea or quality of life compared to usual standard of care [131, 133, 134, 136, 137], except for evidence of sildenafil effect in severe PH [125].

Hypoxic pulmonary vasoconstriction is not the sole driver for COPD with severe PH [15]. This theory reflects results from long-term effects of targeted PH-therapy in COPD-PH where deterioration of gas exchange was shown in some studies [138, 139] and others found no significant or only moderate deterioration [125, 136, 137, 140, 141].

Only retrospective studies have assessed survival in COPD-PH, where it was shown that mostly patients with COPD associated with severe PH survive longer when treated with targeted PH-therapy (mostly PDE-5 inhibitors) [123, 124].

References

1. Agustí A, Celli BR, Criner GJ, Halpin D, Anzueto A, Barnes P, et al. Global initiative for chronic obstructive lung disease 2023 report: GOLD executive summary. Eur Resp J [Internet]. 2023 [cited 2023 Aug 22];61(4). Available from: https://erj.ersjournals.com/content/61/4/2300239.
2. Eddahibi S, Chaouat A, Morrell N, Fadel E, Fuhrman C, Bugnet AS, et al. Polymorphism of the serotonin transporter gene and pulmonary hypertension in chronic obstructive pulmonary disease. Circulation. 2003;108(15):1839–44.
3. Ulrich S, Hersberger M, Fischler M, Nussbaumer-Ochsner Y, Treder U, Russi EW, et al. Genetic polymorphisms of the serotonin transporter, but not the 2a receptor or nitric oxide synthetase, are associated with pulmonary hypertension in chronic obstructive pulmonary disease. Respiration. 2010;79(4):288–95.
4. Neubert L, Borchert P, Stark H, Hoefer A, Vogel-claussen J, Warnecke G, et al. Molecular profiling of vascular remodeling in chronic pulmonary disease. Am J Pathol. 2020;190(7):1382–96.
5. Gordon C, Gudi K, Krause A, Sackrowitz R, Harvey BG, Strulovici-Barel Y, et al. Circulating endothelial microparticles as a measure of early lung destruction in cigarette smokers. Am J Respir Crit Care Med. 2011;184(2):224–32.
6. Song Q, Chen P, Liu XM. The role of cigarette smoke-induced pulmonary vascular endothelial cell apoptosis in COPD. Respir Res. 2021;22(1):39.
7. Doiron D, de Hoogh K, Probst-Hensch N, Fortier I, Cai Y, de Matteis S, et al. Air pollution, lung function and COPD: results from the population-based UK Biobank study. Eur Respir J. 2019;54(1):1802140.
8. Sin DD, Doiron D, Agusti A, Anzueto A, Barnes PJ, Celli BR, et al. Air pollution and COPD: GOLD 2023 committee report. Eur Resp J [Internet]. 2023 [cited 2024 Jan 21];61(5). Available from: https://erj.ersjournals.com/content/61/5/2202469.
9. Simonneau G, Montani D, Celermajer DS, Denton CP, Gatzoulis MA, Krowka M, et al. Haemodynamic definitions and updated clinical classification of pulmonary hypertension. Eur Respir J. 2019;53(1):1801913.
10. Cook DP, Xu M, Martucci VL, Annis JS, Aldrich MC, Hemnes AR, et al. Clinical insights into pulmonary hypertension in chronic obstructive pulmonary disease. Pulm Circ. 2022;12(1):e12006.
11. Cuttica MJ, Kalhan R, Shlobin OA, Ahmad S, Gladwin M, MacHado RF, et al. Categorization and impact of pulmonary hypertension in patients with advanced COPD. Respir Med. 2010;104(12):1877–82.
12. Minai OA, Fessler H, Stoller JK, Criner GJ, Scharf SM, Meli Y, et al. Clinical characteristics and prediction of pulmonary hypertension in severe emphysema. Respir Med. 2014;108(3):482–90.

13. Stenmark KR, Fagan KA, Frid MG. Hypoxia-induced pulmonary vascular remodeling. Circ Res. 2006;99(7):675–91.
14. Peinado VI, Barberà JA, Ramirez J, Gomez FP, Roca J, Jover L, et al. Endothelial dysfunction in pulmonary arteries of patients with mild COPD. Am J Phys. 1998;274(6):L908–13.
15. Piccari L, Blanco I, Torralba Y, Arismendi E, Gistau C, Ramírez A, et al. Mechanisms of hypoxaemia in severe pulmonary hypertension associated with COPD. Eur Respir J. 2023;62(1):2300463.
16. Scharf SM, Iqbal M, Keller C, Criner G, Lee S, Fessler HE. Hemodynamic characterization of patients with severe emphysema. Am J Resp Critical Care Med. 2002.
17. Bishop JM, Cross KW. Use of the physiological variables to predict pulmonary arterial pressure in patients with chronic respiratory disease: multicentre study. Eur Heart J. 1981;2(6):509–17.
18. Ashutosh K, Mead G, Dunsky M. Early effects of oxygen administration and prognosis in chronic obstructive pulmonary disease and cor pulmonale. Am Rev Respir Dis. 1983;127(4):399–404.
19. Lee JH, Oh YM, Seo JB, Lee YK, Kim WJ, Sheen SS, et al. Pulmonary artery pressure in chronic obstructive pulmonary disease without resting hypoxaemia. Int J Tuberc Lung Dis. 2011;15(6):830–7.
20. Nakamura A, Kasamatsu N, Hashizume I, Shirai T, Hanzawa S, Momiki S, et al. Effects of hemoglobin on pulmonary arterial pressure and pulmonary vascular resistance in patients with chronic emphysema. Respiration. 2000;67(5):502–6.
21. Wright JL, Lawson L, Paré PD, Hooper RO, Peretz DI, Nelems JMB, et al. The structure and function of the pulmonary vasculature in mild chronic obstructive pulmonary disease. Am Rev Resp Dis [Internet]. 2015 [cited 2024 Jan 17]. Available from: https://www.atsjournals.org/doi/epdf/10.1164/arrd.1983.128.4.702?role=tab.
22. Thabut G, Dauriat G, Stern JB, Logeart D, Levy A, Marrash-Chahla R, et al. Pulmonary hemodynamics in advanced COPD candidates for lung volume reduction surgery or lung transplantation. Chest. 2005;127(5):1531–6.
23. Eberhardt R, Gerovasili V, Kontogianni K, Gompelmann D, Ehlken N, Herth FJF, et al. Endoscopic lung volume reduction with endobronchial valves in patients with severe emphysema and established pulmonary hypertension. Respiration. 2014;89(1):41–8.
24. Opitz I, Ulrich S. Pulmonary hypertension in chronic obstructive pulmonary disease and emphysema patients: prevalence, therapeutic options and pulmonary circulatory effects of lung volume reduction surgery. J Thoracic Dis [Internet]. 2018 [cited 2024 Jan 17];10(Suppl 23). Available from: https://jtd.amegroups.org/article/view/23102.
25. Butler J, Schrijen F, Henriquez A, Polu JM, Albert RK. Cause of the raised wedge pressure on exercise in chronic obstructive pulmonary disease. Am Rev Respir Dis. 1988;138(2):350–4.
26. Schrijen FV, Henriquez A, Carton D, Delorme N, Butler J. Pulmonary vascular resistance rises with lung volume on exercise in obstructed airflow disease. Clin Physiol. 1989;9(2):143–50.
27. Akcay M, Yeter E, Durmaz T, Keles T, Akar Bayram N, Uyar M, et al. Treatment of acute chronic obstructive pulmonary disease exacerbation improves right ventricle function. Eur J Echocardiogr. 2010;11(6):530–6.
28. Bunel V, Guyard A, Dauriat G, Danel C, Montani D, Gauvain C, et al. Pulmonary arterial histologic lesions in patients with COPD with severe pulmonary hypertension. Chest. 2019;156(1):33–44.
29. Wright JL, Petty T, Thurlbeck WM. Analysis of the structure of the muscular pulmonary arteries in patients with pulmonary hypertension and COPD: National Institutes of Health Nocturnal Oxygen Therapy Trial. Lung. 1992;170(2):109–24.
30. Barberà JA, Peinado VI, Santos S. Pulmonary hypertension in chronic obstructive pulmonary disease. Eur Respir J. 2003;21(5):892–905.
31. Kubo K, Ge RL, Koizumi T, Fujimoto K, Yamanda T, Haniuda M, et al. Pulmonary artery remodeling modifies pulmonary hypertension during exercise in severe emphysema. Respir Physiol. 2000;120(1):71–9.

32. Wilkinson M, Langhorne CA, Heath D, Barer GR, Howard P. A pathophysiological study of 10 cases of hypoxic cor pulmonale. Q J Med. 1988;66(249):65–85.
33. Liu SQ, Fung YC. Changes in the structure and mechanical properties of pulmonary arteries of rats exposed to cigarette smoke. Am Rev Resp Dis [Internet]. 2012 [cited 2024 Jan 17]. Available from: https://www.atsjournals.org/doi/epdf/10.1164/ajrccm/148.3.768?role=tab.
34. Loscalzo J. Endothelial dysfunction in pulmonary hypertension. N Engl J Med. 1992;327(2):117–9.
35. Santos S, Peinado VI, Ramírez J, Morales-Blanhir J, Bastos R, Roca J, et al. Enhanced expression of vascular endothelial growth factor in pulmonary arteries of smokers and patients with moderate chronic obstructive pulmonary disease. Am J Respir Crit Care Med. 2003;167(9):1250–6.
36. Wright JL, Tai H, Dai J, Churg A. Cigarette smoke induces rapid changes in gene expression in pulmonary arteries. Lab Investig. 2002;82(10):1391–8.
37. Wright JL, Tai H, Churg A. Cigarette smoke induces persisting increases of vasoactive mediators in pulmonary arteries. Am J Respir Cell Mol Biol. 2004;31(5):501–9.
38. Giaid A, Yanagisawa M, Langleben D, Michel RP, Levy R, Shennib H, et al. Expression of endothelin-1 in the lungs of patients with pulmonary hypertension. N Engl J Med. 1993;328(24):1732–9.
39. Roland M, Bhowmik A, Sapsford RJ, Seemungal TAR, Jeffries DJ, Warner TD, et al. Sputum and plasma endothelin-1 levels in exacerbations of chronic obstructive pulmonary disease. Thorax. 2001;56(1):30–5.
40. Maruyama K, Ye CL, Woo M, Venkatacharya H, Lines LD, Silver MM, et al. Chronic hypoxic pulmonary hypertension in rats and increased elastolytic activity. Am J Phys Heart Circ Phys. 1991;261(6):H1716–26.
41. Rabinovitch M. Pathobiology of pulmonary hypertension. Annual Rev Pathol Mech Dis. 2007;2(1):369–99.
42. Zaidi SHE, You XM, Ciura S, Husain M, Rabinovitch M. Overexpression of the serine elastase inhibitor elafin protects transgenic mice from hypoxic pulmonary hypertension. Circulation. 2002;105(4):516–21.
43. Marciniak SJ, Lomas DA. What can naturally occurring mutations tell us about the pathogenesis of COPD? Thorax. 2009;64(4):359–64.
44. Gross P, Pfitzer EA, Tolker E, Babyak MA, Kaschak M. Experimental emphysema: its production with papain in normal and silicotic rats. Arch Environ Health. 1965;11:50–8.
45. Wright JL, Farmer SG, Churg A. A neutrophil elastase inhibitor reduces cigarette smoke-induced remodelling of lung vessels. Eur Respir J. 2003;22(1):77–81.
46. Yildiz P, Oflaz H, Cine N, Erginel-Ünaltuna N, Erzengin F, Yilmaz V. Gene polymorphisms of endothelial nitric oxide synthase enzyme associated with pulmonary hypertension in patients with COPD. Respir Med. 2003;97(12):1282–8.
47. Chaouat A, Savale L, Chouaid C, Tu L, Sztrymf B, Canuet M, et al. Role for interleukin-6 in COPD-related pulmonary hypertension. Chest. 2009;136(3):678–87.
48. Hurdman J, Condliffe R, Elliot CA, Davies C, Hill C, Wild JM, et al. ASPIRE registry: assessing the spectrum of pulmonary hypertension identified. Eur Respir J. 2012;39(4):945–55.
49. Wright JL, Churg A. Cigarette smoke causes physiologic and morphologic changes of emphysema in the guinea pig. Am Rev Respir Dis. 1990;142(6_pt_1):1422–8.
50. Wright JL, Churg A. Effect of long-term cigarette smoke exposure on pulmonary vascular structure and function in the guinea pig. Exp Lung Res. 1991;17(6):997–1009.
51. Matsuoka S, Washko GR, Yamashiro T, Estepar RSJ, Diaz A, Silverman EK, et al. Pulmonary hypertension and computed tomography measurement of small pulmonary vessels in severe emphysema. Am J Respir Crit Care Med. 2010;181(3):218–25.
52. Alkhanfar D, Shahin Y, Alandejani F, Dwivedi K, Alabed S, Johns C, et al. Severe pulmonary hypertension associated with lung disease is characterised by a loss of small pulmonary vessels on quantitative computed tomography. ERJ Open Res. 2022;8(2):00503–2021.

53. Mineo TC, Pompeo E, Rogliani P, Dauri M, Turani F, Bollero P, et al. Effect of lung volume reduction surgery for severe emphysema on right ventricular function. Am J Respir Crit Care Med. 2002;165(4):489–94.
54. Weg IL, Rossoff L, McKEON K, Michael Graver L, Scharf SM. Development of pulmonary hypertension after lung volume reduction surgery. Am J Respir Crit Care Med. 1999;159(2):552–6.
55. Criner GJ, Scharf SM, Falk JA, Gaughan JP, Sternberg AL, Patel NB, et al. Effect of lung volume reduction surgery on resting pulmonary hemodynamics in severe emphysema. Am J Respir Crit Care Med. 2007;176(3):253–60.
56. Fishman AP, Fritts HW, Cournand A. Effects of breathing carbon dioxide upon the pulmonary circulation. Circulation. 1960;22(2):220–5.
57. Enson Y, Giuntini C, Lewis ML, Morris TQ, Ferrer MI, Harvey RM. The influence of hydrogen ion concentration and hypoxia on the pulmonary circulation. J Clin Invest. 1964;43(6):1146–62.
58. Lim TP, Brownlee WE. Pulmonary hemodynamics in obstructive lung disease. Dis Chest. 1968;53(2):113–25.
59. Martinez C, Wallenhorst C, Teal S, Cohen AT, Peacock AJ. Incidence and risk factors of chronic thromboembolic pulmonary hypertension following venous thromboembolism, a population-based cohort study in England. Pulm Circ. 2018;8(3):2045894018791358.
60. Kamenskaya O, Loginova I, Chernyavskiy A, Edemskiy A, Lomivorotov VV, Karaskov A. Chronic obstructive pulmonary disease in patients with chronic thromboembolic pulmonary hypertension: prevalence and implications for surgical treatment outcome. Clin Respir J. 2018;12(7):2242–8.
61. Paulus WJ, Tschöpe C. A novel paradigm for heart failure with preserved ejection fraction: comorbidities drive myocardial dysfunction and remodeling through coronary microvascular endothelial inflammation. J Am Coll Cardiol. 2013;62(4):263–71.
62. Gan WQ, Man SFP, Senthilselvan A, Sin DD. Association between chronic obstructive pulmonary disease and systemic inflammation: a systematic review and a meta-analysis. Thorax. 2004;59(7):574–80.
63. Barnes PJ. Senescence in COPD and its comorbidities. Annu Rev Physiol. 2017;79(1):517–39.
64. Wilhelmsen L, Rosengren A, Eriksson H, Lappas G. Heart failure in the general population of men—morbidity, risk factors and prognosis. J Intern Med. 2001;249(3):253–61.
65. Rutten FH, Cramer MJM, Grobbee DE, Sachs APE, Kirkels JH, Lammers JWJ, et al. Unrecognized heart failure in elderly patients with stable chronic obstructive pulmonary disease. Eur Heart J. 2005;26(18):1887–94.
66. McCullough PA, Hollander JE, Nowak RM, Storrow AB, Duc P, Omland T, et al. Uncovering heart failure in patients with a history of pulmonary disease: rationale for the early use of B-type natriuretic peptide in the emergency department. Acad Emerg Med. 2003;10(3):198–204.
67. Sin DD, Man SFP. Why are patients with chronic obstructive pulmonary disease at increased risk of cardiovascular diseases? Circulation. 2003;107(11):1514–9.
68. Sin DD, Man SFP. Chronic obstructive pulmonary disease as a risk factor for cardiovascular morbidity and mortality. Proc Am Thorac Soc. 2005;2(1):8–11.
69. Vasan RS, Sullivan LM, Roubenoff R, Dinarello CA, Harris T, Benjamin EJ, et al. Inflammatory markers and risk of heart failure in elderly subjects without prior myocardial infarction. Circulation. 2003;107(11):1486–91.
70. Barr RG, Bluemke DA, Ahmed FS, Carr JJ, Enright PL, Hoffman EA, et al. Percent emphysema, airflow obstruction, and impaired left ventricular filling. New Engl J Med. 2010;217–27.
71. Watz H, Waschki B, Meyer T, Kretschmar G, Kirsten A, Claussen M, et al. Decreasing cardiac chamber sizes and associated heart dysfunction in COPD: role of hyperinflation. Chest. 2010;138(1):32–8.
72. García AR, Piccari L. Emerging phenotypes of pulmonary hypertension associated with COPD: a field guide. Curr Opin Pulm Med. 2022;28(5):343–51.

73. Olsson KM, Corte TJ, Kamp JC, Montani D, Nathan SD, Neubert L, et al. Pulmonary hypertension associated with lung disease: new insights into pathomechanisms, diagnosis, and management. Lancet Respir Med. 2023;11(9):820–35.
74. de Leeuw PWD, Dees A. Fluid homeostasis in chronic obstructive lung disease. Eur Respir J. 2003;22(46 suppl):33s–40s.
75. Humbert M, Kovacs G, Hoeper MM, Badagliacca R, Berger RMF, Brida M, et al. 2022 ESC/ERS Guidelines for the diagnosis and treatment of pulmonary hypertension. Eur Respir J. 2023;61(1):2200879.
76. Alkukhun L, Baumgartner M, Budev M, Dweik RA, Tonelli AR. Electrocardiographic differences between COPD patients evaluated for lung transplantation with and without pulmonary hypertension. COPD: J Chron Obstruct Pulmon Dis. 2014;11(6):670–80.
77. Hurdman J, Condliffe R, Elliot C, Swift A, Rajaram S, Davies C, et al. Pulmonary hypertension in COPD: results from the ASPIRE registry. Eur Respir J. 2013;41(6):1292–301.
78. Kovacs G, Avian A, Bachmaier G, Troester N, Tornyos A, Douschan P, et al. Severe pulmonary hypertension in COPD: impact on survival and diagnostic approach. Chest. 2022;162(1):202–12.
79. Blanco I, Valeiro B, Torres-Castro R, Barberán-García A, Torralba Y, Moisés J, et al. Effects of pulmonary hypertension on exercise capacity in patients with chronic obstructive pulmonary disease. Arch Bronconeumol. 2019;56(8):499–505.
80. Oki Y, Kaneko M, Fujimoto Y, Sakai H, Misu S, Mitani Y, et al. Usefulness of the 6-minute walk test as a screening test for pulmonary arterial enlargement in COPD. COPD. 2016;11(1):2869–75.
81. Torres-Castro R, Gimeno-Santos E, Vilaró J, Roqué-Figuls M, Moisés J, Vasconcello-Castillo L, et al. Effect of pulmonary hypertension on exercise tolerance in patients with COPD: a prognostic systematic review and meta-analysis. Eur Respir Rev. 2021;30(160):200321.
82. Skjørten I, Hilde JM, Melsom MN, Hisdal J, Hansteen V, Steine K, et al. Cardiopulmonary exercise test and PaO2 in evaluation of pulmonary hypertension in COPD. COPD. 2017;13:91–100.
83. Fisher MR, Criner GJ, Fishman AP, Hassoun PM, Minai OA, Scharf SM, et al. Estimating pulmonary artery pressures by echocardiography in patients with emphysema. Eur Respir J. 2007;30(5):914–21.
84. Arcasoy SM, Christie JD, Ferrari VA, St M, Sutton J, Zisman DA, et al. Echocardiographic assessment of pulmonary hypertension in patients with advanced lung disease. Am J Respir Crit Care Med. 2003;167:735–40.
85. Rodríguez DA, Sancho-Muñoz A, Rodó-Pin A, Herranz A, Gea J, Bruguera J, et al. Right ventricular response during exercise in patients with chronic obstructive pulmonary disease. Heart Lung Circ. 2017;26(6):631–4.
86. Swift AJ, Dwivedi K, Johns C, Garg P, Chin M, Currie BJ, et al. Diagnostic accuracy of CT pulmonary angiography in suspected pulmonary hypertension. Eur Radiol. 2020;30(9):4918–29.
87. Kiely DG, Levin DL, Hassoun PM, Ivy D, Jone P, Bwika J, et al. Statement on imaging and pulmonary hypertension from the Pulmonary Vascular Research Institute (PVRI). Pulm Circ. 2019;9(3):1–32.
88. Dwivedi K, Sharkey M, Condliffe R, Uthoff JM, Alabed S, Metherall P, et al. Pulmonary hypertension in association with lung disease: quantitative CT and artificial intelligence to the rescue? State-of-the-art review. Diagnostics. 2021;11(4):1–20.
89. Alkhanfar D, Dwivedi K, Alandejani F, Shahin Y, Alabed S, Johns C, et al. Non-invasive detection of severe PH in lung disease using magnetic resonance imaging. Front Cardiovasc Med [Internet]. 2023 [cited 2023 Dec 6];10. Available from: https://www.frontiersin.org/articles/10.3389/fcvm.2023.1016994.
90. Galiè N, Humbert M, Vachiery JL, Gibbs S, Lang I, Torbicki A, et al. 2015 ESC/ERS Guidelines for the diagnosis and treatment of pulmonary hypertension. Eur Respir J. 2015;46(4):903–75.

91. Nathan SD, Barbera JA, Gaine SP, Harari S, Martinez FJ, Olschewski H, et al. Pulmonary hypertension in chronic lung disease and hypoxia. Eur Respir J. 2019;53(1):1801914.
92. Zeder K, Avian A, Bachmaier G, Douschan P, Foris V, Sassmann T, et al. Elevated pulmonary vascular resistance predicts mortality in COPD patients. Eur Respir J. 2021;58(2):2100944.
93. Olsson KM, Hoeper MM, Pausch C, Grünig E, Huscher D, Pittrow D, et al. Pulmonary vascular resistance predicts mortality in patients with pulmonary hypertension associated with interstitial lung disease: results from the COMPERA registry. Eur Respir J. 2021;58(2):2101483.
94. Piccari L, Wort SJ, Meloni F, Rizzo M, Price LC, Martino L, et al. The effect of borderline pulmonary hypertension on survival in chronic lung disease. Respiration. 2022;101(8):717–27.
95. Chen W, Thomas J, Sadatsafavi M, FitzGerald JM. Risk of cardiovascular comorbidity in patients with chronic obstructive pulmonary disease: a systematic review and meta-analysis. Lancet Respir Med. 2015;3(8):631–9.
96. Vachiéry JL, Tedford RJ, Rosenkranz S, Palazzini M, Lang I, Guazzi M, et al. Pulmonary hypertension due to left heart disease. Eur Resp J. 2018;1801897.
97. Kovacs G, Avian A, Pienn M, Naeije R, Olschewski H. Reading pulmonary vascular pressure tracings. How to handle the problems of zero leveling and respiratory swings. Am J Respir Crit Care Med. 2014;190(3):252–7.
98. Weitzenblum E, Sautegeau A, Ehrhart M, Mammosser M, Pelletier A. Long-term oxygen therapy can reverse the progression of pulmonary hypertension in patients with chronic obstructive pulmonary disease. Am Revue Resp Dis. 1985.
99. Medical Research Council Working Party. Long term domiciliary oxygen therapy in chronic hypoxic cor pulmonale complicating chronic bronchitis and emphysema: report of the Medical Research Council Working Party. Lancet. 1981;317(8222):681–6.
100. Zhang L, Liu Y, Zhao S, Wang Z, Zhang M, Zhang S, et al. The incidence and prevalence of pulmonary hypertension in the COPD population: a systematic review and meta-analysis. COPD. 2022;17:1365–79.
101. Chaouat A, Bugnet ASS, Kadaoui N, Schott R, Enache I, Ducoloné A, et al. Severe pulmonary hypertension and chronic obstructive pulmonary disease. Am J Respir Crit Care Med. 2005;172(2):189–94.
102. Kovacs G, Agusti A, Barberà JA, Celli B, Criner G, Humbert M, et al. Pulmonary vascular involvement in chronic obstructive pulmonary disease. is there a pulmonary vascular phenotype? Am J Respir Crit Care Med. 2018;198(8):1000–11.
103. Hilde JM, Skjorten I, Hansteen V, Melsom MN, Hisdal J, Humerfelt S, et al. Haemodynamic responses to exercise in patients with COPD. Eur Respir J. 2013;41(5):1031–41.
104. Chaouat A, Weitzenblum E, Krieger J, Ifoundza T, Oswald M, Kessler R. Association of chronic obstructive pulmonary disease and sleep apnea syndrome. Am J Respir Crit Care Med. 1995;151(1):82–6.
105. Sanders MH, Newman AB, Haggerty CL, Redline S, Lebowitz M, Samet J, et al. Sleep and sleep-disordered breathing in adults with predominantly mild obstructive airway disease. Am J Respir Crit Care Med. 2003;167(1):7–14.
106. Adrish M, Nannaka VB, Cano EJ, Bajantri B, Diaz-Fuentes G. Significance of NT-pro-BNP in acute exacerbation of COPD patients without underlying left ventricular dysfunction. COPD. 2017;12:1183–9.
107. Cheng Y, Li L, Tu X, Pei R. The main pulmonary artery to the ascending aorta diameter ratio (PA/A) as a predictor of worse outcomes in hospitalized patients with AECOPD. COPD. 2022;17:1157–65.
108. Takahashi T, Yoshihisa A, Sugimoto K, Yokokawa T, Misaka T, Kaneshiro T, et al. Associations between diabetes mellitus and pulmonary hypertension in chronic respiratory disease patients. PLoS ONE. 2018;13(10):e0205008.
109. Nathan SD, Barnett SD, King CS, Provencher S, Barbera JA, Pastre J, et al. Impact of the new definition for pulmonary hypertension in patients with lung disease: an analysis of the United Network for Organ Sharing database. Pulm Circ. 2021;11(1):1–7.

110. Portillo K, Torralba Y, Blanco I, Burgos F, Rios J, Roca J, et al. Pulmonary hemodynamic profile in chronic obstructive pulmonary disease. Int J Chron Obstruct Pulmon Dis. 2015;10:1313–20.
111. Scharf SM, Iqbal M, Keller C, Criner G, Lee S, Fessler HE. Hemodynamic characterization of patients with severe emphysema. Am J Respir Crit Care Med. 2002;166(3):314–22.
112. Aguirre-Franco C, Torres-Duque CA, Salazar G, Casas A, Jaramillo C, Gonzalez-Garcia M. Prevalence of pulmonary hypertension in COPD patients living at high altitude. Pulmonology. 2022;000(xxxx):1–7.
113. Hoeper MM, Humbert M, Souza R, Idrees M, Kawut SM, Sliwa-Hahnle K, et al. A global view of pulmonary hypertension. Lancet Respir Med. 2016;4(4):306–22.
114. Gall H, Felix JF, Schneck FK, Milger K, Sommer N, Voswinckel R, et al. The Giessen Pulmonary Hypertension Registry: survival in pulmonary hypertension subgroups. J Heart Lung Transplant. 2017;36(9):957–67.
115. Hemnes AR, Leopold JA, Radeva MK, Beck GJ, Abidov A, Aldred MA, et al. Clinical characteristics and transplant- free survival across the spectrum of pulmonary vascular disease. J Am Coll Cardiol. 2022;80(7):697–718.
116. Sassmann T, Douschan P, Foris V, Tröster N, Zeder K, Brcic L, et al. Abnormal pulmonary hemodynamics during exercise is associated with exercise capacity in COPD. Respir Res. 2022;23(1):331.
117. Gupta KK, Roy B, Chaudhary SC, Mishra A, Patel ML, Singh J, et al. Prevalence of pulmonary artery hypertension in patients of chronic obstructive pulmonary disease and its correlation with stages of chronic obstructive pulmonary disease, exercising capacity, and quality of life. J Family Med Prim Care. 2018;7(1):53–7.
118. Gredic M, Blanco I, Kovacs G, Helyes Z, Ferdinandy P, Olschewski H, et al. Pulmonary hypertension in chronic obstructive pulmonary disease. Br J Pharmacol. 2021;178(1):132–51.
119. Bloch KE, Sooronbaev TM, Ulrich S, Lichtblau M, Furian M. Counseling patients with chronic obstructive pulmonary disease traveling to high altitude. High Alt Med Biol. 2023;24(3):158–66.
120. Lichtblau M, Saxer S, Mayer L, Sheraliev U, Mademilov M, Furian M, et al. Effect of acetazolamide on pulmonary vascular haemodynamics in patients with COPD going to altitude: a randomised, placebo-controlled, double-blind trial. ERJ Open Res. 2023;9(2):00412–2022.
121. Lichtblau M, Furian M, Aeschbacher SS, Bisang M, Ulrich S, Saxer S, et al. Dexamethasone improves pulmonary hemodynamics in COPD-patients going to altitude: a randomized trial. Int J Cardiol. 2019;283:159–64.
122. Furian M, Lichtblau M, Aeschbacher SS, Estebesova B, Emilov B, Sheraliev U, et al. Effect of dexamethasone on nocturnal oxygenation in lowlanders with chronic obstructive pulmonary disease traveling to 3100 meters: a randomized clinical trial. JAMA Netw Open. 2019;2(2):e190067.
123. Lange TJ, Baron M, Seiler I, Arzt M, Pfeifer M. Outcome of patients with severe PH due to lung disease with and without targeted therapy. Cardiovasc Ther. 2014;32(5):202–8.
124. Tanabe N, Taniguchi H, Tsujino I, Sakamaki F, Emoto N, Kimura H, et al. Multi-institutional retrospective cohort study of patients with severe pulmonary hypertension associated with respiratory diseases. Respirology. 2015;20(5):805–12.
125. Vitulo P, Stanziola A, Confalonieri M, Libertucci D, Oggionni T, Rottoli P, et al. Sildenafil in severe pulmonary hypertension associated with chronic obstructive pulmonary disease: a randomized controlled multicenter clinical trial. J Heart Lung Transplant. 2017;36(2):166–74.
126. Nocturnal Oxygen Therapy Trial Group. Continuous or nocturnal oxygen therapy in hypoxemic chronic obstructive lung disease. Ann Intern Med [Internet]. 2008 [cited 2024 Jan 15]. Available from: https://www.acpjournals.org/doi/10.7326/0003-4819-93-3-391.
127. Barberà JA, Blanco I. Pulmonary hypertension in patients with chronic obstructive pulmonary disease: advances in pathophysiology and management. Drugs. 2009;69(9):1153–71.
128. Timms RM, Khaja FU, Williams GW. Hemodynamic response to oxygen therapy in chronic obstructive pulmonary disease. Ann Intern Med. 1985;102(1):29–36.

129. Barberà JA, Roger N, Roca J, Rodriguez-Roisin R, Rovira I, Higenbottam TW. Worsening of pulmonary gas exchange with nitric oxide inhalation in chronic obstructive pulmonary disease. Lancet. 1996;347(8999):436–40.
130. Long-Term Oxygen Treatment Trial Research Group. A randomized trial of long-term oxygen for COPD with moderate desaturation. N Engl J Med. 2016;375(17):1617–27.
131. Chen X, Tang S, Liu K, Li Q, Kong H, Zeng X, et al. Therapy in stable chronic obstructive pulmonary disease patients with pulmonary hypertension: a systematic review and meta-analysis. J Thoracic Dis [Internet]. 2015 [cited 2024 Jan 21];7(3). Available from: https://jtd.amegroups.org/article/view/4132.
132. Park J, Song JH, Park DA, Lee JS, Lee SD, Oh YM. Systematic review and meta-analysis of pulmonary hypertension specific therapy for exercise capacity in chronic obstructive pulmonary disease. J Korean Med Sci. 2013;28(8):1200–6.
133. Prins KW, Duval S, Markowitz J, Pritzker M, Thenappan T. Chronic use of PAH-specific therapy in World Health Organization Group III Pulmonary Hypertension: a systematic review and meta-analysis. Pulm Circ. 2017;7(1):145–55.
134. Valerio G, Bracciale P, Grazia D'agostino A. Effect of bosentan upon pulmonary hypertension in chronic obstructive pulmonary disease. Ther Adv Respir Dis. 2009;3(1):15–21.
135. Rietema H, Holverda S, Bogaard HJ, Marcus JT, Smit HJ, Westerhof N, et al. Sildenafil treatment in COPD does not affect stroke volume or exercise capacity. Eur Respir J. 2008;31(4):759–64.
136. Blanco I, Santos S, Gea J, Güell R, Torres F, Gimeno-Santos E, et al. Sildenafil to improve respiratory rehabilitation outcomes in COPD: a controlled trial. Eur Respir J. 2013;42(4):982–92.
137. Goudie AR, Lipworth BJ, Hopkinson PJ, Wei L, Struthers AD. Tadalafil in patients with chronic obstructive pulmonary disease: a randomised, double-blind, parallel-group, placebo-controlled trial. Lancet Respir Med. 2014;2(4):293–300.
138. Stolz D, Rasch H, Linka A, Di Valentino M, Meyer A, Brutsche M, et al. A randomised, controlled trial of bosentan in severe COPD. Eur Respir J. 2008;32(3):619–28.
139. Lederer DJ, Bartels MN, Schluger NW, Brogan F, Jellen P, Thomashow BM, et al. Sildenafil for chronic obstructive pulmonary disease: a randomized crossover trial. COPD: J Chron Obstruct Pulmon Dis. 2012;9(3):268–75.
140. Pichl A, Sommer N, Bednorz M, Seimetz M, Hadzic S, Kuhnert S, et al. Riociguat for treatment of pulmonary hypertension in COPD: a translational study. Eur Resp J [Internet]. 2019 [cited 2024 Jan 21];53(6). Available from: https://erj.ersjournals.com/content/53/6/1802445.
141. Calcaianu G, Canuet M, Schuller A, Enache I, Chaouat A, Kessler R. Pulmonary arterial hypertension-specific drug therapy in COPD patients with severe pulmonary hypertension and mild-to-moderate airflow limitation. Respiration. 2016;91(1):9–17.
142. Andersen KH, Iversen M, Kjaergaard J, Mortensen J, Nielsen-Kudsk JE, Bendstrup E, Videbaek R, Carlsen J. Prevalence, predictors, and survival in pulmonary hypertension related to end-stage chronic obstructive pulmonary disease. J Heart Lung Transplant. 2012;31(4):373–80. https://doi.org/10.1016/j.healun.2011.11.020. Epub 2012 Jan 9. PMID: 22226804.
143. Cuttica MJ, Kalhan R, Shlobin OA, Ahmad S, Gladwin M, Machado RF, Barnett SD, Nathan SD. Categorization and impact of pulmonary hypertension in patients with advanced COPD. Respir Med. 2010;104(12):1877–82. https://doi.org/10.1016/j.rmed.2010.05.009. Epub 2010 Jun 14. PMID: 20547449.
144. Thabut G, Dauriat G, Stern JB, Logeart D, Lévy A, Marrash-Chahla R, Mal H. Pulmonary hemodynamics in advanced COPD candidates for lung volume reduction surgery or lung transplantation. Chest. 2005;127(5):1531–6. https://doi.org/10.1378/chest.127.5.1531. PMID: 15888824.
145. Hilde JM, Skjørten I, Hansteen V, Melsom MN, Hisdal J, Humerfelt S, Steine K. Haemodynamic responses to exercise in patients with COPD. Eur Respir J. 2013;41(5):1031–41. https://doi.org/10.1183/09031936.00085612. Epub 2012 Aug 16. PMID: 22903957.

146. Portillo K, Torralba Y, Blanco I, Burgos F, Rodriguez-Roisin R, Rios J, Roca J, Barberà JA. Pulmonary hemodynamic profile in chronic obstructive pulmonary disease. Int J Chron Obstruct Pulmon Dis. 2015;10:1313–20. https://doi.org/10.2147/COPD.S78180. Erratum in: Int J Chron Obstruct Pulmon Dis. 2015;10:2377. PMID: 26203238; PMCID: PMC4507485.
147. Nathan SD, Barnett SD, King CS, Provencher S, Barbera JA, Pastre J, Shlobin OA, Seeger W. Impact of the new definition for pulmonary hypertension in patients with lung disease: an analysis of the United Network for Organ Sharing database. Pulm Circ. 2021;11(2):2045894021999960. https://doi.org/10.1177/2045894021999960. PMID: 33868639; PMCID: PMC8020109.
148. Zhang L, Liu Y, Zhao S, Wang Z, Zhang M, Zhang S, Wang X, Zhang S, Zhang W, Hao L, Jiao G. The incidence and prevalence of pulmonary hypertension in the COPD population: a systematic review and meta-analysis. Int J Chron Obstruct Pulmon Dis. 2022;17:1365–79. https://doi.org/10.2147/COPD.S359873. PMID: 35711174; PMCID: PMC9196913.

Chapter 9
Pulmonary Hypertension Complicating Interstitial Lung Disease: Current Concepts and Controversies

Christopher S. King and Christopher Thomas

Introduction

The poor prognosis of pulmonary hypertension in interstitial lung disease (ILD-PH) has been recognized for two decades, but for much of this time clinicians demonstrated little enthusiasm toward proactive diagnosis of the disorder [1]. This was largely rooted in a nihilistic attitude stemming from the lack of a clearly effective therapy. This changed with the 2021 publication of the INCREASE trial, the first randomized, controlled trial to conclusively demonstrate the efficacy of pulmonary vasodilator therapy in ILD-PH [2]. Since that publication, there has been an explosion of interest in the topic. Despite a renewed enthusiasm toward the diagnosis and treatment of ILD-PH, numerous questions remain unanswered. In this review, we will cover the information that is known about ILD-PH and highlight areas of uncertainty. The authors will also offer a proposed diagnostic and treatment algorithm. Finally, currently enrolling clinical trials will be reviewed and future questions requiring investigation will be discussed.

C. S. King (✉) · C. Thomas
Advanced Lung Disease and Lung Transplant Program, Inova Fairfax Medical Center, Falls Church, VA, USA
e-mail: Christopher.King@inova.org; Christopher.thomas@inova.org

F. N. Rahaghi et al. (eds.), *The Pulmonary Vasculature in Chronic Lung Disease*, Respiratory Medicine, https://doi.org/10.1007/978-3-032-03581-3_9

Definition of Pulmonary Hypertension Associated with Interstitial Lung Disease

The 7th World Symposium on Pulmonary Hypertension (WSPH) classifies pulmonary hypertension (PH) into five groups based upon the etiology [3]. Group 3 PH consists of PH due to chronic lung diseases (CLD) or hypoxia, including chronic obstructive pulmonary disease and ILD [3]. Historically, Group 3 PH was defined hemodynamically as a mean pulmonary artery pressure (mPAP) ≥ 25 mmHg and pulmonary artery occlusion pressure (PAOP) ≤ 15 mmHg. The 6th WSPH updated this definition to PH due to CLD with a resting mPAP > 20 mmHg with an accompanying pulmonary vascular resistance of ≥ 3 Wood units (WU) and a PAOP ≤ 15 mmHg [4]. They went on to define severe Group 3 PH as mPAP ≥ 35 mmHg or mPAP ≥ 25 mmHg with a low cardiac index (CI) (mPAP ≥ 25 mmHg with a CI < 2.0 L/min/m^2 [4]. They justified the selection of this definition by citing a prior document which argued that "severe" PH accounted for only a small percentage of patients with Group 3 PH and those meeting this hemodynamic threshold had worse exercise tolerance and greater exertional desaturation despite having similar or better lung function on pulmonary function testing (PFTs) [5].

The definition of Group 3 PH was updated once again by the 2022 European Society Cardiology (ESC)/European Respiratory Society (ERS) Guidelines on the diagnosis and treatment of pulmonary hypertension [6]. The 2022 ESC/ERS guidelines defined pre-capillary PH as is seen in CLD-PH as mPAP > 20 mmHg, PAOP ≤ 15 mmHg, and PVR > 2 WU [6]. The rationale for the change in PVR threshold was that a PVR of 2 was the upper limit of normal PVR and the lowest "prognostically relevant threshold" [6]. The ESC/ERS guidelines went on to update the definition of "severe" disease to CLD-PH with a PVR ≥ 5 Wood units. They based this decision on two studies demonstrating PVR > 5 Wood units as prognostically significant in patients with CLD [7, 8]. The 7th WSPH elected to maintain the same definition of PH, but did not provide a specific definition for "severe" ILD-PH, rather stating severity of ILD-PH is a continuum and should take into consideration hemodynamic values and RV function [3]. The implications of the evolving definition of Group 3 PH are unclear. Presumably, an increased number of patients with ILD will meet the definition of ILD-PH, but whether this will translate into institution of treatment or improved outcomes for these patients remains to be seen. Table 9.1 summarizes the evolution of definitions of Group 3 PH.

The hemodynamic definition of Group 3 PH is not the only aspect to have changed over time. Previously, patients with CLD with precapillary hemodynamics could be classified as either Group 1 or Group 3 PH. The 6th WSPH recommended consideration of the patient's hemodynamics, pulmonary function testing, the presence of risk factors for pulmonary arterial hypertension (PAH), and the extent of parenchymal lung disease on CT imaging (Table 9.2). Presence of risk factors for PAH and more severe PH favored a diagnosis of group 1 PH, while more severe parenchymal lung disease on CT or impairment on PFT (forced vital capacity

Table 9.1 Hemodynamic definitions of WHO Group 3 pulmonary hypertension

WHO meeting, Geneva	1975	PH	mPAP ≥ 25 mmHg PAOP ≤ 15 mmHg
6th World symposium on pulmonary hypertension	2019	PH	mPAP > 20 mmHg PAOP ≤ 15 mmHg PVR > 3 Wood units
		Severe PH	mPAP ≥ 35 mmHg or mPAP ≥ 25 mmHg with a CI < 2.0 L/min/M^2
ESC/ERS guidelines	2022	PH	mPAP > 20 mmHg PAOP ≤ 15 mmHg PVR > 2 Wood units
		Severe PH	mPAP > 20 mmHg PAOP ≤ 15 mmHg PVR > 5 Wood units

Abbreviations: *WHO* World Health Organization, *PH* pulmonary hypertension, *mPAP* mean pulmonary artery pressure, *PAOP* pulmonary artery occlusion pressure, *PVR* pulmonary vascular resistance, *CI* cardiac index, *ESC* European Society of Cardiologists, *ERS* European Respiratory Society

Table 9.2 Criteria that favor WHO Group 1 versus Group 3 pulmonary hypertension in interstitial lung disease

	Group 1	Group 3
Pulmonary function testing	Normal or mild impaired FVC > 70% predicted DLCO disproportionately reduced relative to FVC	Moderate or severely impaired FVC < 70% predicted DLCO proportionately reduced relative to FVC
CT scanning	Absent or mild parenchymal lung disease	Moderate or severe lung disease
Hemodynamic profile	Moderate to severe PH	Mild to moderate PH
PAH risk factors (HIV, CTD, CHD, Familial PH)	Present	Absent

Abbreviations: *WHO* World Health Organization, *FVC* forced vital capacity, *DLCO* diffusing capacity of the lung for carbon monoxide, *PH* pulmonary hypertension, *PAH* pulmonary arterial hypertension, *HIV* human immunodeficiency virus, *CTD* connective tissue disease, *CHD* congenital heart disease

Adapted from the 6th World Symposium on Pulmonary Hypertension

[FVC] < 70% predicted) favors a diagnosis of Group 3 PH [4]. The 7th WSPH recommended new subgroups of Group 3 PH based on clinical diagnosis (e.g., ILD, combined pulmonary fibrosis and emphysema (CPFE), chronic obstructive pulmonary disease (COPD), developmental lung diseases, and other) rather than classifications relying on pulmonary function measurements such as "obstructive lung disease" or "restrictive lung disease" [3]. They also state patients with "significant abnormalities in pulmonary function or relevant parenchymal involvement in high resolution CT (HRCT), particularly pulmonary fibrosis and/or emphysema, classification into Group 3 PH should be favored". [3] This seems to direct clinicians to label patients with any notable ILD as Group 3 PH, however, how much parenchymal involvement is considered "relevant" remains at the discretion of the clinician.

Epidemiology of Pulmonary Hypertension Associated with Interstitial Lung Disease

Over 150 different lung diseases are considered forms of ILD [9]. These disorders are grouped together based on common characteristics including restrictive physiology on PFTs, parenchymal involvement on lung imaging and impaired gas exchange. Despite these commonalities, the myriad of ILDs vary with regard to etiology, histopathological and radiographic pattern, and outcomes [9]. The overwhelming majority of data on the prevalence of ILD-PH comes from the IPF population; however, ILD-PH can complicate other ILDs [10]. Over forty studies have reported on prevalence of PH in IPF, with ranges extending from 3% to 86% [11]. The wide variability in estimated prevalence has multiple causes including the methodology used to establish the diagnosis (TTE vs RHC), the population studied (early diagnosis vs advanced disease), and the definition used. It is estimated that approximately 8–15% of IPF patients have ILD-PH at the time of diagnosis, but the prevalence increases over time, with 30–50% of advanced cases having ILD-PH, and >60% of those with end-stage disease [4, 12, 13]. This has implications clinically, as serial longitudinal screening is required so as to not miss the development of ILD-PH over time.

The bulk of the medical literature on prevalence of ILD-PH utilized a definition of mPAP $\geq$ 25 mmHg. It is unclear how much the shifting definition will increase the prevalence of ILD-PH. An analysis of data from the United Network for Organ Sharing (UNOS) on 8991 IPF patients listed for lung transplant found the prevalence of PH increased from 47.6% to 73.6% when the 6th WSPH definition was applied, however only 36.8% had "pre-capillary" PH [14]. To our knowledge, a similar analysis has not been performed with the new ESC/ERS definition.

As mentioned above, ILD-PH has been reported in other types of ILD including idiopathic NSIP (31%), chronic hypersensitivity pneumonitis (20–44%), connective-tissue disease-associated ILD (CTD-ILD) (3–64%), combined pulmonary fibrosis and emphysema (CPFE) (30–50%), and other idiopathic interstitial pneumonias (IIPs) [15–22]. Given differences in the populations of these studies, it is impossible to comment on the relative propensity of each ILD to develop PH. It is clear that the prevalence of ILD-PH is not inconsequential regardless of the type of ILD, so clinicians should remain vigilant for development of ILD-PH in all forms of ILD.

The majority of patients with ILD-PH have mild to moderate PH with mPAPs of 20–35 mmHg, however 10–20% of patients have more significant PH with mPAP > 35 mmHg [1, 23, 24]. It is unclear if this simply represents a spectrum of disease or alternatively two distinct phenotypes of ILD-PH.

Implications of Development of Pulmonary Hypertension Associated with Interstitial Lung Disease

Development of ILD-PH is associated with substantial morbidity with regard to symptomatology, exercise capacity, and need for supplemental oxygen. In a retrospective study of 79 patients with IPF, Lettieri et al. reported that those with PH had a significantly reduced six-minute walk test (6MWT) distance (143.5 m vs 365.9 m, $p < 0.001$) and a lower oxygen desaturation nadir (80.1% vs. 88.0%, $p < 0.001$) [1]. Registry data also confirms reduced functional capacity in ILD-PH. Data on 363 patients from a prospective French registry of PH patients found that in comparison to patients with PAH, those with ILD-PH were more likely to have New York Heart Association Class III or IV symptoms (82.6% vs 46.9%, $p < 0.001$) and lower 6MWT distances (222 m vs 320 m, $p < 0.001$) [25]. The Comparative, Prospective registry of Newly Initiated Therapies for Pulmonary Hypertension (COMPERA) showed similar results, with ILD-PH patients having lower 6MWT distances (251 m vs 303 m, $p < 0.001$) and more WHO Functional Class IV symptoms (25.7% vs 14.7%) compared to patients with PAH [26]. Cardiopulmonary exercise testing data also demonstrates impaired functional capacity on ILD-PH patients, as evidenced by a significant reduction in maximum work rate, peak O_2 uptake, anaerobic threshold, and peak O_2 pulse in IPF patients with PH diagnosed by a systolic pulmonary artery pressure (sPAP) > 35 mmHg on TTE [27].

In addition to causing patients to feel and function worse, ILD-PH has been shown to substantially attenuate survival in multiple studies. Nadrous et al reported a median survival of only 0.7 years in IPF patients with a sPAP > 50 mmHg on TTE as compared to over 4 years in those with sPAP ≤ 50 mmHg [28]. Song and colleagues reported similar findings in a retrospective analysis of 131 IPF patients—those with a sPAP ≥ 40 mmHg had a 1-year mortality of 61.2% as compared with 19.9% for patients with sPAP < 40 mmHg [29]. Lettieri et al. reported markedly increased 1-year mortality in IPF patients with mPAP > 25 mmHg (28.0% vs 5.5%, $p = 0.002$) [1]. One might argue that perhaps the patients with PH in these studies simply had more advanced parenchymal disease or were further into their clinical course, which could explain the differences in mortality observed. To control for this, Kimura and colleagues analyzed initial evaluation data from 101 consecutive IPF patients, performed a multivariate Cox proportional analysis, and found that mPAP was an independent predictor of survival (HR = 1.064; 95% CI 1.015–1.116, $p = 0.010$) [30].

The effects of ILD-PH on survival do not appear to be limited to IPF patients. An observational study of 47 patients with chronic hypersensitivity pneumonitis found increased mortality in patients with abnormal pulmonary hemodynamics, specifically a PVR ≥ 3.3 Wood units and decreased pulmonary vascular compliance. [31] Chen et al followed 132 patients who met criteria for progressive fibrosing ILD. Those with sPAP > 36.5 mmHg by TTE had substantially worse 5-year survival (38.6% vs 77.4%). [32] Whether ILD-PH has a similar prognosis regardless of etiology of ILD is unclear. Alhamad et al examined a cohort of 340 consecutive ILD patients that underwent RHC, of which 28% had PH and 16% had severe PH [33]. This study found that IPF-PH patients fared worse than CTD-ILD or sarcoid-PH patients. French registry data also suggests PH-IPF patients may have a worse prognosis than CPFE-PH or non-IPF ILD-PH patients with 3-year survival rates of 22.9%, 40.2%, and 30% respectively [25]. This is contraindicated by data from the COMPERA registry, which found no difference in survival between IPF-PH and NSIP-PH [26]. Perhaps some of the variability in outcomes among these disease states has to do with age and associated co-morbidities. Although the exact implications of development of ILD-PH on prognosis for individual ILDs remain elusive, it seems clear that ILD-PH does increase morbidity and mortality regardless of the specific ILD. In fact, development of ILD-PH is such a powerful predictor of mortality in ILD, that diagnosis by either TTE or RHC is considered a criterion for referral and listing for lung transplantation according to International Society of Heart and Lung Transplant (ISHLT) guidelines on candidate selection [34].

One interesting feature of ILD-PH, as compared to other forms of PH, is that even modest increases in mPAP have profound impacts on survival. In fact, the association of mPAP less than 25 mmHg with adverse outcomes in ILD patients was one of the factors which led to the revision of the definition of PH by the 6th WSPH [4]. The retrospective analysis of 101 IPF patients by Kimura, et al mentioned above found that a mPAP > 20 mmHg was the optimal cut point for predicting mortality, with a median survival of 20.8 months for those with mPAP > 20 mmHg vs 37.5 months for mPAP ≤ 20 mmHg [30]. Interestingly, the group with mPAP > 20 mmHg in this trial had a mean PVR of ~ 5 Wood units. Another prospective analysis of 68 IPF patients found markedly different 5-year survival in those with a mPAP < 17 mmHg (62.2%) vs ≥ 17 mmHg (16.7%) [35]. Piccari and colleagues found similarly poor 3-year survival in ILD patients with "borderline PH" (mPAP 21-25 and PVR ≥ 3 Wood units (32%)), "moderate PH" (25–25 mmHg and CI ≥ 2 L/min/m^2 (28%)) and severe pH mPAP ≥ 35 mmHg or mPAP ≥ 25 mmHg and CI < 2 L/min/m^2 (33%) as compared to no PH (58%) [23]. This is in contrast to data from the COMPERA registry, which found that patients with ILD-PH with a PVR > 5 Wood units had significantly worse survival than those with a PVR ≤ 5 Wood units [8]. The COMPERA registry only collected data on patients with hemodynamically diagnosed PH so no comparison could be made between those with a PVR < 5 Wood units and no PH. Moreover, COMPERA cohort consisted of patients with significant hemodynamic impairment with mean PVR of 8.1 WUs [26].

The available data suggests that even mild elevations in mPAP, and consequently elevation in PVR, in ILD patients hold prognostic significance. It also seems likely that the higher the elevation in PVR, the worse the prognosis. It is interesting that such modest elevations in PVR have such profound effects on survival in ILD-PH. This is a departure from the pathophysiology of PAH, where right ventricular dysfunction is the primary driver of mortality. Perhaps with exertion, the effects on the elevation in PVR adversely impact right ventricular function yet we fail to see this on the resting testing that is typically performed to diagnose ILD-PH. It may also be that once it starts, ILD-PH is a progressive process which over time will ultimately lead to RV dysfunction. Lastly, perhaps development of PH spurs progression of lung fibrosis, creating a cyclical downward spiral between pulmonary vascular disease and lung fibrosis [36]. Further study of ILD-PH, including invasive exercise testing and longitudinal follow-up of the natural history of the condition, will be required to answer these important questions.

Pathogenesis of Pulmonary Hypertension Associated with Interstitial Lung Disease

The pathogenesis of both ILD and PH is not fully understood. It is also unclear to what degree, if at all, the mechanisms driving progression of the processes are linked. It is also not clear if all ILD-PH represents a continuum of disease or if severe ILD-PH is a distinct entity stemming from a different pathophysiologic basis.

Traditionally, the primary processes thought to be responsible for development of ILD-PH were hypoxemic pulmonary vasoconstriction and destruction of the pulmonary vascular bed due to fibrosis of the lung parenchyma [37]. Hypoxemic pulmonary vasoconstriction, while generally reversible with supplemental oxygen, can lead to vascular remodeling and PAH if episodes are repeated or sustained [38]. Chronic hypoxemia can also lead to "endothelial nitric oxide synthase (eNOS) uncoupling", a form of endothelial dysfunction where eNOS produces harmful free radicals rather than nitric oxide [39]. eNOS uncoupling can also alter the response of the RV to pressure overload, leading to accelerated development of right ventricular dysfunction [40]. Parenchymal destruction from fibrotic lung disease leads to decreased capacitance of the pulmonary vascular bed through both a decrease in the number of vessels and loss of the ability of the vessels to dilate in response to changes in cardiac output during exercise. Both of these changes lead to an increase in PVR [41, 42].

While hypoxemic pulmonary vasoconstriction and parenchymal bed destruction certainly play a role in the development of ILD-PH, it is clear they are not the only factors at play. Histopathologic examination of ILD-PH lungs has shown vascular remodeling in areas unaffected by pulmonary fibrosis, implying these vascular changes are due to other factors [38]. Furthermore, the lack of correlation between the severity of PH and the severity of restriction on PFTs alludes to other factors driving pathogenesis [41]. Disruption of the nitric oxide pathway and overproduction of the pulmonary vasoconstrictor endothelin-1, pathways responsible for development of PAH, have been documented in ILD-PH [38]. Abnormal angiogenesis resulting in decreased vascularity in fibrotic areas and hypervascularity in nonfibrotic areas has been reported [43]. Increases in tumor necrosis factor α, platelet-derived growth factor, fibroblast growth factor, and profibrotic leukotrienes may drive vascular remodeling and fibrosis [44]. Reduced expression of bone morphogenetic protein receptor type-2 (BMPR2) may play a role in ILD-PH as well [37]. It is believed that decreased BMPR2 activity results in an imbalance in BMP and transforming growth factor β (TGF-β), favoring TGF-β, leading to inflammation and angiogenesis [37]. It is likely that there are genetic differences that explain the development of the above alterations that lead to pulmonary vascular remodeling and ILD-PH in some patients. Gene expression of lung tissue from ILD patients with significant PH (mPAP ≥ 40 mmHg) and without PH were compared [45]. Patients with severe ILD-PH had a gene profile with enhanced myofibroblast proliferation and vascular remodeling, while those with no PH had pro-inflammatory genes [45]. Perhaps in the future, clinicians will be able to accurately molecularly phenotype ILD patients to garner important prognostic information and potentially inform therapeutic approach.

Diagnosis of Pulmonary Hypertension Associated with Interstitial Lung Disease

Due to the overlapping symptomatology of ILD and PH, both of which cause dyspnea on exertion, need for supplemental oxygen, and cough, it can be difficult to discern when ILD-PH develops. To further complicate things, no single diagnostic test short of right heart catheterization can accurately establish the diagnosis, although a number of noninvasive tests can be suggestive of the condition. Clinicians must maintain a high index of suspicion and should use every clinical interaction as an opportunity to screen for development of ILD-PH.

As mentioned above, the symptoms of PH are non-specific and overlap substantially with those of ILD. Common reported early symptoms include fatigue and dyspnea on exertion [46]. As PH progresses, more severe symptoms including chest pain and syncope may develop. Physical exam in insensitive for diagnosis of PH. Associated findings include jugular venous distention, peripheral edema, ascites, right ventricular heave, and loud P2 on cardiac exam, although no single finding can accurately predict the presence of PH. The combined findings of peripheral edema, parasternal heave, and jugular venous distention were suggestive of PH. [47] It should be noted that these physical exam findings are all manifestations of right ventricular failure and only occur with more advanced PH. Therefore, if one waits for physical exam signs to develop in ILD-PH it would lead to substantial delays in diagnosis and miss numerous cases.

While no single non-invasive diagnostic tool can establish the diagnosis, a number of commonly obtained tests can be suggestive of the diagnosis. Somewhat surprisingly, degree of restriction on PFTs measured by plethysmography or spirometry fails to predict ILD-PH [48]. However, DLCO can alert clinicians to the diagnosis of PH in several ways. Severely reduced DLCO (<40%), DLCO reduced out of proportion to lung volumes (FVC/DLCO ratio > 1.6), and changing DLCO (DLCO worsening with stable FVC, DLCO decline of > 15%, or rapidly declining DLCO) were all identified as parameters suggestive of development of ILD-PH on a recent Delphi survey of experts in ILD-PH [49]. DLCO also has prognostic significance in ILD-PH. A multivariate analysis found it to be the only lung function parameter predictive of survival, with ILD-PH patients with DLCO < 32% predicted having 1- and 5-year survival rates of 68% and 13%, respectively [50].

Exercise capacity testing also has utility in the diagnostic evaluation of ILD-PH. 6MWT can be suggestive of development of ILD-PH in a number of ways. Both reduced exercise capacity as measured by 6MWT distance and exertional desaturation are associated with development of ILD-PH and are predictive of increased mortality [33, 51–54]. Impaired heart rate recovery, which is defined as the maximum heart rate minus heart rate at 1 min of recovery < 13 beats per minute, following 6MWT is also associated with PH in patients with IPF [55]. Some studies have demonstrated the ability of cardiopulmonary exercise testing to predict ILD-PH or provide prognostic information in ILD-PH; however, cardiopulmonary exercise testing has less practical utility given the infrequency of performance and logistical difficulties in performing in patients requiring oxygen supplementation during exercise [56]. [57]

Chest imaging is commonly performed in the diagnostic evaluation of patients with ILD and may provide insight into the development of ILD-PH. Akin to the failure of degree of restriction of PFT to predict ILD-PH, the degree of fibrosis on CT imaging has not been consistently demonstrated to predict ILD-PH [58]. Other CT findings can be predictive of ILD-PH however, including a pulmonary artery to aorta ratio > 0.9, as well as a ratio of the RV to the left ventricle > 1 [59–61] (Fig. 9.1). Swift and colleagues developed a CT angiography derived model

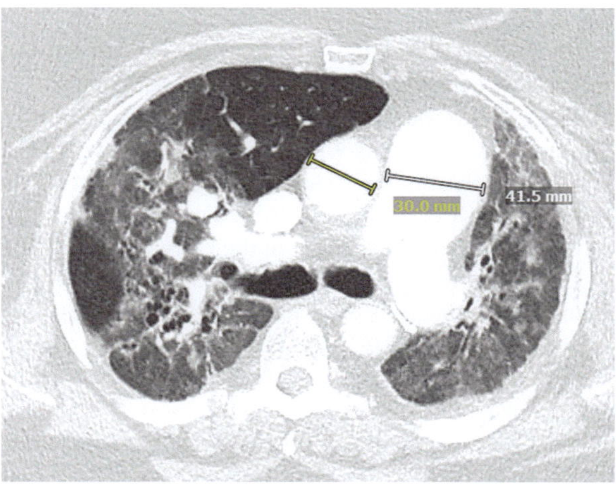

Fig. 9.1 CT findings suggestive of ILD-PH. (**a**) Pulmonary artery to aorta ratio > 0.9 (**b**) RV to LV ratio > 1

incorporating pulmonary artery diameter, right ventricular outflow tract thickness, septal angle and left ventricular area with good performance characteristics for diagnosis of PAH, however this study was not specific to the ILD-PH population [62]. It would be interesting to see if this prediction model performs similarly well in the ILD population.

TTE is the most commonly employed noninvasive screening modality for ILD-PH. The primary means of diagnosis of PH by TTE in the majority of studies over the years has depended on estimation of the right ventricular systolic pressure by measurement of the tricuspid regurgitant jet [41]. Unfortunately, adequate visualization of the RV can be difficult in patients with ILD and can lead to over- or underestimation of right ventricular systolic pressure or failure to provide an estimate at all [13, 63]. Newer studies incorporating a more comprehensive view of the RV, including variables such as RV outflow tract diameter, tricuspid annular plane systolic excursion, have demonstrated improved diagnostic accuracy [63, 64]. Bax and colleagues combined right ventricular systolic pressure with five other indirect markers of PH (right atrial area, early diastolic pulmonary regurgitant velocity, right ventricular fractional area of change, LV eccentricity index, and RV to left ventricle basal diameter) to make a multivariable predictive model with that accurately detected severe PH in ILD patients [65]. Based on the available data, it appears TTE can detect more advanced PH manifesting right ventricular dysfunction with reasonable diagnostic accuracy. Unfortunately, ILD-PH with modest elevations in pulmonary artery pressures still holds prognostic significance yet may fail to produce notable changes in RV size or function, making TTE a suboptimal diagnostic modality for early detection of ILD-PH. The inadequacies of TTE for diagnosis of ILD-PH were highlighted in a study of 265 ILD patients with suspected PH who had both TTE and RHC [66]. In the study, 40% of patients classified as low risk for PH based on TTE findings by European Society of Cardiology/European Respiratory Society guidelines were found to have PH when RHC was performed. This study highlights the need for clinicians to maintain a high index of suspicion in order to facilitate early diagnosis of ILD-PH, even in the face of a normal TTE.

There is limited data to support the use of cardiac MRI for ILD-PH, and this modality is not widely used in clinical practice due to cost and accessibility. Cardiac MRI appears to be well-tolerated in ILD patients and may have a role in assessing RV function in patients with poor TTE windows [67]. A cardiac MRI model using ventricular mass index, systolic septal angle, and PA relative area of change diagnosed severe PH accurately [68]. Further study will be required to determine if cardiac MRI may have a role in the early diagnosis of ILD-PH.

Given that numerous tests can be suggestive of the diagnosis of ILD-PH, many attempts have been made to develop a composite score to non-invasively detect the presence of ILD-PH [65, 69–72]. Unfortunately, the majority of these studies have methodological limitations including failure to confirm PH with RHC and lack of validation in an external cohort. In fact, only four scores have to date been externally validated. The first, by Bax and colleagues, utilizes echocardiographic parameters and is focused on identifying severe ILD-PH and lacks the sensitivity and specificity to detect mild or moderate ILD-PH [65]. Similarly, a score developed by

Zisman et al, which incorporates pulse oximetry and %predicted FVC and %predicted DLCO, was only validated in a cohort of patients with advanced ILD awaiting lung transplant and may miss less severe cases of ILD-PH [73]. The FORD model is based on readily available clinical parameters including FVC to DLCO ratio (F), oxygen saturation nadir on 6MWT (O), race (R), and six-minute walk distance (D) [69]. It demonstrated reasonable accuracy in the derivation and validation cohorts, with areas under the curve (AUC) of 0.75 and 0.69, respectively. Parikh and colleagues recently validated the ILD-PH detection tool [72]. This tool incorporates eight weighted parameters and provides a low, intermediate, or high risk of ILD-PH based on the combined score. The authors report a sensitivity of 93.3%, specificity of 90.9%, and AUC of 0.921 for diagnosing ILD-PH. Tables 9.3 and 9.4 summarizes the FORD and ILD-PH detection score.

Table 9.3 FORD model

Ford score		
Predictor	Category	Points[a]
FVC%/DLCO%	<2	0
	2–3	2
	>3	34
Oxygen nadir on 6MWT	>88	0
	83–88	19
	≤82	33
Race	White	0
	Non-white	20
Distance (on 6MWT)	>350	0
	250–350	9
	<250	13

FVC forced vital capacity, *DLCO* diffusing capacity of the lung for carbon monoxide, *6MWT* six-minute walk test

[a]Total score 0–100 with higher scores having a greater likelihood of ILD-PH

Table 9.4 ILD-PH detection score

ILD-PH detection score	Score
6MWD < 350 m	2
Physical exam for PH	2
DLCO < 40%	2
Supplemental oxygen	2
Elevated BNP	1
Syncope or presyncope	1
PA enlargement on CT Chest	1
CTD or sarcoidosis	1
≤3 Low risk	
4–5 Intermediate risk	
≥6 High risk	

6MWT six-minute walk test, *DLCO* diffusing capacity of the lung for carbon monoxide, *PH* pulmonary hypertension, *BNP* brain natriuretic peptide, *PA* pulmonary artery, *CTD* connective tissue disease

Although multiple non-invasive tests can suggest ILD-PH, the diagnosis can only be established and severity assessed by RHC. Careful attention must be paid to proper performance of RHC, as swings in intra-thoracic pressure can make interpretation of RHC in ILD difficult. Exercise testing or fluid challenge during RHC may be useful in unmasking group 2 PH and should be considered, particularly in patients with cardiovascular comorbidities and/or ECHO parameters suggestive of diastolic dysfunction [74]. RHC is an invasive and time-consuming test, and while rare, can be associated with complications. Despite this, since the advent of effective pharmacologic therapy for ILD-PH, clinicians should be proactive about referring patients for RHC if there is a reasonable likelihood of ILD-PH. Additionally, RHC is required for lung transplant evaluations, so all patients undergoing transplant evaluation will require this test.

It is of paramount importance that clinicians maintain a high index of suspicion and constantly monitor for the onset of ILD-PH. No formal recommendations exist regarding the optimal screening strategy or frequency of screening for ILD-PH. We recommend carefully scrutinizing performed testing for evidence of ILD-PH. Additionally, we typically perform screening TTE on an annual basis for all patients with ILD. Patients with clinical or echocardiographic evidence of ILD-PH should be referred for RHC. Additionally, there should be a low threshold for referral of patients with unexplained worsening clinical status for RHC. Another important point to emphasize is that even if patients do not have ILD-PH initially, there is an increasing incidence of ILD-PH over time as ILD progresses. For that reason, clinicians must remain vigilant for the diagnosis throughout the clinical course. Figure 9.2 summarizes a proposed diagnostic algorithm for screening of ILD-PH.

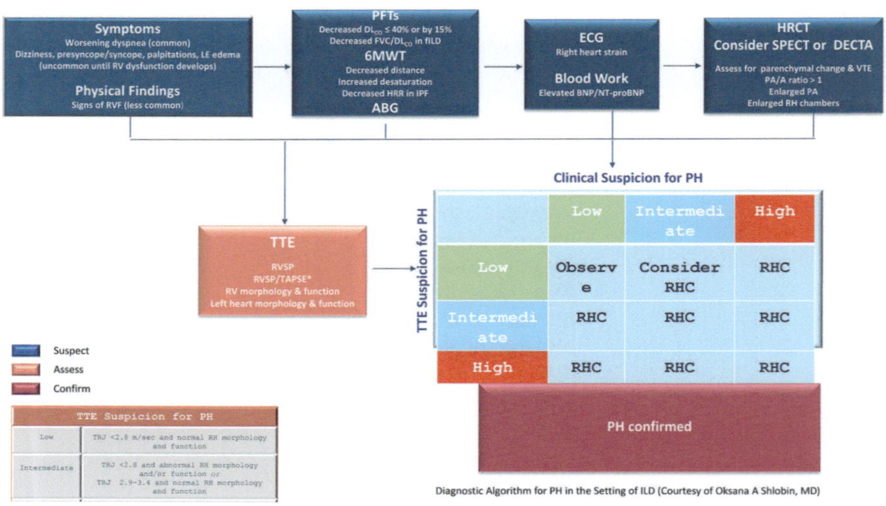

Fig. 9.2 Proposed diagnostic algorithm for screening for ILD-PH. (Courtesy of Oksana A. Shlobin, MD)

Treatment of ILD-PH

The treatment paradigm for ILD-PH, particularly with regard to use of pulmonary vasodilators, remains controversial. The reasons for this are myriad, but the primary reason is a paucity of high-quality randomized clinical trials (RCTs), as well as contradictory data amongst the available studies. In this section, we will attempt to summarize the available literature on the topic and provide a proposed algorithm for treatment of ILD-PH.

Rational arguments can be made both for and against the use of pulmonary vasodilators in ILD-PH. Those favoring treatment will point to the morbidity and mortality of ILD-PH, which seems to be driven primarily by the pulmonary vascular disease. Given this relationship, intuitively one might hypothesize that reducing the pulmonary pressures with treatment and consequently improving RV dysfunction and cardiac output would translate into improved outcomes. Proponents of treatment would also point to the numerous pharmaceutical agents that have been successfully employed in treatment of PAH. Unfortunately, the success seen in treatment of PAH was not realized in many of the trials of ILD-PH. There are numerous potential explanations for this. One hypothesis is that use of non-selective pulmonary vasodilators may undo hypoxic pulmonary vasoconstriction in areas of the lung most severely affected by pulmonary fibrosis, resulting in ventilation/perfusion (V/Q) mismatch. For the most part, this concern has not been observed in clinical trials. A small trial of intravenous epoprostenol did result in increased hypoxemia; however, improvements in oxygenation have been observed in trials of sildenafil and inhaled prostanoids [75, 76]. V/Q mismatch does not absolutely translate into clinical worsening, as the resultant hypoxemia may be correctable with supplemental oxygenation with an end result of improved cardiac output and increased oxygen delivery to tissues. Another potential deleterious result of pulmonary vasodilator therapy in ILD-PH is development of pulmonary edema due to pulmonary venoocclusive lesions in ILD patients. While theoretically a concern, this phenomenon has rarely observed with use of pulmonary vasodilators in ILD-PH. [77, 78]

Given that these potential concerns have largely not been realized in practice, why then has there been a lack of success in the majority of the clinical trials to date? First, conduction of RCTs on a relatively rare condition with poor outcomes can be difficult. Clinicians may elect to treat off-label rather than referring for clinical trials. Also, many trials performed to date utilized echocardiography or DLCO to establish the diagnosis of ILD-PH rather than RHC. This strategy runs the risk of enrolling patients without ILD-PH or with PH due to other etiologies unlikely to have a favorable response to pulmonary vasodilator therapy. Most importantly, severity of PH has not been taken into consideration in the design of many trials. The severity of ILD-PH is a spectrum, with most cases with non-severe PH. Perhaps patients with mild hemodynamic derangements but more severe fibrotic disease are a distinct phenotype, less likely to respond to pulmonary vasodilator therapy, with the elevations in PAPs merely a surrogate for the severity of lung disease. If this is the case, RCTs would have to specifically enroll patients with more severe, maladaptive elevations in PAPs that are out of proportion to the severity of fibrotic lung disease. Alternatively, mild ILD-PH may represent early disease that will progress over time and ultimately would prove pulmonary vasodilator therapy beneficial; however, RCTs fail to follow patients long enough to demonstrate a salutary effect of treatment. There may also be differences in the individual pulmonary vasodilator agents or their delivery mechanisms that could influence the response to pulmonary vasodilators.

With these potential obstacles to successful clinical trial design in mind, we will review the major clinical trials of pulmonary vasodilator therapy in ILD-PH to date, organized by drug class. Endothelin receptor antagonists (ERAs) have been studied in six RCTs [79–84]. Four of these trials did not specifically enroll patients with ILD-PH, but rather focused on functional status and disease progression in a general IPF population. Studies on bosentan and macitentan failed to demonstrate any conclusive benefit in the IPF population [79–81]. The Randomized, Placebo-Controlled Study to Evaluate Safety and Effectiveness of Ambrisentan in IPF (ARTEMIS-IPF) was terminated early for potential harm after enrollment of approximately 500 patients [82]. The Study of Ambrisentan in Subjects with Pulmonary Hypertension Associated With Idiopathic Pulmonary Fibrosis (ARTEMIS-PH), which did include only RHC-proven ILD-PH, was terminated after a subgroup analysis failed to demonstrate any signs of efficacy and suggested harm [84]. Similarly, the Bosentan in Pulmonary Hypertension in Interstitial Lung Disease Treatment Study (B-PHIT) showed no improvement in symptoms, hemodynamics, or functional outcomes in a group of RHC-confirmed ILD-PH treated with bosentan [83]. Given the lack of efficacy demonstrated in the majority of studies, as well as potential harm associated with ambrisentan in the ARTEMIS trial, use of ambrisentan is not recommended in IPF-PH [6]. The authors' practice is to avoid use of all ERAs based on the available data.

The Safety of Riociguat in Patients With Symptomatic Pulmonary Hypertension Associated with Idiopathic Interstitial Pneumonia (RISE-IIP) was a phase IIb study examining the effects of the soluble guanylate cyclase stimulator riociguat in a cohort of RHC-proven PH patients with IIPs, which excluded patients with CTD-related ILD [85]. A small pilot trial of riociguat in ILD-PH demonstrating favorable hemodynamic effects and minimal safety issues served as the impetus for RISE-IIP [86]. Unfortunately, the study failed to yield similar results to this pilot trial and was terminated early for increased serious adverse effects and death in both the treatment group and the cross-over arm of the open-label extension study. On the basis of the RISE-IIP study, use of riociguat is contraindicated in patients with IIP-PH [6].

Studies of the phosphodiesteras-5 (PDE-5) inhibitor sildenafil stand in contrast to the discouraging results of the studies on ERAs and riociguat. The Sildenafil Trial of Exercise Performance in Idiopathic Pulmonary Fibrosis (STEP-IPF) compared sildenafil to placebo in a group of 180 patients with advanced IPF [76]. While the study did not require PH by TTE or RHC, it did require reduced DLCO as an enrollment criteria, making it likely that a large portion of the participants had ILD-PH. The study failed to meet its primary endpoint of improvement in 6MWT of $\geq 20\%$, but demonstrated improvements in a number of secondary endpoints including DLCO, arterial oxygen saturations, and quality of life metrics.

While not an RCT, the COMPERA registry examined patients with ILD-PH initiated on pulmonary vasodilator therapy in a prospective manner [26]. Of the 151 patients included, 88% were treated with PDE-5 inhibitors. Nearly 25% of patients improved functional class and the treated group demonstrated a median 6MWT improvement of 24.5 m. A retrospective, observational cohort study followed 128 patients with RHC-proven PH, 50 of whom were treated with PDE5 inhibitors. They found that survival was significantly longer in those treated with PDE5 inhibitors (median 2.18 years versus 0.94 years, $p = 0.003$) [87]. The aggregate data on sildenafil seems to suggest that its use is unlikely to be harmful and may provide benefit on functional status and quality of life. Ideally, the utility of sildenafil in ILD-PH would be examined in an adequately powered RCT, however it is unlikely that such a trial will ever be undertaken.

Over the years, numerous small series reported on the effects of prostanoid therapy via various delivery mechanisms (inhaled, IV) in ILD-PH with mixed results [75, 88, 89]. In 2021, the landmark INCREASE trial of inhaled treprostinil in ILD-PH was published [90]. This 16-week, phase 3, multicenter, randomized, double-blind study compared placebo to inhaled treprostinil delivered by an iNEB device in 326 patients with ILD-PH. The study met its primary endpoint of improvement in the 6MWT distance at 16 weeks, making it the first RCT of pulmonary vasodilator therapy in PH-ILF to ever conclusively demonstrate benefit. Additionally, inhaled treprostinil improved a number of secondary endpoints including reductions in NT-proBNP and time to clinical worsening. The effects of inhaled treprostinil seem dose-dependent with a follow-up study demonstrating greater benefit in terms of preventing clinical worsening and achieving clinical improvement in patients who titrated to a higher dosage (≥9 breaths per session) [91]. A subsequent post-hoc analysis found that continued treatment with inhaled treprostinil in patients who experienced a first disease progression event reduced the risk for subsequent disease progression events including 15% or greater decline in 6MWT distance, 10% or greater decline in FVC, acute exacerbation of IPF, cardiopulmonary hospitalization, lung transplantation, or death [92]. Based on the available data, inhaled treprostinil has established itself as the first-line and only FDA-approved therapy for ILD-PH.

Proposed Treatment Algorithm

As mentioned above, there remains no universally agreed upon treatment strategy for ILD-PH, however, some general aspects of treatment do seem to garner unanimous support. Although it has not been demonstrated to directly affect the trajectory of ILD-PH, clinicians should institute appropriate treatment of the underlying ILD. Pulmonary rehabilitation should be recommended to combat deconditioning and improve quality of life. [93] Counseling on smoking cessation and appropriate vaccinations should be provided. Patients should be screened for nocturnal desaturation and sleep disordered breathing, and these should be corrected with supplemental oxygen or continuous positive airway pressure (CPAP) as appropriate. Serial screening for exertional desaturation should be performed and if discovered, supplemental oxygen should be prescribed. Diuretic therapy should be prescribed for patients with evidence of volume overload. Clinicians should not lose sight of the fact that ILD-PH is associated with a markedly attenuated life span, even when treated with pulmonary vasodilator therapy. Therefore, timely referral of appropriate candidates for lung transplantation evaluation is recommended.

Recommendations for institution of pulmonary vasodilator therapy are less clear. There has been some evolution in the guidance on treatment of patients with ILD-PH in recent years. Traditionally, a review of the patient's hemodynamics and extent of lung disease by imaging and PFTs was undertaken, with less severe ILD and more severe hemodynamic impairment favoring use of pulmonary vasodilators. The 6th WSPH recommended management of patients with PH and "limited chronic lung disease" according to established PAH guidelines. [4] The 7th WSPH guidelines distanced themselves from this guidance saying "analyses of various registries strongly suggest that the response to therapy is reduced in this group (mild chronic lung disease and PH) in comparison to those with a classic IPAH phenotype." [12] Based on this decreased emphasis on categorization of ILD-PH as "WHO Group 1" phenotype or "WHO Group 3" phenotype, it seems prudent to focus more on the degree of hemodynamic impairment when developing a treatment plan.

The 2022 ESC/ERS PAH guidelines recommend an individualized approach to treatment for ILD-PH and also that treatment is undertaken at experienced PAH centers [6]. Furthermore, they emphasize the importance of referral for lung transplantation in patients with ILD-PH. The authors concur with all these statements, however, the practice patterns of the authors differ somewhat from the latest ESC/ERS treatment guidelines with regard to a few points [6]. The ESC/ERS guidelines provide somewhat confusing guidance at first glance, recommending against use of PAH in lung disease and non-severe PH, but also stating use of inhaled treprostinil may be considered in patients with ILD-PH. It should be noted, however, that there is a small footnote on the recommendation regarding non-severe PH that states "this does not include inhaled trepostinil, which may be considered in patients with PH associated with ILD, regardless of severity." [6] The authors will typically advocate for treatment of patients who met the enrollment criteria of the INCREASE study (mPAP $\geq$ 25 mmHg and PVR $\geq$ 3 WUs) [90]. The INCREASE trial itself is sometimes used as an argument against treatment of non-severe ILD-PH. The origin of this is grounded in an analysis in the supplementary appendix of the INCREASE paper that shows no statistically significant difference in 6MWT distance for patients with PVR < 4 WUs [90]. It should be noted that very few patients with PVR < 4 were included in the INCREASE trial ($n = 52$ of 241 with data to analyze on week 16 6MWT). Given the progressive nature of ILD-PH, it seems likely that treatment may delay the onset of more severe ILD-PH and potentially improve outcomes. This notion is supported by a follow-up manuscript of the INCREASE population which found that patients with a PVR $\leq$ 5 WU without a treatment delay had a lower likelihood of hospitalization, lung disease exacerbation, or death [94]. The authors would not currently recommend use of pulmonary vasodilator therapy in ILD-PH not meeting the inclusion criteria of the INCREASE trial (mPAP 20–25 mmHg and PVR < 3 WUs). These patients should be followed over time to monitor for progression of ILD-PH to a point warranted institution of therapy. Another issue not addressed in the guidelines is how to handle very severe ILD-PH. The authors will use parenteral prostanoids as first-line therapy in patients with very severe ILD-PH with a CI < 2 WU or significant RV dysfunction on an individual basis. Such off-label use has been validated in retrospective case series but should only be undertaken in centers of excellence in PH and requires careful monitoring of the patient. [89]

The authors also deviate from the ESC/ERS guidelines with regard to choice of pulmonary vasodilator. The authors would advocate for inhaled treprostinil as first-line therapy for ILD-PH rather than a PDE-5 inhibitor, both of which received a level IIB recommendation [6]. This decision is based on the fact that INCREASE is the only high-quality RCT to ever conclusively demonstrate improvement with pulmonary vasodilator therapy in ILD-PH. Sildenafil therapy would be reserved for those patients who are intolerant to inhaled treprostinil, or who have ongoing RV dysfunction and PVR elevation despite optimization of inhaled treprostinil. The ESC/ERS guidelines recommend avoidance of riociguat in IIP-PH and ambrisentan in treatment of IPF-PH. While the authors agree with these recommendations, they would extend them to avoidance of use of ERAs at large in ILD-PH due to lack of benefit with bosentan and macitentan. Figure 9.3 provides a proposed treatment algorithm.

A few specific populations warrant special consideration. CTD-ILD-PH appears to be distinct from other forms of ILD-PH with regard to response to pulmonary vasodilator therapy and outcome [12]. An analysis looking at outcomes of treatment ILD-PH patients found 5-year survival rates of 56% in CTD-ILD-PH versus only 15% in IPF-PH [33]. It seems CTD-ILD-PH patients, particularly those with mild ILD, may respond more favorably to pulmonary vasodilator therapy and potentially could delay the need for lung transplantation. Further study is required on this unique population. CPFE patients may also respond differently to pulmonary vasodilator therapy. A post-hoc analysis of the RISE-IIP trial of riociguat in IIP-PH, which was terminated early for harm in the treated group, found that patients with more emphysema than fibrosis may have driven the negative outcomes of the study [95]. Similarly, the PERFECT trial examining the effects of inhaled treprostinil in COPD-PH was terminated early for adverse events and increased mortality in the treatment group [96]. There were however 82 patients (25.2%) with CPFE included in the INCREASE Trial [90]. A subgroup analysis of the trial showed no statistically significant improvement in 6MWT at 16 weeks in this specific population, however, it was underpowered to do so. A post hoc analysis looking at the multiple disease progression events showed that patients with CPFE benefited from the treatment. [92] Based in the available evidence it seems reasonable to trial inhaled trepostinil in CPFE patients with predominantly fibrotic phenotype while cautiously monitoring for adverse effects. Further study of CPFE-PH patients is required to better understand the varying responses of various phenotypes.

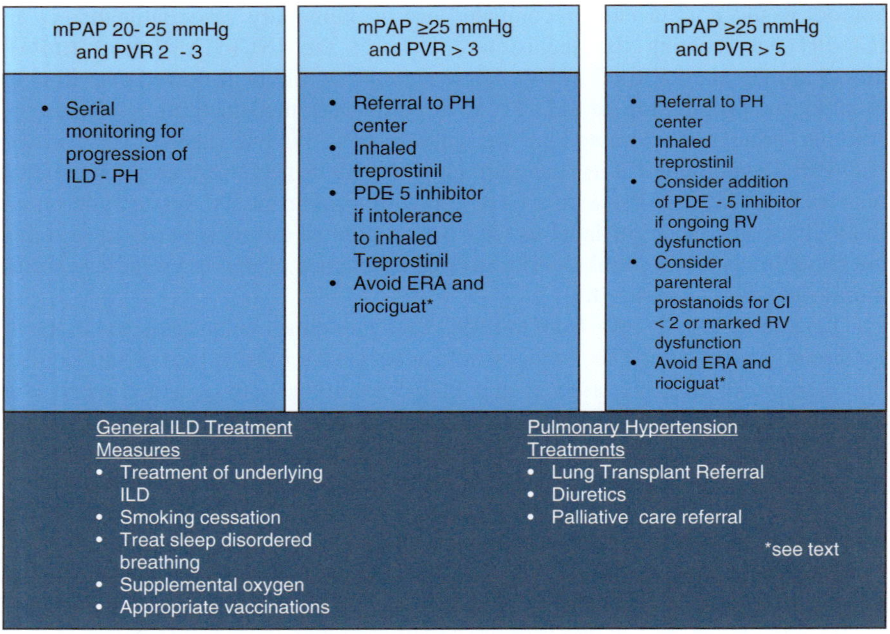

Fig. 9.3 Proposed treatment algorithm for ILD-PH

The Future of ILD-PH

Despite an explosion in interest and research into ILD-PH in recent years, many questions remain unanswered. The natural history and optimal screening algorithm of ILD-PH are incompletely understood. It is hoped that the Pulmonary Hypertension Screening in Patients with Interstitial Lung Disease for Earlier Detection (PHINDER) trial and DeciPHer-ILD registry will lend further insight to these areas [97, 98]. Sotatercept, an activin receptor type IIa-Fc fusion protein, represents an exciting a new treatment pathway in WHO Group 1 PAH [99]. Whether this agent has applicability on ILD-PH requires future study. Several studies of novel agents are underway as well [100]. [101] Hopefully, continued study will increase our understanding of ILD-PH and produce new therapeutic interventions to address this debilitating and deadly condition.

Conclusion

Great advances in the understanding and treatment of ILD-PH have been realized in recent years, yet it remains a deadly condition associated with significant morbidity and markedly reduced survival. Further study is needed to determine how best to screen for ILD-PH and to determine the utility of pulmonary vasodilator therapy in treating less severe ILD-PH. In the meantime, clinicians must maintain a high index of suspicion to diagnose ILD-PH in a timely manner and institute appropriate therapy. In the age of emerging therapeutics such as inhaled prostanoids, clinicians must not lose sight of the full spectrum of care for patients with ILD-PH, which includes oxygen therapy, vaccination, pulmonary rehabilitation, early evaluation for lung transplantation, and palliative care. We hope that continued study of this condition will result in improved therapeutic options and ultimately better outcomes for this challenging patient population.

References

1. Lettieri CJ, Nathan SD, Barnett SD, Ahmad S, Shorr AF. Prevalence and outcomes of pulmonary arterial hypertension in advanced idiopathic pulmonary fibrosis. Chest. 2006;129(3):746–52.
2. Nathan SD, Waxman A, Tapson V. Inhaled treprostinil in group 3 pulmonary hypertension. Reply N Engl J Med. 2021;384(19):1871–2.
3. Kovacs G, Bartolome S, Denton CP, Gatzoulis MA, Gu S, Khanna D, et al. Definition, classification and diagnosis of pulmonary hypertension. Eur Respir J. 2024;64(4).
4. Nathan SD, Barbera JA, Gaine SP, Harari S, Martinez FJ, Olschewski H, et al. Pulmonary hypertension in chronic lung disease and hypoxia. Eur Respir J. 2019;53(1).
5. Seeger W, Adir Y, Barbera JA, Champion H, Coghlan JG, Cottin V, et al. Pulmonary hypertension in chronic lung diseases. J Am Coll Cardiol. 2013;62(25 Suppl):D109–16.
6. Humbert M, Kovacs G, Hoeper MM, Badagliacca R, Berger RMF, Brida M, et al. 2022 ESC/ERS Guidelines for the diagnosis and treatment of pulmonary hypertension. Eur Heart J. 2022;43(38):3618–731.
7. Zeder K, Avian A, Bachmaier G, Douschan P, Foris V, Sassmann T, et al. Elevated pulmonary vascular resistance predicts mortality in COPD patients. Eur Respir J. 2021;58(2).
8. Olsson KM, Hoeper MM, Pausch C, Grunig E, Huscher D, Pittrow D, et al. Pulmonary vascular resistance predicts mortality in patients with pulmonary hypertension associated with interstitial lung disease: results from the COMPERA registry. Eur Respir J. 2021;58(2).
9. Dhont S, Zwaenepoel B, Vandecasteele E, Brusselle G, De Pauw M. Pulmonary hypertension in interstitial lung disease: an area of unmet clinical need. ERJ Open Res. 2022;8(4).
10. Tyagi R, Kant S, Verma SK, Kushwaha RAS, Kumar S, Garg R, et al. Spectrum of interstitial lung diseases and their association with pulmonary hypertension. Monaldi Arch Chest Dis. 2021;92(3).
11. Raghu G, Amatto VC, Behr J, Stowasser S. Comorbidities in idiopathic pulmonary fibrosis patients: a systematic literature review. Eur Respir J. 2015;46(4):1113–30.
12. Shlobin OA, Adir Y, Barbera JA, Cottin V, Harari S, Jutant EM, et al. Pulmonary hypertension associated with lung diseases. Eur Respir J. 2024;64(4)
13. Nathan SD, Shlobin OA, Ahmad S, Koch J, Barnett SD, Ad N, et al. Serial development of pulmonary hypertension in patients with idiopathic pulmonary fibrosis. Respiration. 2008;76(3):288–94.
14. Nathan SD, Barnett SD, King CS, Provencher S, Barbera JA, Pastre J, et al. Impact of the new definition for pulmonary hypertension in patients with lung disease: an analysis of the United Network for Organ Sharing database. Pulm Circ. 2021;11(2):2045894021999960.
15. Nikkho SM, Richter MJ, Shen E, Abman SH, Antoniou K, Chung J, et al. Clinical significance of pulmonary hypertension in interstitial lung disease: a consensus statement from

the Pulmonary Vascular Research Institute's innovative drug development initiative-Group 3 pulmonary hypertension. Pulm Circ. 2022;12(3):e12127.
16. King CS, Brown AW, Shlobin OA, Weir N, Libre M, Franco-Palacios D, et al. Prevalence and impact of WHO group 3 pulmonary hypertension in advanced idiopathic nonspecific interstitial pneumonia. Eur Respir J. 2018;52(1).
17. Cottin V, Nunes H, Mouthon L, Gamondes D, Lazor R, Hachulla E, et al. Combined pulmonary fibrosis and emphysema syndrome in connective tissue disease. Arthritis Rheum. 2011;63(1):295–304.
18. Walscher J, Gross B, Morisset J, Johannson KA, Vasakova M, Bruhwyler J, et al. Comorbidities and survival in patients with chronic hypersensitivity pneumonitis. Respir Res. 2020;21(1):12.
19. Todd NW, Lavania S, Park MH, Iacono AT, Franks TJ, Galvin JR, et al. Variable prevalence of pulmonary hypertension in patients with advanced interstitial pneumonia. J Heart Lung Transplant. 2010;29(2):188–94.
20. Oliveira RK, Pereira CA, Ramos RP, Ferreira EV, Messina CM, Kuranishi LT, et al. A haemodynamic study of pulmonary hypertension in chronic hypersensitivity pneumonitis. Eur Respir J. 2014;44(2):415–24.
21. Gunnarsson R, Andreassen AK, Molberg O, Lexberg AS, Time K, Dhainaut AS, et al. Prevalence of pulmonary hypertension in an unselected, mixed connective tissue disease cohort: results of a nationwide, Norwegian cross-sectional multicentre study and review of current literature. Rheumatology (Oxford). 2013;52(7):1208–13.
22. Handa T, Nagai S, Miki S, Ueda S, Yukawa N, Fushimi Y, et al. Incidence of pulmonary hypertension and its clinical relevance in patients with interstitial pneumonias: comparison between idiopathic and collagen vascular disease associated interstitial pneumonias. Intern Med. 2007;46(12):831–7.
23. Piccari L, Wort SJ, Meloni F, Rizzo M, Price LC, Martino L, et al. The effect of borderline pulmonary hypertension on survival in chronic lung disease. Respiration. 2022;101(8):717–27.
24. Shorr AF, Wainright JL, Cors CS, Lettieri CJ, Nathan SD. Pulmonary hypertension in patients with pulmonary fibrosis awaiting lung transplant. Eur Respir J. 2007;30(4):715–21.
25. Chebib N, Mornex JF, Traclet J, Philit F, Khouatra C, Zeghmar S, et al. Pulmonary hypertension in chronic lung diseases: comparison to other pulmonary hypertension groups. Pulm Circ. 2018;8(2):2045894018775056.
26. Hoeper MM, Behr J, Held M, Grunig E, Vizza CD, Vonk-Noordegraaf A, et al. Pulmonary hypertension in patients with chronic fibrosing idiopathic interstitial pneumonias. PLoS One. 2015;10(12):e0141911.
27. Boutou AK, Pitsiou GG, Trigonis I, Papakosta D, Kontou PK, Chavouzis N, et al. Exercise capacity in idiopathic pulmonary fibrosis: the effect of pulmonary hypertension. Respirology. 2011;16(3):451–8.
28. Nadrous HF, Pellikka PA, Krowka MJ, Swanson KL, Chaowalit N, Decker PA, et al. Pulmonary hypertension in patients with idiopathic pulmonary fibrosis. Chest. 2005;128(4):2393–9.
29. Song JW, Song JK, Kim DS. Echocardiography and brain natriuretic peptide as prognostic indicators in idiopathic pulmonary fibrosis. Respir Med. 2009;103(2):180–6.
30. Kimura M, Taniguchi H, Kondoh Y, Kimura T, Kataoka K, Nishiyama O, et al. Pulmonary hypertension as a prognostic indicator at the initial evaluation in idiopathic pulmonary fibrosis. Respiration. 2013;85(6):456–63.
31. Oliveira RKF, Ota-Arakaki JS, Gomes PS, Gimenez A, Messina CMS, Ramos RP, et al. Pulmonary haemodynamics and mortality in chronic hypersensitivity pneumonitis. Eur Respir J. 2018;51(6).
32. Chen X, Guo J, Yu D, Jie B, Zhou Y. Predictors of mortality in progressive fibrosing interstitial lung diseases. Front Pharmacol. 2021;12:754851.
33. Alhamad EH, Cal JG, Alrajhi NN, Alharbi WM. Predictors of mortality in patients with interstitial lung disease-associated pulmonary hypertension. J Clin Med. 2020;9(12).

34. Leard LE, Holm AM, Valapour M, Glanville AR, Attawar S, Aversa M, et al. Consensus document for the selection of lung transplant candidates: an update from the International Society for Heart and Lung Transplantation. J Heart Lung Transplant. 2021;40(11):1349–79.
35. Hamada K, Nagai S, Tanaka S, Handa T, Shigematsu M, Nagao T, et al. Significance of pulmonary arterial pressure and diffusion capacity of the lung as prognosticator in patients with idiopathic pulmonary fibrosis. Chest. 2007;131(3):650–6.
36. Nathan SD. Progress in the treatment of pulmonary hypertension associated with interstitial lung disease. Am J Respir Crit Care Med. 2023;208(3):238–46.
37. Piccari L, Allwood B, Antoniou K, Chung JH, Hassoun PM, Nikkho SM, et al. Pathogenesis, clinical features, and phenotypes of pulmonary hypertension associated with interstitial lung disease: a consensus statement from the Pulmonary Vascular Research Institute's Innovative Drug Development Initiative—Group 3 Pulmonary Hypertension. Pulm Circ. 2023;13(2):e12213.
38. Klinger JR, Group III. Pulmonary hypertension: pulmonary hypertension associated with lung disease: epidemiology, pathophysiology, and treatments. Cardiol Clin. 2016;34(3):413–33.
39. Janaszak-Jasiecka A, Ploska A, Wieronska JM, Dobrucki LW, Kalinowski L. Endothelial dysfunction due to eNOS uncoupling: molecular mechanisms as potential therapeutic targets. Cell Mol Biol Lett. 2023;28(1):21.
40. Zhao YY, Zhao YD, Mirza MK, Huang JH, Potula HH, Vogel SM, et al. Persistent eNOS activation secondary to caveolin-1 deficiency induces pulmonary hypertension in mice and humans through PKG nitration. J Clin Invest. 2009;119(7):2009–18.
41. King CS, Shlobin OA. The trouble with group 3 pulmonary hypertension in interstitial lung disease: dilemmas in diagnosis and the conundrum of treatment. Chest. 2020;158(4):1651–64.
42. Nathan SD, Noble PW, Tuder RM. Idiopathic pulmonary fibrosis and pulmonary hypertension: connecting the dots. Am J Respir Crit Care Med. 2007;175(9):875–80.
43. Corte TJ, Wort SJ, Wells AU. Pulmonary hypertension in idiopathic pulmonary fibrosis: a review. Sarcoidosis Vasc Diffuse Lung Dis. 2009;26(1):7–19.
44. King CS, Nathan SD. Practical considerations in the pharmacologic treatment of idiopathic pulmonary fibrosis. Curr Opin Pulm Med. 2015;21(5):479–89.
45. Mura M, Anraku M, Yun Z, McRae K, Liu M, Waddell TK, et al. Gene expression profiling in the lungs of patients with pulmonary hypertension associated with pulmonary fibrosis. Chest. 2012;141(3):661–73.
46. Shellenberger RA, Imtiaz K, Chellappa N, Gundapanneni L, Scheidel C, Handa R, et al. Physical examination for the detection of pulmonary hypertension: a systematic review. Cureus. 2021;13(9):e18020.
47. Braganza M, Shaw J, Solverson K, Vis D, Janovcik J, Varughese RA, et al. A prospective evaluation of the diagnostic accuracy of the physical examination for pulmonary hypertension. Chest. 2019;155(5):982–90.
48. Nathan SD, Shlobin OA, Ahmad S, Urbanek S, Barnett SD. Pulmonary hypertension and pulmonary function testing in idiopathic pulmonary fibrosis. Chest. 2007;131(3):657–63.
49. Rahaghi FF, Kolaitis NA, Adegunsoye A, de Andrade JA, Flaherty KR, Lancaster LH, et al. Screening strategies for pulmonary hypertension in patients with interstitial lung disease: a multidisciplinary Delphi study. Chest. 2022;162(1):145–55.
50. Rose L, Prins KW, Archer SL, Pritzker M, Weir EK, Misialek JR, et al. Survival in pulmonary hypertension due to chronic lung disease: influence of low diffusion capacity of the lungs for carbon monoxide. J Heart Lung Transplant. 2019;38(2):145–55.
51. Lettieri CJ, Nathan SD, Browning RF, Barnett SD, Ahmad S, Shorr AF. The distance-saturation product predicts mortality in idiopathic pulmonary fibrosis. Respir Med. 2006;100(10):1734–41.
52. Lama VN, Flaherty KR, Toews GB, Colby TV, Travis WD, Long Q, et al. Prognostic value of desaturation during a 6-minute walk test in idiopathic interstitial pneumonia. Am J Respir Crit Care Med. 2003;168(9):1084–90.

53. Yoo DK, Zompatori M, Barrile A, Rossi G, D'Amato D, Sergiacomi G, et al. Associated pulmonary hypertension is an independent contributor to exercise intolerance in chronic fibrosing interstitial pneumonias. Respiration. 2018;96(6):543–51.
54. Minai OA, Santacruz JF, Alster JM, Budev MM, McCarthy K. Impact of pulmonary hemodynamics on 6-min walk test in idiopathic pulmonary fibrosis. Respir Med. 2012;106(11):1613–21.
55. Swigris JJ, Olson AL, Shlobin OA, Ahmad S, Brown KK, Nathan SD. Heart rate recovery after six-minute walk test predicts pulmonary hypertension in patients with idiopathic pulmonary fibrosis. Respirology. 2011;16(3):439–45.
56. Glaser S, Obst A, Koch B, Henkel B, Grieger A, Felix SB, et al. Pulmonary hypertension in patients with idiopathic pulmonary fibrosis—the predictive value of exercise capacity and gas exchange efficiency. PLoS One. 2013;8(6):e65643.
57. Armstrong HF, Schulze PC, Bacchetta M, Thirapatarapong W, Bartels MN. Impact of pulmonary hypertension on exercise performance in patients with interstitial lung disease undergoing evaluation for lung transplantation. Respirology. 2014;19(5):675–82.
58. Zisman DA, Karlamangla AS, Ross DJ, Keane MP, Belperio JA, Saggar R, et al. High-resolution chest CT findings do not predict the presence of pulmonary hypertension in advanced idiopathic pulmonary fibrosis. Chest. 2007;132(3):773–9.
59. Yagi M, Taniguchi H, Kondoh Y, Ando M, Kimura T, Kataoka K, et al. CT-determined pulmonary artery to aorta ratio as a predictor of elevated pulmonary artery pressure and survival in idiopathic pulmonary fibrosis. Respirology. 2017;22(7):1393–9.
60. Shin S, King CS, Puri N, Shlobin OA, Brown AW, Ahmad S, et al. Pulmonary artery size as a predictor of outcomes in idiopathic pulmonary fibrosis. Eur Respir J. 2016;47(5):1445–51.
61. Bax S, Jacob J, Ahmed R, Bredy C, Dimopoulos K, Kempny A, et al. Right ventricular to left ventricular ratio at CT pulmonary angiogram predicts mortality in interstitial lung disease. Chest. 2020;157(1):89–98.
62. Swift AJ, Dwivedi K, Johns C, Garg P, Chin M, Currie BJ, et al. Diagnostic accuracy of CT pulmonary angiography in suspected pulmonary hypertension. Eur Radiol. 2020;30(9):4918–29.
63. Nowak J, Hudzik B, Jastrzebski D, Niedziela JT, Rozentryt P, Wojarski J, et al. Pulmonary hypertension in advanced lung diseases: echocardiography as an important part of patient evaluation for lung transplantation. Clin Respir J. 2018;12(3):930–8.
64. Prins KW, Rose L, Archer SL, Pritzker M, Weir EK, Olson MD, et al. Clinical determinants and prognostic implications of right ventricular dysfunction in pulmonary hypertension caused by chronic lung disease. J Am Heart Assoc. 2019;8(2):e011464.
65. Bax S, Bredy C, Kempny A, Dimopoulos K, Devaraj A, Walsh S, et al. A stepwise composite echocardiographic score predicts severe pulmonary hypertension in patients with interstitial lung disease. ERJ Open Res. 2018;4(2).
66. Keir GJ, Wort SJ, Kokosi M, George PM, Walsh SLF, Jacob J, et al. Pulmonary hypertension in interstitial lung disease: limitations of echocardiography compared to cardiac catheterization. Respirology. 2018;23(7):687–94.
67. Kamide H, Kato S, Hayakawa K, Fukui K, Kitamura H, Ogura T, et al. Impairment of right ventricular strain evaluated by cardiovascular magnetic resonance feature tracking in patients with interstitial lung disease. Int J Cardiovasc Imaging. 2021;37(3):1073–83.
68. Alkhanfar D, Dwivedi K, Alandejani F, Shahin Y, Alabed S, Johns C, et al. Non-invasive detection of severe PH in lung disease using magnetic resonance imaging. Front Cardiovasc Med. 2023;10:1016994.
69. Nathan SD, Chandel A, Wang Y, Xu J, Shao L, Watkins TR, et al. Derivation and validation of a noninvasive prediction tool to identify pulmonary hypertension in patients with IPF: evolution of the model FORD. J Heart Lung Transplant. 2024;43(4):547–53.
70. Joseph P, Savarimuthu S, Zhao J, Yan X, Oakland HT, Cullinan M, et al. Noninvasive determinants of pulmonary hypertension in interstitial lung disease. Pulm Circ. 2023;13(1):e12197.

71. Trushenko NV, Suvorova OA, Nekludova GV, Levina IA, Chikina SY, Nikolenko AM, et al. Predictors of pulmonary hypertension and right ventricular dysfunction in patients with hypersensitivity pneumonitis. Life (Basel). 2023;13(6).
72. Parikh R, O'Sullivan DM, Farber HW. The PH-ILD Detection tool: External validation and use in patients with ILD. Pulm Circ. 2023;13(3):e12273.
73. Zisman DA, Karlamangla AS, Kawut SM, Shlobin OA, Saggar R, Ross DJ, et al. Validation of a method to screen for pulmonary hypertension in advanced idiopathic pulmonary fibrosis. Chest. 2008;133(3):640–5.
74. Ewert R, Heine A, Muller-Heinrich A, Bollmann T, Obst A, Desole S, et al. Exercise and fluid challenge during right heart catheterisation for evaluation of dyspnoea. Pulm Circ. 2020;10(3).
75. Ghofrani HA, Wiedemann R, Rose F, Schermuly RT, Olschewski H, Weissmann N, et al. Sildenafil for treatment of lung fibrosis and pulmonary hypertension: a randomised controlled trial. Lancet. 2002;360(9337):895–900.
76. Idiopathic Pulmonary Fibrosis Clinical Research N, Zisman DA, Schwarz M, Anstrom KJ, Collard HR, Flaherty KR, et al. A controlled trial of sildenafil in advanced idiopathic pulmonary fibrosis. N Engl J Med. 2010;363(7):620–8.
77. Colombat M, Mal H, Groussard O, Capron F, Thabut G, Jebrak G, et al. Pulmonary vascular lesions in end-stage idiopathic pulmonary fibrosis: histopathologic study on lung explant specimens and correlations with pulmonary hemodynamics. Hum Pathol. 2007;38(1):60–5.
78. Cottin V. Treatment of pulmonary hypertension in interstitial lung disease: do not throw out the baby with the bath water. Eur Respir J. 2013;41(4):781–3.
79. Raghu G, Million-Rousseau R, Morganti A, Perchenet L, Behr J, Group MS. Macitentan for the treatment of idiopathic pulmonary fibrosis: the randomised controlled MUSIC trial. Eur Respir J. 2013;42(6):1622–32.
80. King TE Jr, Behr J, Brown KK, du Bois RM, Lancaster L, de Andrade JA, et al. BUILD-1: a randomized placebo-controlled trial of bosentan in idiopathic pulmonary fibrosis. Am J Respir Crit Care Med. 2008;177(1):75–81.
81. King TE Jr, Brown KK, Raghu G, du Bois RM, Lynch DA, Martinez F, et al. BUILD-3: a randomized, controlled trial of bosentan in idiopathic pulmonary fibrosis. Am J Respir Crit Care Med. 2011;184(1):92–9.
82. Raghu G, Behr J, Brown KK, Egan JJ, Kawut SM, Flaherty KR, et al. Treatment of idiopathic pulmonary fibrosis with ambrisentan: a parallel, randomized trial. Ann Intern Med. 2013;158(9):641–9.
83. Corte TJ, Keir GJ, Dimopoulos K, Howard L, Corris PA, Parfitt L, et al. Bosentan in pulmonary hypertension associated with fibrotic idiopathic interstitial pneumonia. Am J Respir Crit Care Med. 2014;190(2):208–17.
84. Cottin V, Price LC, Valenzuela C. The unmet medical need of pulmonary hypertension in idiopathic pulmonary fibrosis. Eur Respir J. 2018;51(1).
85. Nathan SD, Behr J, Collard HR, Cottin V, Hoeper MM, Martinez FJ, et al. Riociguat for idiopathic interstitial pneumonia-associated pulmonary hypertension (RISE-IIP): a randomised, placebo-controlled phase 2b study. Lancet Respir Med. 2019;7(9):780–90.
86. Hoeper MM, Halank M, Wilkens H, Gunther A, Weimann G, Gebert I, et al. Riociguat for interstitial lung disease and pulmonary hypertension: a pilot trial. Eur Respir J. 2013;41(4):853–60.
87. Dawes TJW, McCabe C, Dimopoulos K, Stewart I, Bax S, Harries C, et al. Phosphodiesterase 5 inhibitor treatment and survival in interstitial lung disease pulmonary hypertension: a Bayesian retrospective observational cohort study. Respirology. 2023;28(3):262–72.
88. Olschewski H, Ghofrani HA, Walmrath D, Schermuly R, Temmesfeld-Wollbruck B, Grimminger F, et al. Inhaled prostacyclin and iloprost in severe pulmonary hypertension secondary to lung fibrosis. Am J Respir Crit Care Med. 1999;160(2):600–7.
89. Saggar R, Khanna D, Vaidya A, Derhovanessian A, Maranian P, Duffy E, et al. Changes in right heart haemodynamics and echocardiographic function in an advanced phenotype

of pulmonary hypertension and right heart dysfunction associated with pulmonary fibrosis. Thorax. 2014;69(2):123–9.
90. Waxman A, Restrepo-Jaramillo R, Thenappan T, Ravichandran A, Engel P, Bajwa A, et al. Inhaled treprostinil in pulmonary hypertension due to interstitial lung disease. N Engl J Med. 2021;384(4):325–34.
91. Nathan SD, Deng C, King CS, DuBrock HM, Elwing J, Rajagopal S, et al. Inhaled treprostinil dosage in pulmonary hypertension associated with interstitial lung disease and its effects on clinical outcomes. Chest. 2023;163(2):398–406.
92. Nathan SD, Tapson VF, Elwing J, Rischard F, Mehta J, Shapiro S, et al. Efficacy of inhaled treprostinil on multiple disease progression events in patients with pulmonary hypertension due to parenchymal lung disease in the INCREASE Trial. Am J Respir Crit Care Med. 2022;205(2):198–207.
93. Ryerson CJ, Cayou C, Topp F, Hilling L, Camp PG, Wilcox PG, et al. Pulmonary rehabilitation improves long-term outcomes in interstitial lung disease: a prospective cohort study. Respir Med. 2014;108(1):203–10.
94. Weatherald J, Nathan SD, El-Kersh K, Argula RG, DuBrock HM, Rischard FP, et al. Inhaled treprostinil in patients with pulmonary hypertension associated with interstitial lung disease with less severe haemodynamics: a post hoc analysis of the INCREASE study. BMJ Open Respir Res. 2024;11(1).
95. Nathan SD, Cottin V, Behr J, Hoeper MM, Martinez FJ, Corte TJ, et al. Impact of lung morphology on clinical outcomes with riociguat in patients with pulmonary hypertension and idiopathic interstitial pneumonia: a post hoc subgroup analysis of the RISE-IIP study. J Heart Lung Transplant. 2021;40(6):494–503.
96. Nathan SD, Argula R, Trivieri MG, Aziz S, Gay E, Medarov B, et al. Inhaled treprostinil in pulmonary hypertension associated with COPD: PERFECT study results. Eur Respir J. 2024;63(6).
97. https://clinicaltrials.gov/study/NCT05776225?term=phinder&rank=1;Pages on 11/16/2024.
98. https://clinicaltrials.gov/study/NCT06025578?term=ph-ild&aggFilters=phase:3 snrrtt;Pages on 11/15/2024.
99. Hoeper MM, Badesch DB, Ghofrani HA, Gibbs JSR, Gomberg-Maitland M, McLaughlin VV, et al. Phase 3 trial of sotatercept for treatment of pulmonary arterial hypertension. N Engl J Med. 2023;388(16):1478–90.
100. https://clinicaltrials.gov/study/NCT06475781?term=ph-ild&aggFilters=status:not%20rec&rank=4;Pages on 11/15/2024.
101. https://clinicaltrials.gov/study/NCT06635850?term=ph-ild&aggFilters=status:not%20rec&rank=2;Pages on 11/15/2024.

Chapter 10
Pulmonary Hypertension Associated with Sarcoidosis

Alexander Liu, Vasilis Kouranos, and Laura C. Price

Abbreviations

PA	Pulmonary artery
PAP	Pulmonary arterial pressure
PASP	Pulmonary arterial systolic pressure
PAWP	Pulmonary arterial wedge pressure
PET	Positron emission tomography
PH	Pulmonary hypertension
PVR	Pulmonary vascular resistance
RHC	Right heart catheterisation
SAPH	Sarcoidosis-associated pulmonary hypertension
TTE	Transthoracic echocardiography

A. Liu
Department of Cardiology, Royal Brompton Hospital, Part of Guy's and St Thomas' NHS Foundation Trust, London, UK
e-mail: alexander.liu2@nhs.net

V. Kouranos
Interstitial Lung Disease Team, Royal Brompton Hospital, Part of Guy's and St Thomas' NHS Foundation Trust, London, UK

National Heart and Lung Institute, Imperial College London, London, UK
e-mail: vasileios.kouranos@nhs.net

L. C. Price (✉)
National Heart and Lung Institute, Imperial College London, London, UK

National Pulmonary Hypertension Service, Royal Brompton Hospital, Part of Guy's and St Thomas' NHS Foundation Trust, London, UK
e-mail: lauraclaireprice@nhs.net

F. N. Rahaghi et al. (eds.), *The Pulmonary Vasculature in Chronic Lung Disease*, Respiratory Medicine, https://doi.org/10.1007/978-3-032-03581-3_10

Introduction

Sarcoidosis is a multisystem inflammatory disease of unclear aetiology, as characterised by the formation of non-caseating granuloma in affected tissues [1]. Pulmonary involvement in sarcoidosis is very common, present in up to 90% of cases, and can affect both the airways, nodes and the lung parenchyma [2]. Development of pulmonary hypertension (PH) in patients with sarcoidosis is not only well recognised but also associated with reduced functional capacity, quality of life [3] and both fatal and non-fatal complications [4]. Indeed, patients with sarcoidosis-associated pulmonary hypertension (SAPH) have up to a seven-fold greater mortality risk, as compared to sarcoidosis patients without PH [4].

The pathophysiology of SAPH is varied and remains incompletely understood [4]. The diagnostic and management strategies for SAPH rely largely on those established in non-sarcoid patients with PH [5]. In this chapter, we will discuss the epidemiology, pathophysiology and the contemporary diagnostic and therapeutic strategies for SAPH.

Definitions of PH

Although several surrogate non-invasive markers are available for the suggestion of PH, the reference standard method for definitive PH diagnosis and phenotyping requires assessment using right heart catheterisation (RHC) [5].

PH is now defined by a mean pulmonary arterial pressure (mPAP) of greater than 20 mmHg measured during RHC studies [5]. PH can be further categorised into pre-capillary, post-capillary, combined pre- and post-capillary or exercise-related [5]. Pre-capillary PH is defined as mPAP $>$ 20 mmHg, with normal pulmonary arterial wedge pressure (PAWP $\leq$ 15 mmHg) and elevated pulmonary vascular resistance (PVR $>$ 2 Wood Units [WU]) [5]. Post-capillary PH is defined as mPAP $>$ 20 mmHg, with elevated PAWP ($>$15 mmHg) and normal PVR ($\leq$2 WU) [5]. Combined pre- and post-capillary PH is defined as mPAP $>$ 20 mmHg, with both elevated PAWP ($>$15 mmHg) and PVR ($>$2 WU) [5]. Exercise PH is defined as elevated mPAP/cardiac output slope between rest and stress ($>$3 mmHg/L/min) [5]. The haemodynamic definitions of PH subtypes are illustrated in Fig. 10.1.

Epidemiology of SAPH

The prevalence of SAPH is heavily dependent on the mode of diagnosis and the criteria and/or methods used to make the diagnosis (Table 10.1). The prevalence may vary depending on the method and timing of diagnosis, with factors such as mPAP used, the baseline population and the stage of sarcoidosis disease severity [6]. Recent studies estimating the prevalence of SAPH are shown in Table 10.1.

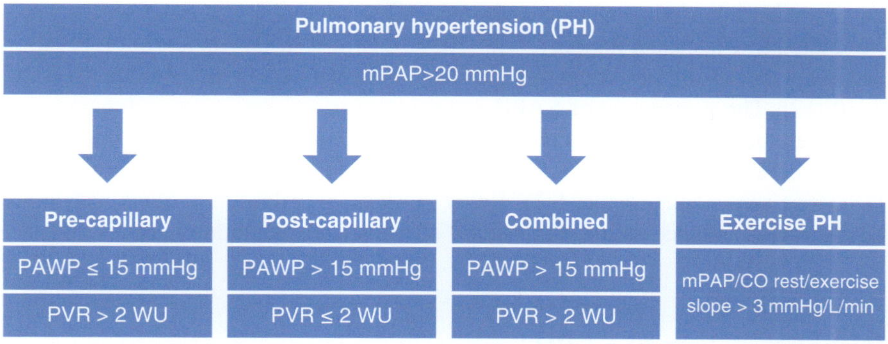

Fig. 10.1 Haemodynamic definitions of pulmonary hypertension (PH). *mPAP* mean pulmonary arterial pressure, *PAWP* pulmonary arterial wedge pressure, *PVR* pulmonary vascular resistance

Table 10.1 Studies estimating the prevalence of sarcoidosis associated pulmonary hypertension

Authors	Study design	N	Site	SAPH testing	Prevalence
Huitema et al. 2019 [6]	Single centre prospective, all-comers	399	Netherland	TTE ± RHC	2.9%
Pabst et al. 2013 [7]	Single centre prospective, all-comers	111	Germany	TTE ± RHC	3.6%
Alhamad et al. 2010 [8]	Multicentre retrospective, all-comers	96	Saudi Arabia	TTE	20%
Bourbonnais et al. 2008 [9]	Single centre prospective, all-comers	141	USA	TTE ± RHC	14%
Handa et al. 2006 [10]	Single centre prospective, all-comers	246	Japan	TTE	5.7%
Shorr et al. 2005 [11]	Registry, retrospective, advanced	363	USA	RHC	73.8%

N number of patients included in the study, *RHC* right heart catheterisation studies, *TTE* transthoracic echocardiography

The PULmonary hypertension in pulmonary SARcoidosis (PULSAR) study included 399 sarcoidosis patients referred to a Dutch tertiary centre (90.5% Caucasian) [6], in whom screening was performed using clinical and transthoracic echocardiographic (TTE) data [6]. Patients with intermediate and high probability for PH based on TTE underwent invasive RHC assessment with PH being defined as a mPAP > 25 mmHg [6]. The prevalence of PH in this patient cohort was around 2.9% [6]. Other studies with smaller sample sizes have presented higher prevalence of PH in patients with sarcoidosis [7, 8, 12], ranging from 3.6% [7] to over 20% [8].

Despite the recent research efforts, the true prevalence of PH in sarcoidosis patients remains unclear, owing predominantly to a lack of data from large multicentre studies or registries. Most existing studies investigating the prevalence of SAPH have also been based on a PH criterion of mPAP > 25 mmHg, which has recently been revised to a lower level (>20 mmHg) [5]. Furthermore, studies based on non-Caucasian patients have reported higher prevalence of SAPH than those conducted in Caucasian patients [6, 8–10, 12]. However, this apparent observation is largely based on single-centred studies with relatively small sample sizes [6, 8–10, 12]. The prevalence of SAPH in regard to variations in other demographic characteristics such as age, gender, and geographic locations also remain unclear. Like in other PH-ILD settings including IPF where PH tends to progress over time [13], case series suggest that SAPH may be more prevalent in patients with more advanced sarcoidosis, including those before lung transplantation [11].

Pathophysiology of SAPH

The development of SAPH is multi-factorial and the full range of World Health Organisation (WHO) classification of PH subtypes can occur in sarcoidosis patients [14]. Broadly as an aide memoir, SAPH can be considered in the following contexts: (i) in the presence (or absence) of pulmonary parenchymal disease; (ii) in the presence of left sided cardiac disease; (iii) in the context of veno-occlusive disease; (iv) associated with thromboembolic diseases; (v) related to extrinsic factors such as pulmonary vascular compression; and/or (vi) linked to other co-morbidities such as anaemia and liver disease. The main pathophysiological contributions are summarised in Fig. 10.2.

SAPH and Parenchymal Lung Disease

Although SAPH occurs more frequently in patients with fibrotic lung disease, the severity of PH does not correlate well with the degree of fibrotic lung damage [14]. The disruption of the alveolar capillary bed with fibrotic replacement, along with chronic hypoxia, leads to pre-capillary PH in patients with sarcoidosis [11, 14]. However, SAPH can also occur in patients with little or no parenchymal lung damage [14], which indicates that other factors, such as left-sided cardiac disease or pulmonary vascular pathology, may play a more important role in these cases.

Obstructive sleep apnoea (OSA) can also occur more commonly in patients with sarcoidosis, especially in those taking regular corticosteroid therapy or those with concurrent congestive heart failure [4]. Since OSA is a known risk factor for the development of PH, it may contribute to the pathogenesis of SAPH [4].

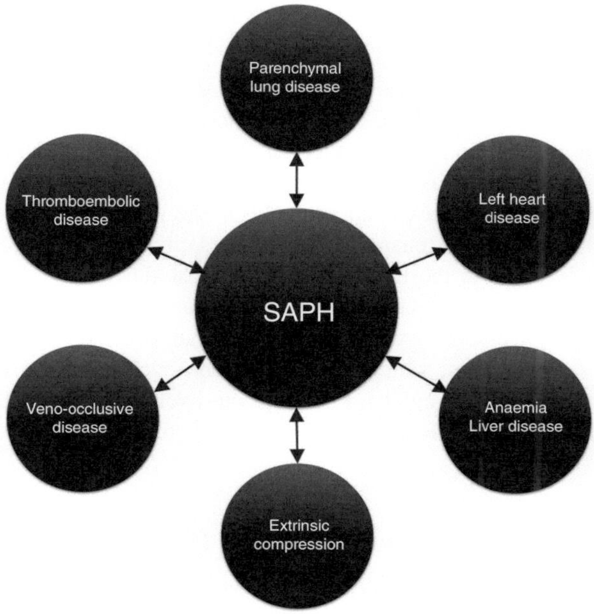

Fig. 10.2 Summary of main contributory factors to sarcoidosis-associated pulmonary hypertension (SAPH)

SAPH with Left-Sided Cardiac Disease

The involvement of left-sided cardiac disease can lead to post-capillary or combined SAPH. Left-sided cardiac disease in SAPH may be either related to cardiac involvement of sarcoidosis or due to non-sarcoid aetiologies such as ischaemic or valvular heart disease [4].

Cardiac involvement occurs in about a quarter of patients with sarcoidosis and can present in a number of ways, including with heart failure, ventricular arrhythmias, high-grade atrioventricular blocks or at post-mortem [15]. Both left ventricular (LV) systolic and diastolic dysfunction can occur in cardiac sarcoidosis (CS) [15], which lead to retrograde pressure transmission towards the pulmonary vasculature, leading to an elevated PAWP [4]. This "back pressure" from the LV dysfunction can also cause chronic vasoconstrictive changes in the pulmonary vasculature, leading to increased PVR and elements of combined pre- and post-capillary PH [16].

SAPH can also be associated with right ventricular (RV) dysfunction in sarcoidosis [4, 14]. Although RV dysfunction can occur in CS in the presence of left heart disease, isolated RV involvement is much rarer [17]. RV dysfunction in sarcoidosis occurs primarily due to three mechanisms: (i) due to direct cardiac involvement of sarcoidosis, either isolated or as extension of LV disease; (ii) due to congestion and volume overload as a result of LV dysfunction; or (iii) due to pulmonary disease involving parenchymal and/or vascular pathologies [4, 14, 15].

SAPH and Veno-occlusive Disease

Veno-occlusive disease is associated with pre-capillary PH and in the context of sarcoidosis patients, the pathogenesis may be related to non-caseating granuloma formation in the pulmonary vessel walls [18]. From autopsy studies, granulomatous involvement has been reported in the entire pulmonary vasculature, from the elastic pulmonary arteries and arterioles to the venules [18]. The distribution of the granuloma can be extensive, in many cases circumferentially affecting all layers from the adventitia to the intima, leading to vascular fibrosis [18]. Granulomatous involvement was also evident in the pulmonary lymphatic capillaries and collecting lymphatic vessels, as well as in the blood supply to the pulmonary vasculature itself, the vasa vasorum, which can mimic veno-occlusive disease [18]. The combination of pulmonary vascular wall fibrosis and veno-occlusive disorders in sarcoidosis leads to elevated PVR and pre-capillary PH [4, 14].

SAPH and Thromboembolic Disease

Sarcoidosis is associated with a heightened risk of venous thromboembolism (VTE) [19–21], which may be due to the chronic and/or systemic inflammation that renders patients in a hypercoagulable state [4]. Data from population-based studies from the United States and the United Kingdom suggest the elevated risk of VTE in sarcoidosis patients to be two to three-fold [20, 21]. Patients with SAPH and VTE are prone to both large central pulmonary emboli as well as smaller, sub-segmental peripheral thrombi, which may not always be easily apparent on non-invasive pulmonary imaging [4].

SAPH and Extrinsic Factors

Extrinsic factors contributing to SAPH can be broadly categorised as pulmonary and extra-pulmonary in origin. Pulmonary causes mainly hinge on the presence of external compression of major pulmonary vascular branches by enlarged and fibrosed hilar and mediastinal lymph nodes that are often present in pulmonary or multi-systems sarcoidosis [4, 14, 22]. This external compression leads to pulmonary vascular luminal stenoses, blood flow limitations, and ensuing PH [22]. Non-pulmonary factors contributing to SAPH are mainly comprised of anaemia-related high cardiac output heart failure or, rarely, chronic liver disease [4].

Diagnosis and Assessment of SAPH

The screening workup for SAPH involves a combination of clinical assessment, functional and imaging investigations [14]. Establishing the presence of SAPH based on clinical history and examination findings alone can be challenging, owing to the frequent presence of con-commitment and confounding pathologies, such as parenchymal lung disease and cardiac failure [4]. In patients first diagnosed with sarcoidosis, a significant delay in establishing a diagnosis of SAPH has been documented, from 12.6 years [23] to up to 17 years [24]. This prolonged diagnostic delay is married with the fact that most patients have already developed more severe forms of SAPH at the time of diagnosis, based on the index RHC measurements [14]. The simplified screening and diagnostic modalities for SAPH are summarised in Fig. 10.3.

Symptomology and Clinical Examination

The symptoms associated with SAPH, such as dyspnoea, chest discomfort and palpitations, can be non-specific and indeed are also common manifestations of sarcoidosis and/or other cardiovascular co-morbidities [4]. However, the worsening of symptoms, oxygenation and gas transfer, out of proportion to measures of lung fibrosis, or the development of RV failure and/or systemic congestion in patients with previously stable sarcoidosis disease history would warrant consideration of SAPH as a contributor to the deterioration [4]. Indeed, driven by the importance of establishing SAPH diagnosis early in the disease natural history, clinicians should have both a heightened clinical vigilance and a low threshold to proceed to SAPH screening in stable sarcoidosis patients who develop new symptomatic deterioration [4, 14].

The occurrence of syncope, whether upon exertion or at rest, would be concerning and should prompt not only screening for exercise PH, but also high-grade atrioventricular blocks and/or ventricular arrhythmias in patients with sarcoidosis and potential cardiac involvement [5, 15].

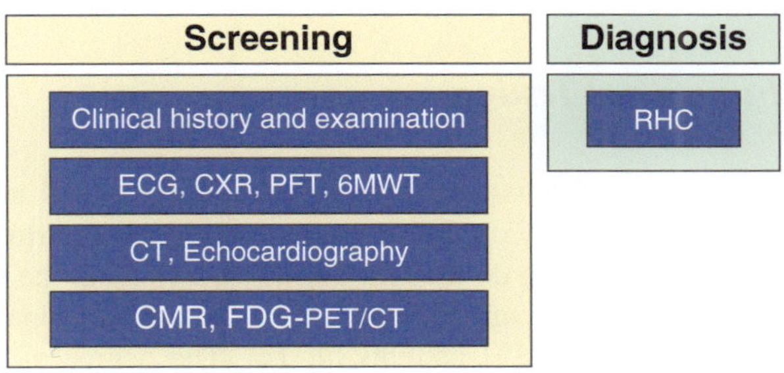

Fig. 10.3 Summary of the methods for the screening and diagnosis of sarcoidosis-associated pulmonary hypertension

Clinical signs on physical examination in a patient with SAPH can be similar to that with PH in general, which might include a loud pulmonary component of the second heart sound (P2), elevated jugular venous pressure (JVP) and/or peripheral oedema consistent with RV failure [4]. An RV heave might be felt at the precordium consistent with RV hypertrophy and/or strain [4]. However, the appearance of these signs consistent with RV failure and/or strain tend to indicate late-stage SAPH, whereby adverse cardiac remodelling has taken place [4].

Electrocardiogram (ECG)

ECG changes suggestive of PH include p-wave pulmonale, right axis deviation, features of RV hypertrophy or strain and right bundle branch block [5]. ECG features are non-specific for PH [5] and their presence is likely to increase the overall risk in patients with PAH [25]. Abnormalities on ECG should raise the clinical suspicion of possible presence of PH in sarcoidosis patients but are non-specific, forming part of an initial screening process along with clinical history, examination and other modalities. A 12-lead ECG is also important to exclude acute arrhythmia in breathless patients—patients with significant PH often develop atrial arrhythmias due to atrial stretch and scarring, which can otherwise be asymptomatic.

Chest X-Ray (CXR)

CXR abnormalities tend to represent advanced parenchymal lung disease which are associated with SAPH [10]. However, SAPH can occur in the absence of parenchymal lung disease [4], which renders CXR a relatively unreliable tool for this purpose. The presence of CXR findings suggestive of parenchymal disease should lead to further investigation with computed tomography (CT). The role of CXR therefore remains a screening tool for sarcoid-related lung parenchymal disease, rather than SAPH itself, and a negative CXR does not rule out the presence of SAPH. Cardiomegaly and right atrial enlargement can be obvious in late cases however.

Functional Testing

Since most patients diagnosed with sarcoidosis will undergo pulmonary function testing (PFT) early on, PFT represents an ideal opportunity to assess the likelihood of a patient having concurrent SAPH [4, 14]. Both the forced vital capacity (FVC) and the diffusing capacity of the lung for carbon monoxide (DLCO) are known to be reduced in SAPH patients [4, 14]. The degree of DLCO reduction in SAPH patients is often disproportionally worse than the severity of lung fibrosis [14], and a correlation has been reported between a low DLCO level (<60% predicted) and elevated pulmonary arterial pressures [9]. Moreover, reduced DLCO level on PFT has also been associated with estimated pulmonary artery systolic pressures (PASP) on TTE [26]. Corte et al reported in a mixed fibrotic IIP population that a KCO <50% or a 15% fall in KCO (diffusing capacity of carbon monoxide/alveolar volume) was even more specific than DLCO at predicting PH and also mortality [27].

The 6-minute walk test (6MWT) is also a simple and non-invasive screening method for the functional deficits often present in SAPH [14]. Like PFTs, abnormal parameters from 6MWT are not specific for SAPH per se, but do offer useful clues as to the probability of a sarcoidosis patient having PH [4]. Due to reduced exertional capacity in SAPH, patients often demonstrate reduced performance during a 6MWT [4], and the presence of oxygen desaturation below 90% on 6MWT in sarcoidosis patients is associated with a ~12-fold increased risk of co-existing SAPH [4, 14].

Prognostically, the combination of significantly reduced DLCO (<35% predicted) and 6MWD (<300 m) is linked to reduced transplant-free survival in SAPH patients [23].

Computed Tomography (CT)

Chest CT and CT pulmonary angiography (CTPA) form part of the first-line imaging workup investigations for SAPH [4, 14]. CT offers good spatial resolution for the assessment of pulmonary arterial anatomy, cardiac chamber size and lung parenchymal structural assessment [4]. When timed correctly with the intravenous contrast injection, CTPA also allows a one-stop assessment of central and segmental pulmonary thromboembolic disease as well as vascular compression [28]. Newer dual energy CTPA techniques also allow assessment of distal vasculature and provide perfusion maps. The significantly reduced radiation exposure with fine-tuned modern-day scanners means that serial CTPA scanning can also be used to monitor disease progression in sarcoidosis and offer important insights into SAPH pathophysiology.

The assessment of pulmonary arterial (PA) diameter and its relationship with other surrounding structures form important surrogate markers of SAPH on CT [4]. Conventionally, a ratio of the main PA diameter and the ascending aortic diameter (at the right PA level) of >1.0 (i.e. the main PA being wider than the ascending aorta) has been correlated with the presence of PH [29]. Similarly, a ratio of RV to LV diameters of >1.0 (i.e. the RV being wider than the LV) has also been linked with PH [14]. In patients with established Scadding stage IV sarcoidosis, an elevated PA diameter corrected for body surface area was found to be a predictor for SAPH [30]. Although CT cannot provide a definitive diagnosis of SAPH, abnormal findings should prompt further investigation for PH.

Echocardiography

TTE is a useful screening tool for PH and is commonly used in sarcoidosis patients due to its dual usefulness in the assessment of cardiac involvement. TTE utilises the tricuspid regurgitation (TR) velocity and inferior vena cava status to provide an estimation of the pulmonary arterial systolic pressures (PASP). The PASP, along with other TTE features, acts as a surrogate marker to offer a probability of pulmonary hypertension. The use of TTE has been firmly integrated into the ESC guidelines for PH screening [5].

A few limitations remain on the use of TTE for SAPH screening. Firstly, TR jets are not always present which are required for PASP estimation, rendering TTE at times unreliable [4]. Secondly, TTE estimation of PASP is further unreliable in patients with co-existing lung fibrosis, which would be problematic in a significant proportion of sarcoidosis patients [14]. Thirdly, TTE assessment depends on the presence of good transthoracic windows, which is not always available in patients with pulmonary disease [4]. Lastly, there is little evidence supporting the use of TTE for the screening of asymptomatic sarcoidosis patients [14].

Cardiovascular Magnetic Resonance (CMR) and Positron Emission Tomography (PET)

CMR is considered the reference standard multi-parametric method for assessing cardiac volumes, systolic function and myocardial scar [31]. In the assessment of PH, CMR offers more detailed assessment of RV size and function, as well as an assessment of PA/aortic diameters and RV:LV ratios [31]. CMR provides detailed assessments of LV volumes, systolic function and myocardial tissue characterisation, which are not only useful for the detection of left-sided cardiac disease but also form part of the advanced imaging workup for cardiac sarcoidosis [15]. Late gadolinium enhancement (LGE) imaging enables assessment of both LV and RV fibrosis which can offer important clues as to the underlying aetiology of LV and/or RV dysfunction [31].

Although CMR excels in providing high spatial resolution for cardiac imaging, it has a lower temporal resolution than Doppler TTE for the assessment of cardiac valvular function [32]. CMR is not used for the estimation of PASP nor pulmonary arterial acceleration times which the TTE can provide in the screening for PH. There is currently limited evidence for the routine use of CMR for the direct assessment of early SAPH beyond the detection of cardiac involvement of sarcoidosis [14].

18F-fluorodeoxyglucose (FDG)-PET/CT, along with CMR, form the cornerstone of advanced imaging workup for cardiac sarcoidosis [15]. PA and RV uptake of FDG has also been reported in pulmonary arterial hypertension (PAH) and RV failure, as surrogate markers of increased pulmonary and vascular tissue metabolism and inflammation [33, 34], which is potentially useful for monitoring response to therapy [35, 36]. FDG uptake may also play a role in the early detection of SAPH [37], however it must be emphasised that FDG-PET imaging is not currently in routine practice for this purpose. Recent evidence also suggests that FDG uptake in the PA, as detected using PET/CMR imaging, is linked with PH [38], which also requires further clinical validation.

Invasive Assessment of SAPH

RHC assessment is the reference standard for the diagnosis of SAPH and should be considered in any sarcoidosis patient with clinical suspicion for PH after non-invasive screening [14]. It is best performed in the absence of decompensated congestive heart failure or recent respiratory deteriorations such as acute chest infections [4, 14]. Although a reasonable proportion (~25%) of patients with SAPH can display acute vaso-responsiveness to inhaled nitric oxide or prostacyclin [39], the degree of responsiveness is a poor predictor of therapeutic response—for example to sildenafil [40] and calcium channel antagonists [41]. Therefore, unlike in patients with idiopathic PAH, routine vaso-reactivity testing during RHC is not recommended [14]. At RHC, sometimes a fluid challenge or leg elevation can unmask LV diastolic dysfunction [5].

Figure 10.4 provides an illustration of a SAPH patient.

Management Strategies

The clinical management of patients with SAPH depends on the underlying pathophysiological process, and since one or more different mechanisms for PH could be present in any given patient, the therapeutic strategies should also be tailored to the individual [4]. Effective therapy for SAPH is also not only about the instigation of disease modifying drugs, rather, it requires a robust structure that facilitates the referral of patients to expert centres, timely assessment and workup of patients, multi-disciplinary team meetings providing input for complex cases and holistic considerations for the psycho-social aspect of patients with a chronic and often debilitating illness.

Multidisciplinary Approach in the Diagnosis and Management

As a multi-system disease with a variety of different possible pathophysiological mechanisms, it is strongly recommended that the diagnosis and management of SAPH are performed by a multi-disciplinary team (MDT). This would enable review of clinical information, non-invasive imaging data, histological data and

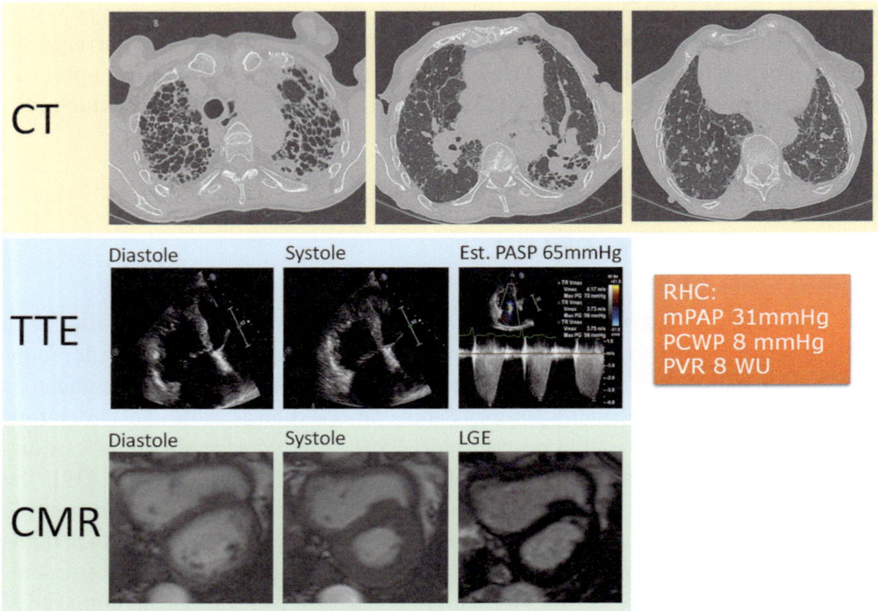

Fig. 10.4 A patient with sarcoidosis-associated pulmonary hypertension. This patient has pulmonary sarcoidosis and chronic thromboembolism who developed pre-capillary pulmonary hypertension. On computed tomography (CT) of the chest, there were extensive lung parenchymal fibrotic changes, with dilatation of the proximal pulmonary arteries. On transthoracic echocardiography (TTE), the right ventricle was dilated, with a high velocity tricuspid regurgitant (TR) jet and an elevated estimated pulmonary arterial systolic pressure (PASP) of 65 mmHg. The cardiovascular magnetic resonance (CMR) imaging showed dilated right ventricle with both systolic and diastolic septal flattening. There was no significant myocardial fibrosis on late gadolinium enhancement (LGE) imaging. The right heart catheter (RHC) study measurements were consistent with pre-capillary pulmonary hypertension. *mPAP* mean pulmonary arterial pressure, *PCWP* pulmonary capillary wedge pressure, *PVR* pulmonary vascular resistance, *WU* wood units

invasive RHC information by various experts in the same sitting, to arrive at a joint decision in diagnosis, assessment of severity and management planning in consensus. Such a standardised approach eliminates any regional or physician-specific variations, and in doing so is in the best interest of the patient. The MDT approach also enables streamlining of communication channels between healthcare providers and the patient. In particular, for therapeutic strategies based on clinical experience, rather than robust clinical trials, an MDT approach would enable patients to benefit from certain treatments, such as immunosuppression, on a case-to-case basis with the joint opinions of an expert panel.

Mechanistic Considerations

From a mechanistic viewpoint, effective treatment of SAPH relies upon elucidating the underlying driver of disease. In patients with SAPH and pulmonary vascular dysfunction, pulmonary vasodilator therapy, targeting the major pathways of endothelial dysfunction, can be considered with the aim to relieve both pulmonary vasoconstriction and vascular remodelling [4]. In those with SAPH and left heart disease, treatment can be focused on optimising the management of cardiac sarcoidosis or other causes of LV systolic and/or diastolic dysfunction [4]. SAPH patients with evidence of parenchymal lung damage may benefit from treatment of hypoxia, hypercapnia and any associated sleep apnoea [14]. Management of thromboembolic disease is paramount where present in SAPH patients which would usually long-term anticoagulation, with monitoring for bleeding complications including haemoptysis. In very rare cases with minimal lung fibrosis, patients may be referred for pulmonary endarterectomy or balloon pulmonary angioplasty [14]. Interventional therapeutic measures such as pulmonary arterial [42] or venous [43] stenting may be beneficial for the management of extrinsic pulmonary vascular compression due to sarcoid adenopathy or mediastinitis. Optimisation of anaemia and liver disease, if present, can be beneficial from the co-morbidity management perspective [4, 14]. Finally, lung transplantation should be considered in patients when SAPH is diagnosed, which although may pose a high perioperative risk, longer term survival is more impacted by fibrosis severity and age than the presence of severe PH pre-transplant [44].

Therapeutic Structure

From a therapeutic structure viewpoint, timely referral to a tertiary specialist centre with experience in managing SAPH patients is essential for optimising the diagnostic and therapeutic strategies. It can enable prompt expert clinical evaluation as well as offer one-stop workup of patients which minimises delays in reaching a diagnosis and initiating appropriate treatment. Expert-led follow-up of SAPH patients can provide continuity of care for the patients. The tertiary centres are also hubs for the clinical training of future experts in SAPH and the conduct of clinical research which can help to propel the field forward.

Management of SAPH may be complex if more than one underlying pathophysiological process is present, for instance, patients with concomitant granulomatous vascular pathology and lung parenchymal disease. In such cases, management guided by a consensus decision reached by a multi-disciplinary team (MDT) meeting, with review of the clinical data and investigations by a panel of experts, would be particularly beneficial.

Drug Therapies

Pulmonary hypertension therapies have been used in patients with sarcoidosis [14]. Although randomised prospective clinical trial data in this setting is very limited, evidence from clinical registries suggest that up to 72–77% of patients with SAPH are treated with PAH therapies [14, 23]. This practice is supported by the UK commissioners where SAPH is considered PAH-like in aetiology, whereas the use of pulmonary vasodilators in SAPH is off-label in other countries [14]. Patients with small pulmonary vein disease or Group 2 PH can develop pulmonary oedema with PAH therapies [14], despite some studies suggesting these drugs are well tolerated.

Studies generally suggest that pulmonary vasodilators can lead to improved haemodynamic parameters, exercise capacity, functional status and reductions in brain natriuretic peptides [4, 14]. However, these drugs have not been shown to confer prognostic value in terms of reducing mortality in SAPH patients [4, 14]. The response to vasodilator therapies also appears little affected by the presence of lung fibrosis, despite lung fibrosis being a prognostic factor in patients with sarcoidosis [4, 14].

There is a current paucity of randomised controlled trials for drug therapies in SAPH patients and most of the evidence behind the clinical use of targeted therapies are based on small retrospective studies or registries [4, 14]. The remainder of the chapter will discuss the current evidence behind the specific drug therapies in SAPH.

Endothelin Receptor Antagonists

In a double-blind randomised controlled trial, RHC-confirmed SAPH patients treated with bosentan ($n = 23$; maximal dose 125 mg bd) for 16 weeks had significant falls in both mPAP and PVR, whilst patients treated with placebo ($n = 12$) had no significant changes in these haemodynamic parameters [45]. However, there was no significant change in 6MWT in either treatment group, suggesting that haemodynamic changes do not always translate to improvements in functional status [45]. Two patients (9%) in the bosentan-treated group required escalation of supplemental oxygen therapy at the end of the treatment period [45].

In a prospective, open-label, proof of concept trial, 21 patients with SAPH were treated with ambrisentan at a starting dose of 5 mg/day for 4 weeks with subsequent escalation to 10/mg day for 20 weeks [46]. There was a high dropout rate of 52% during the study [46]. There was no association with significant improvements in 6WMT, dyspnoea, diffusion capacity, natriuretic peptides or quality of life [46]. In the patients who completed 24-week ambrisentan therapy, there was a trend towards improvements in quality of life and functional class which did not reach statistical significance [46].

In a retrospective review of 6 patients with severe SAPH treated with macitentan (in combination with sildenafil in 4 patients), the therapy was well tolerated in 5 patients with improvement in functional capacity in 4 patients [47].

Phosphodiesterase 5 Inhibitors (PDE5i)

Although there are no randomised controlled trial data on the use of PDE5i, retrospective studies have supported their use in SAPH patients, often in combination with other PH therapies. In a single-centred retrospective study of 25 patients with end-stage pulmonary sarcoidosis referred for lung transplantation, sildenafil treatment was associated with reductions in mPAP and PVR improvement in cardiac output and cardiac index, without significant changes in 6MWT results [48]. In another study, treatment with sildenafil mono-therapy or in combination with other pulmonary vasodilators led to improvements in 6MWT, natriuretic peptide levels and TR severity on echocardiography [49].

Neutral findings were reported for tadalafil in a two-centred open-label study involving 12 SAPH patients, with a high dropout rate of 5/12 (42%) [50]. In particular, treatment with tadalafil did not lead to significant changes in 6MWT results nor natriuretic peptide levels [50].

Guanylate Cyclase Stimulator

The potential clinical use of riociguat (a soluble guanylate cyclase stimulator) in the treatment of SAPH patients was the subject of a recent double-blind placebo-controlled trial in 16 patients, performed on a 1:1 randomisation basis (riociguat vs placebo) [51]. The primary end point was defined by the time taken to reach the first adverse endpoint, including all-cause mortality, hospitalisation due to worsening cardiopulmonary status attributable to disease progression, incline in 6MWD test by >50 m, or worsening functional class [51]. After the 1-year study period, the primary endpoint was reached in 5/8 of placebo-treated patients and 0/8 of the riociguat-treated patients [51]. Whilst 6MWT distance worsened in the placebo-treated group, it improved in the riociguat-treated group [51]. Riociguat therapy was not associated with significant adverse events [51].

Prostacyclin-Based Therapy

The tolerability of prostacyclin therapy in SAPH patients, even in those with significant fibrosis and severe gas exchange impairment, is generally good according to retrospective studies, which may lead to improvement in functional capacity, serum natriuretic peptides and measured haemodynamic parameters [14, 39]. In one study, Kimberly et al also reported assessment at baseline RHC using acute vasoresponder testing at RHC which showed a 25% fall in PVR in most patients who went onto long-term IV therapy, leading to an improvement in WHO functional class [39]. Although inhaled iloprost can induce cough in a proportion of patients, an open-label, prospective study of 15 patients showed that it is associated with reduced mPAP and PVR, as well as improvements in quality of life [52]. More recently, inhaled treprostinil was shown to significantly increase exercise tolerance and improve exacerbation rates in patients with ILD-PH (excluding patients with sarcoidosis) in the INCREASE trial [53]. Based on these results, the SAPPHIRE study is currently examining the impact on PVR (primary outcome) and other clinical outcomes at 16 weeks following treatment with inhaled treprostinil in patients with Scadding IV sarcoidosis and pre-capillary PH defined by mPAP $\geq$ 25 mmHg, PCWP $\leq$ 15 mmHg and PVR > 3 Wood units [54].

Combination Therapy

Upfront combination therapy with ambrisentan and tadalafil (AMBITON protocol) was tested in 3 patients with SAPH, with improvements in haemodynamic and functional improvements in all patients [55]. Sequential combination therapy with macitentan followed by tadalafil was reported to improve haemodynamics, exercise capacity and functional class in a 46-year-old patient with SAPH [56], with secondary corticosteroid-based immunosuppression. These findings, based on these small patient groups, require wider validation.

Immunosuppressive Therapy

Immunosuppressive therapy including corticosteroids has been used alone [57] or in combination with PAH-based drugs in the management of SAPH [58]. Theoretically, reducing the degree of vascular inflammation, lymphadenopathy and possibly retarding the fibrotic process with immunosuppressive therapy is expected to be beneficial in the management of SAPH. However, there is little clinical evidence to suggest that immunosuppressive therapy leads to improvements in haemodynamic parameters or functional capacity in SAPH [4, 24].

Conclusion

SAPH is a disease associated with significant morbidity and mortality. Screening and diagnosis of SAPH and identifying the disease phenotype is important and will determine the treatment of SAPH, which may involve oxygen and diuretics, in some cases PAH drug therapy and immunosuppression as well as pulmonary vascular stenting in compressive phenotypes. Future randomised clinical trials are required to further understand the role of monotherapy or combination PAH drug therapies in SAPH with the aim to improve symptoms, exercise tolerance, quality of life and prognosis of patients.

References

1. Churg A, Carrington CB, Gupta R. Necrotizing sarcoid granulomatosis. Chest. 1979;76(4):406–13. https://doi.org/10.1378/chest.76.4.406.
2. Baughman RP, Lower EE, Gibson K. Pulmonary manifestations of sarcoidosis. Presse medicale (Paris, France : 1983). 2012;41(6 Pt 2):e289–302. https://doi.org/10.1016/j.lpm.2012.03.019 [published Online First: 2012/05/15].
3. Lawrie A, Hamilton N, Wood S, et al. Healthcare resource utilization and quality of life in patients with sarcoidosis-associated pulmonary hypertension. Pulm Circ. 2022;12(4).
4. Duong H, Bonham CA. Sarcoidosis-associated pulmonary hypertension: pathophysiology, diagnosis, and treatment. Clin Pulm Med. 2018;25(2):52–60. https://doi.org/10.1097/cpm.0000000000000252. [published Online First: 2018/10/09]
5. Humbert M, Kovacs G, Hoeper MM, et al. 2022 ESC/ERS Guidelines for the diagnosis and treatment of pulmonary hypertension: Developed by the task force for the diagnosis and treatment of pulmonary hypertension of the European Society of Cardiology (ESC) and the European Respiratory Society (ERS). Endorsed by the International Society for Heart and Lung Transplantation (ISHLT) and the European Reference Network on rare respiratory diseases (ERN-LUNG). Eur Heart J. 2022;43(38):3618–731. https://doi.org/10.1093/eurheartj/ehac237.
6. Huitema MP, Bakker ALM, Mager JJ, et al. Prevalence of pulmonary hypertension in pulmonary sarcoidosis: the first large European prospective study. 2019;54(4):1900897. https://doi.org/10.1183/13993003.00897-2019
7. Pabst S, Hammerstingl C, Grau N, et al. Pulmonary arterial hypertension in patients with sarcoidosis: the Pulsar single center experience. Adv Exp Med Biol. 2013;755:299–305. https://doi.org/10.1007/978-94-007-4546-9_38. [published Online First: 2012/07/25]
8. Alhamad EH, Idrees MM, Alanezi MO, et al. Sarcoidosis-associated pulmonary hypertension: clinical features and outcomes in Arab patients. Ann Thoracic Med. 2010;5(2):86–91. https://doi.org/10.4103/1817-1737.62471. [published Online First: 2010/06/29]
9. Bourbonnais JM, Samavati L. Clinical predictors of pulmonary hypertension in sarcoidosis. Eur Respir J. 2008;32(2):296–302. https://doi.org/10.1183/09031936.00175907. [published Online First: 2008/04/04]
10. Handa T, Nagai S, Miki S, et al. Incidence of pulmonary hypertension and its clinical relevance in patients with sarcoidosis. Chest. 2006;129(5):1246–52. https://doi.org/10.1378/chest.129.5.1246. [published Online First: 2006/05/11]
11. Shorr AF, Helman DL, Davies DB, et al. Pulmonary hypertension in advanced sarcoidosis: epidemiology and clinical characteristics. Eur Respir J. 2005;25(5):783–8. https://doi.org/10.1183/09031936.05.00083404. [published Online First: 2005/05/03]

12. Kaptan Özen D, Mutlu B, Kocakaya D, et al. Pulmonary hypertension in patients with sarcoidosis: a single-center experience. Anatol J Cardiol. 2021;25(1):36–41. https://doi.org/10.14744/AnatolJCardiol.2020.88054. [published Online First: 2021/01/01]
13. Nathan SD. Pulmonary hypertension in interstitial lung disease. 2008;62(s160):21–8. https://doi.org/10.1111/j.1742-1241.2008.01624.x.
14. Samaranayake CB, McCabe C, Wort SJ, et al. Sarcoidosis associated pulmonary hypertension: an update. Curr Opin Pulm Med. 2021;27(5):285–95. https://doi.org/10.1097/mcp.0000000000000793. [published Online First: 2021/06/16]
15. Kouranos V, Sharma R. Cardiac sarcoidosis: state-of-the-art review. Heart. 2021;107(19):1591–9. https://doi.org/10.1136/heartjnl-2019-316442. [published Online First: 2021/03/07]
16. Guazzi M, Borlaug BA. Pulmonary hypertension due to left heart disease. Circulation. 2012;126(8):975–90. https://doi.org/10.1161/circulationaha.111.085761. [published Online First: 2012/08/22]
17. Patel MB, Mor-Avi V, Murtagh G, et al. Right heart involvement in patients with sarcoidosis. Echocardiography (Mount Kisco, NY). 2016;33(5):734–41. https://doi.org/10.1111/echo.13163. [published Online First: 2016/01/17]
18. Takemura T, Matsui Y, Saiki S, et al. Pulmonary vascular involvement in sarcoidosis: a report of 40 autopsy cases. Hum Pathol. 1992;23(11):1216–23. https://doi.org/10.1016/0046-8177(92)90288-e. [published Online First: 1992/11/01]
19. Swigris JJ, Olson AL, Huie TJ, et al. Increased risk of pulmonary embolism among US decedents with sarcoidosis from 1988 to 2007. Chest. 2011;140(5):1261–6. https://doi.org/10.1378/chest.11-0324. [published Online First: 2011/05/14]
20. Ungprasert P, Crowson CS, Matteson EL. Association of sarcoidosis with increased risk of VTE: a population-based study, 1976 to 2013. Chest. 2017;151(2):425–30. https://doi.org/10.1016/j.chest.2016.09.009. [published Online First: 2016/10/01]
21. Crawshaw AP, Wotton CJ, Yeates DG, et al. Evidence for association between sarcoidosis and pulmonary embolism from 35-year record linkage study. Thorax. 2011;66(5):447–8. https://doi.org/10.1136/thx.2010.134429. [published Online First: 2010/09/15]
22. Damuth TE, Bower JS, Cho K, et al. Major pulmonary artery stenosis causing pulmonary hypertension in sarcoidosis. Chest. 1980;78(6):888–91. https://doi.org/10.1378/chest.78.6.888. [published Online First: 1980/12/01]
23. Shlobin OA, Kouranos V, Barnett SD, et al. Physiological predictors of survival in patients with sarcoidosis-associated pulmonary hypertension: results from an international registry. Eur Respir J. 2020;55(5) https://doi.org/10.1183/13993003.01747-2019. [published Online First: 2020/03/07]
24. Boucly A, Cottin V, Nunes H, et al. Management and long-term outcomes of sarcoidosis-associated pulmonary hypertension. Eur Respir J. 2017;50(4) https://doi.org/10.1183/13993003.00465-2017. [published Online First: 2017/10/21]
25. Minhas J, Moutchia J, Al-Naamani N, et al. Electrocardiographic abnormalities and their association with outcomes in randomized clinical trials of pulmonary arterial hypertension. Ann Am Thoracic Soci. 2024. https://doi.org/10.1513/AnnalsATS.202307-609OC [published Online First: 2024/01/19].
26. Mirsaeidi M, Omar HR, Baughman R, et al. The association between BNP, 6MWD test, DLCO% and pulmonary hypertension in sarcoidosis. Sarcoidosis Vasculitis Diffuse Lung Dis. 2016;33(4):317–20. [published Online First: 2017/01/13].
27. Corte TJ, Wort SJ, MacDonald PS, et al. Pulmonary function vascular index predicts prognosis in idiopathic interstitial pneumonia. Respirology (Carlton, Vic). 2012;17(4):674–80. https://doi.org/10.1111/j.1440-1843.2011.02121.x. [published Online First: 2012/01/04]
28. Stein PD, Fowler SE, Goodman LR, et al. Multidetector computed tomography for acute pulmonary embolism. 2006;354(22):2317–27. https://doi.org/10.1056/NEJMoa052367.
29. Ng CS, Wells AU, Padley SP. A CT sign of chronic pulmonary arterial hypertension: the ratio of main pulmonary artery to aortic diameter. J Thorac Imaging. 1999;14(4):270–8. https://doi.org/10.1097/00005382-199910000-00007.

30. Huitema MP, Spee M, Vorselaars VM, et al. Pulmonary artery diameter to predict pulmonary hypertension in pulmonary sarcoidosis. Eur Respir J. 2016;47(2):673–6. https://doi.org/10.1183/13993003.01319-2015. [published Online First: 2015/10/24]
31. Kelle S, Bucciarelli-Ducci C, Judd RM, et al. Society for Cardiovascular Magnetic Resonance (SCMR) recommended CMR protocols for scanning patients with active or convalescent phase COVID-19 infection. J Cardiovasc Magn Reson. 2020;22(1):61. https://doi.org/10.1186/s12968-020-00656-6. [published Online First: 2020/09/04]
32. Han Y, Chen T, Bryant J, et al. Society for Cardiovascular Magnetic Resonance (SCMR) guidance for the practice of cardiovascular magnetic resonance during the COVID-19 pandemic. J Cardiovasc Magn Reson. 2020;22(1):26. https://doi.org/10.1186/s12968-020-00628-w. [published Online First: 2020/04/29]
33. Ahmadi A, Ohira H, Mielniczuk LM. FDG PET imaging for identifying pulmonary hypertension and right heart failure. Curr Cardiol Rep. 2015;17(1):555. https://doi.org/10.1007/s11886-014-0555-7. [published Online First: 2014/12/17]
34. Hagan G, Southwood M, Treacy C, et al. (18)FDG PET imaging can quantify increased cellular metabolism in pulmonary arterial hypertension: a proof-of-principle study. Pulm Circ. 2011;1(4):448–55. https://doi.org/10.4103/2045-8932.93543. [published Online First: 2012/04/25]
35. Zhao L, Ashek A, Wang L, et al. Heterogeneity in lung 18FDG uptake in pulmonary arterial hypertension. 2013;128(11):1214–24. doi:https://doi.org/10.1161/CIRCULATIONAHA.113.004136.
36. Marsboom G, Wietholt C, Haney CR, et al. Lung ^{18}F-fluorodeoxyglucose positron emission tomography for diagnosis and monitoring of pulmonary arterial hypertension. Am J Respir Crit Care Med. 2012;185(6):670–9. https://doi.org/10.1164/rccm.201108-1562OC. [published Online First: 2012/01/17]
37. Ovadia M. Pulmonary arterial 18F-FDG uptake in sarcoidosis. 2022;15(1):121–25. doi:https://doi.org/10.1016/j.jcmg.2021.08.014.
38. Maier A, Liao SL, Lescure T, et al. Pulmonary artery (18)F-fluorodeoxyglucose uptake by PET/CMR as a marker of pulmonary hypertension in sarcoidosis. JACC Cardiovasc Imaging. 2022;15(1):108–20. https://doi.org/10.1016/j.jcmg.2021.05.023. [published Online First: 2021/07/19]
39. Fisher KA, Serlin DM, Wilson KC, et al. Sarcoidosis-associated pulmonary hypertension: outcome with long-term epoprostenol treatment. Chest. 2006;130(5):1481–8. https://doi.org/10.1378/chest.130.5.1481. [published Online First: 2006/11/14]
40. Milman N, Svendsen CB, Iversen M, et al. Sarcoidosis-associated pulmonary hypertension: acute vasoresponsiveness to inhaled nitric oxide and the relation to long-term effect of sildenafil. Clin Respir J. 2009;3(4):207–13. https://doi.org/10.1111/j.1752-699X.2008.00120.x. [published Online First: 2010/03/20]
41. Preston IR, Klinger JR, Landzberg MJ, et al. Vasoresponsiveness of sarcoidosis-associated pulmonary hypertension. Chest. 2001;120(3):866–72. https://doi.org/10.1378/chest.120.3.866. [published Online First: 2001/09/14]
42. Hamilton-Craig CR, Slaughter R, McNeil K, et al. Improvement after angioplasty and stenting of pulmonary arteries due to sarcoid mediastinal fibrosis. Heart Lung Circ. 2009;18(3):222–5. https://doi.org/10.1016/j.hlc.2007.12.006. [published Online First: 2008/04/02]
43. Condado JF, Babaliaros V, Henry TS, et al. Pulmonary stenting for the treatment of sarcoid induced pulmonary vascular stenosis. Sarcoidosis Vasculitis Diffuse Lung Dis. 2016;33(3):281–7. [published Online First: 2016/10/21]
44. Le Pavec J, Valeyre D, Gazengel P, et al. Lung transplantation for sarcoidosis: outcome and prognostic factors. Eur Respir J. 2021;58(2) https://doi.org/10.1183/13993003.03358-2020. [published Online First: 2021/01/23]
45. Baughman RP, Culver DA, Cordova FC, et al. Bosentan for sarcoidosis-associated pulmonary hypertension: a double-blind placebo controlled randomized trial. Chest. 2014;145(4):810–7. https://doi.org/10.1378/chest.13-1766.

46. Judson MA, Highland KB, Kwon S, et al. Ambrisentan for sarcoidosis associated pulmonary hypertension. Sarcoidosis Vasculitis Diffuse Lung Dis. 2011;28(2):139–45. [published Online First: 2011/11/29]
47. Mathijssen H, Huitema MP, Bakker ALM, et al. Safety of macitentan in sarcoidosis-associated pulmonary hypertension: a case-series. Sarcoidosis Vasculitis Diffuse Lung Dis. 2020;37(1):74–8. https://doi.org/10.36141/svdld.v37i1.9292. [published Online First: 2020/10/24]
48. Milman N, Burton CM, Iversen M, et al. Pulmonary hypertension in end-stage pulmonary sarcoidosis: therapeutic effect of sildenafil? J Heart Lung Transplant. 2008;27(3):329–34. https://doi.org/10.1016/j.healun.2007.11.576. [published Online First: 2008/03/18]
49. Keir GJ, Walsh SL, Gatzoulis MA, et al. Treatment of sarcoidosis-associated pulmonary hypertension: a single centre retrospective experience using targeted therapies. Sarcoidosis Vasculitis Diffuse Lung Dis. 2014;31(2):82–90. [published Online First: 2014/08/01]
50. Ford HJ, Baughman RP, Aris R, et al. Tadalafil therapy for sarcoidosis-associated pulmonary hypertension. Pulm Circ. 2016;6(4):557–62. https://doi.org/10.1086/688775. [published Online First: 2017/01/17]
51. Baughman RP, Shlobin OA, Gupta R, et al. Riociguat for sarcoidosis-associated pulmonary hypertension: results of a 1-year double-blind, placebo-controlled trial. Chest. 2022;161(2):448–57. https://doi.org/10.1016/j.chest.2021.07.2162. [published Online First: 2021/08/08]
52. Baughman RP, Judson MA, Lower EE, et al. Inhaled iloprost for sarcoidosis associated pulmonary hypertension. Sarcoidosis Vasculitis Diffuse Lung Dis. 2009;26(2):110–20. [published Online First: 2010/06/22]
53. Waxman A, Restrepo-Jaramillo R, Thenappan T, et al. Inhaled treprostinil in pulmonary hypertension due to interstitial lung disease. N Engl J Med. 2021;384(4):325–34. https://doi.org/10.1056/NEJMoa2008470. [published Online First: 2021/01/14]
54. (SAPPHIRE) ITiSPWPH. https://classic.clinicaltrials.gov/ct2/show/NCT03814317. Accessed 25 Jan 2024.
55. Abston E, Hon S, Lawrence R, et al. Treatment of newly diagnosed sarcoid-associated pulmonary hypertension with ambrisentan and tadalafil combination therapy. Sarcoidosis Vasculitis Diffuse Lung Dis. 2020;37(2):234–8. https://doi.org/10.36141/svdld.v37i2.9343. [published Online First: 2020/10/24]
56. Sumimoto K, Taniguchi Y, Emoto N, et al. Combination therapy with pulmonary arterial hypertension targeted drugs and immunosuppression can be a useful strategy for sarcoidosis-associated pulmonary hypertension: a case report. Eur Heart J Case Rep. 2021;5(1):ytaa454. https://doi.org/10.1093/ehjcr/ytaa454. [published Online First: 2021/02/09]
57. Nunes H, Humbert M, Capron F, et al. Pulmonary hypertension associated with sarcoidosis: mechanisms, haemodynamics and prognosis. Thorax. 2006;61(1):68. https://doi.org/10.1136/thx.2005.042838.
58. Baughman RP, Shlobin OA, Wells AU, et al. Clinical features of sarcoidosis associated pulmonary hypertension: results of a multi-national registry. Respir Med. 2018;139:72–8. https://doi.org/10.1016/j.rmed.2018.04.015. [published Online First: 2018/06/03]

Chapter 11
PVD Associated with ARDS and Post-COVID Syndromes

Vaughn Craddock, Sahil Pandya, Leslie Spikes, and Navneet Kaur Dhillon

An Overview of ARDS and Pathophysiology

Diagnosis of ARDS

ARDS is a cause of acute respiratory failure in which damage to epithelial and endothelial cells within the lungs leads to hypoxemia, hypercapnia, and pulmonary edema. In 2023, the diagnosis of ARDS was expanded to create a more encompassing definition based on current practices, namely with the increased utilization of heated high-flow nasal cannula (HHFNC) [1]. Building on the previous Berlin Criteria [2], the new definition defines ARDS as an "acute, diffuse, inflammatory lung injury precipitated by a predisposing risk factor, such as pneumonia, nonpulmonary infection, trauma, transfusion, burn, aspiration, or shock." This definition includes ultrasound findings to coincide with previously defined radiology findings, maintains acuity of onset (<1 week), and defines severity in both intubated and non-intubated patients based on the degree of supplemental oxygen support. Non-intubated patients require supplemental oxygen support that is defined as >30 L/min or non-invasive ventilation (NIV) with at least 5 cm H_2O of end-expiratory pressure [1]. This definition may have implications in the identification of more indolent phenotypes of ARDS and has potential implications on therapeutic strategies and considerations.

V. Craddock · S. Pandya · L. Spikes · N. K. Dhillon (✉)
Division of Pulmonary, Critical Care and Sleep Medicine, Department of Internal Medicine, University of Kansas Medical Center, Kansas City, Kansas, KS, USA
e-mail: spandya2@kumc.edu; lspikes@kumc.edu; ndhillon@kumc.edu

F. N. Rahaghi et al. (eds.), *The Pulmonary Vasculature in Chronic Lung Disease*, Respiratory Medicine, https://doi.org/10.1007/978-3-032-03581-3_11

Alveolar Epithelial and Endothelial Barrier Integrity Contribute to ARDS Pathophysiology

ARDS has a variety of direct (intrapulmonary) and indirect (extrapulmonary) etiologies, making it difficult to uniformly characterize [3]. In general, immune dysregulation, oxidative stress, and the accumulation of leukocytes within the lungs disrupt the alveolar epithelium and alveolar-capillary barrier, leading to the accumulation of fluid and macromolecules within the alveolar airspace (pulmonary edema) [4–7].

The alveolar epithelium consists of two types of cells. Type I alveolar epithelial cells (AECI) are thin, squamous epithelial cells that permit gas exchange and provide a barrier against microbial pathogens [3, 5, 8]. Type II alveolar epithelial cells (AECII) are cuboidal epithelial cells involved in tissue repair and regeneration, ion transport and fluid reabsorption, and surfactant production [4, 9]. Surfactant is composed of phospholipids and protein and is important for microbial clearance and reducing alveolar surface tension. If AECIIs are damaged, decreased surfactant production results in increased surface tension, which draws alveolar walls inwards and contributes to alveolar collapse (i.e., atelectasis). The alveolar-capillary barrier consists of a single layer of microvascular endothelial cells that surround the alveolar epithelium. Sandwiched between these two layers is a thin area of the interstitium, composed of elastic fibers and bundles of collagen that provide structural support to the alveolus [10]. AECs and endothelial cells, respectively, are linked tightly together by tight junction proteins that regulate paracellular fluid and ion transport between the blood, pulmonary interstitium, and alveolar compartment [4, 11]. This apparatus forms a well-regulated system that prevents undesired fluid and macromolecules of the blood from spilling into the alveolar compartment. In settings of infection or severe inflammation, however, this system can be significantly impaired and result in protein-rich edema with fibrin deposition in the alveoli.

While there are a multitude of factors involved in ARDS pathophysiology, it is speculated that early lung injury and inflammation are initiated by pattern recognition receptors (PRRs) from various cell types within pulmonary tissue that respond to exogenous pathogen-associated molecular patterns (PAMPs) from bacteria and viruses or endogenous damage-associated molecular patterns (DAMPs) from damaged tissue [5, 12]. Some viruses, such as influenza A and SARS-CoV-2, directly cause apoptosis and necrosis of AECII [13–15]. Indirectly, activation of TLR and other PRR signaling pathways leads to the transcription of NF-kB and IRFs, further potentiating the innate immune response [12, 16]. Expression of NF-kB leads to the production of many pro-inflammatory molecules that contribute to immune activation and alveolar epithelial cell injury [6, 12, 17–20]. In response to acute inflammation, endothelial paracellular permeability increases as a result of changes in tight-junction protein expression, which allows for fluid to accumulate in the alveolar airspace [21]. Additionally, broad immune activation leads to the expression of chemoattractants involved in the recruitment of neutrophils to the inflamed tissue [7, 12, 17].

It is well established that neutrophils are at the center of ARDS pathophysiology and are positively correlated with disease severity [5, 7, 22–25]. While classic neutrophil chemoattractants, such as IL-8 and TGF-β1, are elevated in acute lung injury (ALI) and ARDS, recruitment of neutrophils to the lungs in ARDS is still not fully understood [7, 12, 22, 25–27]. In addition to fighting pathogens, neutrophils cause devastating tissue damage by facilitating the production of reactive oxygen species (ROS), potentiating inflammation, and releasing neutrophil extracellular traps (NETs) [7]. ROS are, in part, a result of NADPH-oxidase complex (NOX2) on the surface of activated neutrophil membranes. The dysfunction of aerobic respiration and the electron transport chain within mitochondria is also a key contributor to the accumulation of ROS in hypoxic environments [28]. NOX2 reduces oxygen to hydrogen peroxide, which can yield hydroxyl radicals and cause phospholipid membrane damage and cell death to both the alveolar epithelium and microvascular endothelium [3, 7, 29]. As high numbers of activated neutrophils migrate through endothelial cells to reach the alveolar airspace, it is conceivable that local hydroxyl radicals produced by the activity of neutrophil-associated NOX2 can damage endothelial cell membranes. This could be one of the many ways that the endothelial barrier is disrupted in ARDS. NETs, on the other hand, are chromatin-like structures composed of nucleic acid, histones, and proteins [30]. Most notably, NETs contain neutrophil elastase (a serine protease), which is implicated in the pathophysiology of chronic pulmonary emphysema [31]. Neutrophil elastase likely contributes to the acute breakdown of the interstitium and diffuse alveolar damage (DAD), a histological hallmark of ARDS [32].

In summary, it is the combination of direct tissue injury, intense inflammation, and neutrophil recruitment to alveolar tissue that results in direct damage to alveolar epithelial and microvascular endothelial cells (Fig. 11.1). Alveolar damage in ALI and ARDS severely impairs gas exchange in the lungs, leading to hypoxemia and hypercapnia. We will now explore in detail how these mechanisms impact the pulmonary vasculature.

The Pulmonary Vascular Disease in ARDS

The definitive diagnosis of pulmonary hypertension (PH) in ARDS remains challenging—as the majority of these patients remain too unstable to tolerate a right heart catheterization (RHC) at the onset of illness. That being said, the clinical implications of developing changes in pulmonary vascular resistance (PVR) are well recognized at the physiologic level. The increase in PVR related to hypoxic vasoconstriction ultimately leads to RV dysfunction and subsequent RV failure [33]. This is primarily a Group 3 PH process, given that hypoxia is the primary mechanism for vascular-mediated changes. Signals of developing PH in the acute setting include: elevated PASP measured indirectly via echocardiography, refractory hypoxia despite optimal mechanical ventilatory strategies, and signs of progressive volume overload despite aggressive diuretic strategies [34]. Calcainu et al [35]

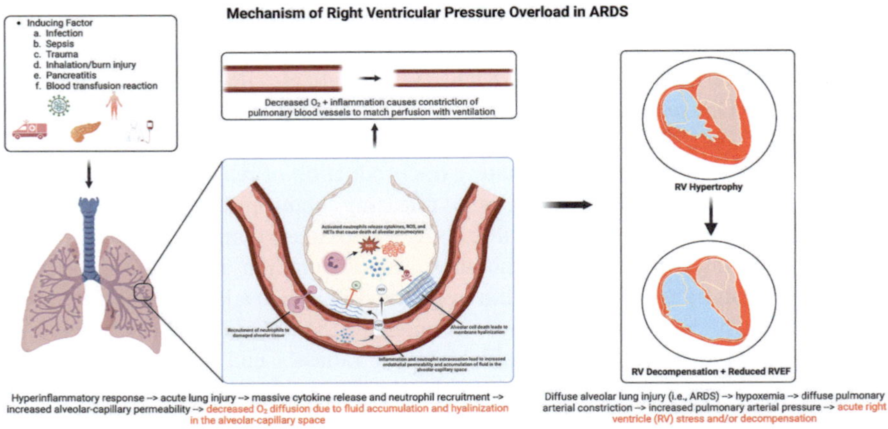

Fig. 11.1 ARDS is a consequence of massive inflammation, most often induced by severe infection, trauma, inhalation or burn injuries, pancreatitis, and/or blood transfusion reactions. A hyperinflammatory response can occur due to acute lung injury or may cause acute lung injury. In either case, neutrophils are recruited to alveolar tissue where they release immune-activating cytokines, reactive oxygen species (ROS), and neutrophil extracellular traps (NETs). Inflammatory cytokines (e.g., TNF-alpha, IL-1, and IL-6) increase capillary permeability, which leads to fluid accumulation from the bloodstream within the alveolar-capillary space. ROS and NETs can cause alveolar cell damage and death which promotes membrane hyalinization. Both fluid accumulation and membrane hyalinization limit the oxygen diffusing capacity of the alveolar membrane, leading to decreased diffusion of oxygen into the bloodstream. Resulting hypoxemia causes constriction of pulmonary arteries and increases stress (afterload) on the right ventricle (RV), which may result in RV decompensation. BioRender was used to generate this schematic

analyzed a small cohort of 38 patients who all received RHC during their hospitalization with ARDS. They found that PVR > 3 and Diastolic Pulmonary Gradient >7 were associated with a higher severity of illness. Despite these findings and heterogenous exposure to pulmonary vasodilators, acute treatment of hypoxia-mediated pulmonary vasoconstriction has never been shown to improve mortality [36]. In the context of the COVID-19 pandemic, significant research was dedicated to evaluating outcomes of rescue therapies related to refractory hypoxemia. A large cohort study by Al Sulaiman et al [37] demonstrated that the use of inhaled Nitric Oxide (iNO) improved oxygenation and pulmonary pressures in the first 48 h of treatment, but had no impact on mortality and had a signal towards worsening acute kidney injury, length of stay, and pneumonia.

There is data to suggest that inhaled prostacyclins may have the ability to provide transient improvement in oxygenation in ARDS; however, these studies have also not been able to show lasting mortality benefits whereby the benefits consistently outweigh the treatment-related risks [38]. Emerging data that needs further exploration is related to potential sub-phenotypes of ARDS (pre-existing systolic cardiac dysfunction) that may benefit more robustly from these therapies, especially if introduced early [39]. In the absence of pre-existing PH, survivors of ARDS largely have normalization of PASP via echocardiography 6–12 months post-hospitalization. This may not be true, however, of those who have pre-existing cardiac conditions or develop significant pulmonary fibrosis after their acute insult [40]. Because of these data points, the decision to utilize inhaled vasodilators remains hypothesis-generating but without consistent supportive evidence.

Epidemiologically, in mild to moderate ARDS, Squara et al [41] found an elevated mean pulmonary arterial pressure at 48 h of diagnosis of ARDS. Those with lower P/F ratios (indicating greater severity of illness) tended to have higher mPAP compared to those who had higher P/F ratios. Thereafter, several studies have been published finding mixed results in terms of mPAP truly being an independent predictor of mortality in these patients [42, 43]. Additionally, given the decline in the use of pulmonary arterial catheters in the management of sepsis in the ICU, access to this data has markedly declined, namely because having it has not demonstrated a substantial change in outcomes. Thus, although the development of PH likely has a prognostic value in ARDS, its acute treatment has not been reliably shown to improve long-term outcomes based on the current data available.

ARDS-Associated V/Q Mismatch and Pulmonary Vasoconstriction

Ventilation-perfusion (V/Q) coupling describes the efficiency of gas exchange that occurs within the alveolar compartment and, put simply, considers the inhalation of oxygen, exhalation of carbon dioxide, and blood flow through the pulmonary vasculature [44]. V/Q mismatch may occur when gas exchange and/or blood flow through the pulmonary vessels is impaired, such as in pulmonary embolism. V/Q mismatch can also occur because of pathologic remodeling of the pulmonary interstitium (i.e., pulmonary fibrosis) or alveoli (i.e., emphysema), as well as in acute settings such as ARDS.

ARDS-related V/Q mismatch is highly unpredictable and may result from poor ventilation, poor perfusion, or both concurrently. As described above, dysfunction of alveolar epithelial cells and the alveolar-capillary barrier results in atelectasis and pulmonary edema. Ventilation may be severely impaired in regions of the lungs that are most injured, which can result in hypoxemia and hypercapnia. Small pulmonary arterioles are highly sensitive to low oxygen levels in the blood and will respond by constricting to slow down blood flow and match perfusion with ventilation [45]. Hypoxia causes inhibition of voltage-gated K^+ channels within pulmonary arterial smooth muscle cells (PASMCs), which results in depolarization of PASMC membranes and accumulation of cytosolic free Ca^{2+}, triggering vasoconstriction [46, 47]. In response to the shear stress caused by PASMC constriction, pulmonary arterial endothelial cells (PAECs) release nitric oxide (NO) which counteracts PASMC contraction by activating soluble guanylyl cyclase to increase cGMP, an important inducer of vasodilation [48]. Simultaneously, hypoxia-inducible factor (HIF) proteins are key modulators of cellular responses to hypoxia and facilitate several mechanisms of crosstalk between PAECs and PASMCs. Activation of HIF-1α is shown to increase the production of endothelin-1 (ET-1) by endothelial cells, a mediator of pulmonary arterial vasoconstriction that is implicated in the pathophysiology of other pulmonary vascular diseases, including pulmonary arterial hypertension [49, 50]. ET-1 stimulates ET_A receptors on PASMCs to induce vasoconstriction while concurrently stimulating ET_B receptors on PAECs to stimulate NO production and release to induce vasodilation [51]. In ARDS, damage to PAECs due to shear stress, ROS, and massive inflammation can result in decreased NO production (e.g., endothelial dysfunction) and prolonged constriction of pulmonary vessels. In combination with reduced ventilation, dysregulated perfusion of alveoli can lead to unpredictable V/Q matching.

Endothelial Activation and Dysfunction in ARDS-Associated V/Q Mismatch

In addition to regulating fluid homeostasis between the bloodstream and the pulmonary interstitium, PAECs are important influencers of pulmonary hemodynamics and hemostasis. It is not surprising that endothelial activation, damage, and dysfunction are highly implicated in ARDS pathophysiology. Endothelial cells are activated by acute-phase reactants and pro-inflammatory cytokines, including TNF-α, IL-1, and IL-6 [52, 53]. Endothelial activation leads to modulated expression of tight junctions (i.e., increased endothelial permeability), expression of leukocyte adhesion molecules (LAMs) for the recruitment and transmigration of immune cells, a dramatic shift from anti-thrombotic to pro-thrombotic phenotypes, and cytokine production. Surrounding alveoli, we discussed above that increased permeability of PAECs contributes to pulmonary edema. Concurrently, expression of LAMs like E-selectin and ICAM-1 facilitates neutrophil rolling and adhesion to the endothelium, and thus aids in the accumulation of neutrophils in vascular and alveolar tissue [54, 55]. Of note is the shift to pro-thrombotic phenotypes by PAECs following activation.

In relatively minor injuries to tissue and blood vessels, inflammation is tame, and endothelial cells have a more gradual activation timeline. However, in more severe, rapid episodes of tissue injury, endothelial cells activate rather abruptly which increases the risk of dysregulated responses to tissue injury and makes it harder to step on the brakes. Abrupt activation of endothelial cells by inflammation increases the fusion and exocytosis of lysosomal storage vesicles called Weibel-Palade bodies (WPBs). These vesicles are preformed bodies composed primarily of P-selectin and von Willebrand factor (vWF) [56]. P-selectin is also expressed by platelets and binds to P-selectin glycoprotein ligand-1 (PSGL-1) on neutrophils, suggesting that P-selectin contributes to the recruitment of neutrophils to areas of tissue injury with a concurrently high risk of clotting [57]. vWF, on the other hand, is the first step in primary hemostasis that adheres to platelets to initiate clotting. High levels of clotting and complement factors also lead to the consumption and loss of anti-thrombotic and anti-inflammatory factors that reside on the endothelial membrane surface under physiologic conditions, such as thrombomodulin and heparan sulfate [52]. To support these molecular mechanisms, patients with direct ARDS have a higher risk and prevalence of venous thromboembolism (VTE), that is, deep vein thrombosis or pulmonary embolism [58, 59]. Therefore, high levels of endothelial activation within the lungs during ARDS lead to an increased risk of clots within the pulmonary vasculature that can further disrupt V/Q matching and increase resistance against the right ventricle.

Interestingly, it was also discovered that IL-8, a potent neutrophil chemoattractant, can be found in WBPs [60, 61]. In addition to increased clotting, this suggests another mechanism by which endothelial activation may contribute to ARDS pathophysiology: via the recruitment of neutrophils following the release of IL-8 and P-selectin-containing WPBs. It was previously demonstrated in mice that an inability to synthesize WPBs, and thus express P-selectin on the endothelial surface, results in reduced adhesion of leukocytes to endothelial tissue [62]. Additionally, porcine models have demonstrated an increased expression of WPBs and vWF in pulmonary arteries relative to the endothelium of other organs [63]. If these results are translatable to human tissue, then they may suggest another explanation for how endothelial cells contribute to ARDS pathophysiology and why neutrophil recruitment to pulmonary vascular and alveolar tissue is so sensitive in ARDS. It may also be important to note that desmopressin, along with its therapeutic analog vasopressin (which is commonly administered in patients with ARDS shock for hemodynamic support), stimulates the release of WPBs, vWF, and factor VIII [64]. One might be curious if vasopressin consequently increases the risk of clotting, however, at least one study of 175 patients in each arm found that vasopressin infusions do not increase the risk of VTE in patients with shock [65]. Nonetheless, the release of these vesicles may still contribute to ARDS pathophysiology via clotting or neutrophil recruitment.

Right Ventricular Dysfunction and Acute Cor Pulmonale in ARDS

Hypoxia-induced pulmonary vasoconstriction is a vital homeostatic mechanism for diverting intrapulmonary blood from regions of low oxygen to regions of normal oxygen and is usually not physiologically problematic in cases of focal atelectasis or pneumonia. However, if intrapulmonary shifting occurs more globally, then too much of the lungs' vascular system may become compromised, and diffuse constriction of pulmonary arterioles overwhelmingly increases pulmonary arterial pressure and, thus, right ventricular systolic pressure (RVSP) (Fig. 11.1). Considering that the RV is a much lower pressure system compared to the left ventricle (LV), it may be possible for right heart decompensation to occur acutely in cases of

ARDS. RV failure secondary to pathologic pulmonary remodeling and subsequent diffuse intrapulmonary shifting of blood flow is referred to as acute *cor pulmonale* and is the most concerning clinical endpoint that may result from increased RVSP.

Acute COVID-19 and Pulmonary Vasculature

Lung Injury and ARDS in Acute COVID-19

Since its emergence in December 2019, COVID-19 has caused significant disease and mortality that has had lasting effects on global health care, economic, and social systems. ARDS and respiratory failure are among the most common clinical outcomes in hospitalized patients with acute COVID-19 [66, 67]. SARS-CoV-2, the virus responsible for COVID-19, invades host cells through interactions between the Spike (S) protein on the virus' membrane and ACE2 receptors on host cell membranes [68]. ACE2 is abundantly expressed on lung epithelial cells, most importantly type II alveolar epithelial cells (AECII) [69]. Invasion of AECII by the virus leads to their dysfunction and death, yielding decreased surfactant production and atelectasis. Consequently, atelectasis decreases lung compliance and increases the pressure required to inflate the lungs with air. If lung expansion is impaired, then less oxygen is inhaled, and less carbon dioxide is exhaled. Trapping of carbon dioxide (i.e., hypercapnia) leads to acidosis of the blood and metabolic dysfunction, and decreased oxygen in the blood (i.e., hypoxemia) causes constriction of pulmonary arterioles to shift blood to more oxygenated areas of the lung. If the virus is not controlled by the immune response and instead allowed to spread diffusely throughout lung tissue, the respiratory system fails, and systemic hypoxemia ensues. It is estimated that as much as 24% of patients with SARS-CoV-2 pneumonia develop atelectasis, and the larger the area of atelectasis in a patient's lungs the more severe the disease and the higher the risk of mortality [70].

In addition to atelectasis, SARS-CoV-2 can instigate an exaggerated inflammatory immune response, known as a cytokine storm. The mechanism is not completely understood, but it is thought that crosstalk between epithelial and immune cells of infected tissues leads to an untamed hyperinflammatory response. In response to infection, the innate immune system releases proinflammatory cytokines IL-1, IL-6, IL-8, IL-12, IL-17, and TNF-α [71]. Most notably, IL-8 and IL-17 are important chemoattractants for neutrophils, the drivers of lung damage in ARDS. IL-8 is demonstrated to be a reliable marker of COVID-19 disease severity [72]. Additionally, a study by Wu et al. [73] found that SARS-CoV-2 variants with open reading frame 8 (ORF8) gene deletion cause a milder disease compared to variants with intact ORF8. This is fascinating because ORF8 encodes for a viral cytokine that behaves similarly to IL-17A, only it has a much stronger and broader activating effect on IL-17R [73].

IL-17 levels are highly correlated with lung injury. One study of 210 patients by Xie et al. [74] discovered that patients with SNPs in the human gene coding region for IL-17A had varying levels of susceptibility to ARDS. In other words, patients with decreased IL-17 responses were protected from ARDS, while those who had a hyperactive IL-17 response were at increased risk of ARDS and death. IL-17A is associated with acute airway and alveolar inflammation, likely due to its ability to activate neutrophils [75]. As discussed above, activated neutrophils release protease-containing NETs that break down connective tissue in the lungs and cause alveolar destruction. Simultaneously, inflammation leads to increased endothelial permeability which allows for fluid to accumulate in the lungs (pleural edema). In combination with AECII damage and atelectasis, increased endothelial permeability and pleural edema contribute to the development of hypoxemia. While IL-17 contributes to neutrophil-mediated lung injury and ARDS, it is also involved in the pathophysiology of myocarditis and dilated cardiomyopathy, as well as angiogenesis [76, 77].

Some studies have hypothesized that, because SARS-CoV-2 invades host cells via the ACE2 receptor, it might decrease ACE2 expression on the surface of endothelial cells, thus interfering with the renin-angiotensin-aldosterone system (RAAS) [78, 79]. ACE2 is responsible for breaking down angiotensin II, and increased levels of angiotensin II are associated with hypertension, vascular remodeling, inflammation in blood vessels, and cardiac fibrosis [80, 81]. It is suggested that a decrease in ACE2 caused by SARS-CoV-2 causes enhanced vascular remodeling and contributes to disease manifestations seen in acute COVID-19. However, while SARS-CoV-2 may decrease ACE2 expression, it is unclear to what extent the RAAS is actually affected by acute COVID-19. Although ACE2 is highly expressed in pulmonary epithelial cells, it is also expressed throughout many different organs including the brain, kidneys, and GI tract [69]. Therefore, if ACE2 is theoretically decreased in one vital organ, the breakdown of angiotensin II may be compensated for at another site. The distribution of ACE2 expression throughout the body may help explain how SARS-CoV-2 is able to cause damage to multiple different organs, but it is important to remember that there are other factors related to acute lung injury at play that can also cause multiorgan dysfunction, such as hypoxemia and lactic acidosis, in acute COVID-19. Hypotheses around SARS-CoV-2 interference with the RAAS prompted many clinical trials that aimed to test if therapies could intervene with the dysregulated RAAS in acute COVID-19 using angiotensin receptor blockers (e.g., Losartan), but Losartan had no beneficial treatment effect in a meta-analysis conducted by Di Stefano et al. [82]. In theory, increased angiotensin II locally in the lungs caused by SARS-CoV-2 infection could contribute to pulmonary hypertension in acute COVID-19, but it is unknown how significant this physiologic dysregulation would be and how long it would last if other organ systems can compensate for increased blood levels of angiotensin II. That said, ACE2 may protect against the development of ARDS by breaking down other macromolecules that contribute to pulmonary vasodilation [83], so decreased ACE2 may contribute to increased pulmonary pressures due to hypoxemia-induced vasoconstriction of the pulmonary arteries.

Some studies have reported acute increases in pulmonary artery pressures and right ventricular dysfunction in COVID-19 patients [84–88]. Wolters, et al. found 29.7% of patients with acute COVID-19 infections had elevated RVSP on echocardiogram and PH prevalence was estimated at 12% in an earlier Italian population [87]. These changes were likely driven by hypoxia and intrapulmonary shunting as seen in other causes of acute lung injury or ARDS. Limitations of these studies included little previous data on echocardiogram findings before COVID-19 infection and there were no invasive hemodynamic measurements (right heart catheterization) to confirm the presence of pulmonary hypertension.

COVID-19 Coagulopathy

SARS-CoV-2 can also induce hypercoagulability in many patients with acute COVID-19. Hypercoagulability is evidenced by abnormal lab findings, including but not limited to elevated D-Dimer, prolonged prothrombin and activated partial thromboplastin, and high or low platelet counts—however, it probably depends on the stage and severity of disease that these lab findings present [89, 90]. In a systematic review that analyzed 47 candidate studies, it was reported that the pooled estimate of pulmonary embolism (PE) in COVID-19 patients was 32%, and the pooled estimate of deep vein thrombosis (DVT) was 27% [91]. Collectively, PE and DVT are referred to as venous thromboembolism (VTE). Stroke and myocardial infarction are also reported in COVID-19 patients, but not as commonly as VTE [92]. The considerably high incidence of VTE was reported despite at least 36 of the 47 studies administering prophylactic antithrombotic therapy to patients [91]. VTE, especially PE, is the most frequent thrombotic complication of COVID-19 [90, 92–94].

Coagulopathy in COVID-19 is highly complex and multifactorial, so it helps to consider contributing factors to clot risk in COVID-19 in terms of Virchow's Triad. In 1856, Rudolf Virchow proposed that blood clots are more likely to occur in states of decreased perfusion (stasis), endothelial injury, and hypercoagulability [95]. In COVID-19 patients, decreased perfusion likely occurs due to hyperinflammation-induced vasodilation and increased endothelial permeability that allows plasma fluid to leak into extravascular spaces. Endothelial injury is probably a result of inflammation, increased ROS, acidosis, and direct infection by SARS-CoV-2. Hypercoagulability, however, is more complex.

Hyperinflammation is one important factor to consider in COVID-19 hypercoagulability. The interplay between inflammation and hemostasis has long been established [96]. Tissue factor (TF) is an important link between inflammation and thrombosis, and patients with acute COVID-19 are shown to have higher levels of circulating TF [97, 98]. Following blood vessel injury, TF complexes with Factor VIIa to activate the coagulation cascade and form a clot. TF is primarily expressed by cells in the adventitial layer of blood vessels and is exposed only after injury to the inner endothelial lining of a blood vessel [99]. TF is also expressed by other cell types, including monocytes, platelets, and endothelial cells, which increase TF expression and its release on extracellular vesicles (Evs) in response to proinflammatory cytokines [98–100]. As this review is focused on the pulmonary vasculature during COVID-19 ARDS, we will consider the implications of hypercoagulability within the lungs. Significant clot burden in the lungs is a risk factor for hypoxic respiratory failure and mortality in acute COVID-19. Clotting within the pulmonary vasculature may be a consequence of hyperinflammation and direct injury of endothelial cells by SARS-CoV-2, or there could be other physiological factors at play.

It may be that TF is expressed on the surface of endothelial cells within pulmonary vessels at higher levels than other organ sites during acute lung inflammation and injury. Free heme in the blood has been shown to induce TF expression in endothelial cells [101], and patients with severe acute COVID-19 have significant clotting that can cause hemolysis by the mechanical shearing of erythrocytes. In mice with sickle cell disease (SCD), endothelial cells within pulmonary veins express TF following hypoxia exposure, and TF expression by these cells is positively correlated with SCD crisis severity [102]. SCD is characterized by recurrent acute or chronic episodes of hemolysis during times of hypoxemia and pH disturbances in the blood. While the exact pathogenesis of PH in SCD is debated, contributing factors include endothelial injury, acute/chronic inflammation, hypercoagulability and thrombosis, chronic intravascular hemolysis, and altered bioavailability in nitric oxide, making this pathogenesis somewhat similar to COVID-19 infection [103]. Pulmonary pressures can vary widely during times of crises and quiescence. In COVID-19, hemolysis, hypoxemia, and mixed acidosis can all be observed, sometimes simultaneously. Perhaps by increased TF expression and clotting in the pulmonary microvasculature, more blood is diverted toward more oxygenated areas for better perfusion. However, during acute COVID-19 if the virus spreads diffusely throughout the lungs, this mechanism may overcompensate and create overwhelming pressures in the pulmonary vasculature synergistically with hypoxia-induced vasoconstriction (discussed above).

In addition to TF, there are broader mechanisms by which hyperinflammation leads to hypercoagulability. It is simplest to again think of it in terms of Virchow's Triad: stasis of blood flow, endothelial injury, and hypercoagulability. TNF-α and IL-1 are acute phase reactants that activate endothelial cells and induce expression of adhesive proteins, such as intercellular adhesion molecule-1 (ICAM-1), which promote rolling and adhesion of leukocytes and initiate their extravasation into extravascular tissue [104]. In combination with cytokine-induced changes in tight-junction protein expression, leukocyte transmigration through the vascular endothelium increases endothelial permeability and leakage of intravascular fluid into the extravascular space, which decreases forward blood flow. Thus, inflammation causes blood stasis. Additionally, SARS-CoV-2 has been shown to induce IL-1-mediated activation of the NLRP3 inflammasome which leads to endotheliitis and endothelial apoptosis [105]. Further, a study by Joffre et al. [106] demonstrated that SARS-CoV-2 can infect and replicate within pulmonary microvascular endothelial cells; however, other studies contradict these findings. Nevertheless, the Spike protein released by infected lung epithelial cells or in circulation may promote endothelial activation, cell injury, and death. Given the proximity to alveolar cells where the advent of infection often occurs, it is fair to assume that most endothelial cells infected with SARS-CoV-2 are likely within the pulmonary vasculature. Whenever the vascular endothelium is injured and apoptotic, it exposes underlying collagen which binds vWF to activate the clotting cascade. vWF is released in Weibel-Palade Bodies (WBPs) by endothelial cells in response to endothelial inflammation/activation [56]. In addition, TF expression may be increased on activated endothelial cells or are exposed on adventitial cells following endothelial injury to promote Factor VIIa complexing and coagulation activation as well. It is also important to consider the normal anticoagulant function of undamaged endothelial tissue. The endothelium is coated with glycocalyx, a matrix of glycoproteins and proteoglycans that serve a variety of functions, including repulsion of circulating erythrocytes from interacting with endothelial cells, maintenance of endothelial integrity and prevention of extravascular edema, and antithrombosis [107]. When the glycocalyx is disturbed, this too may predispose to clotting.

In addition to hyperinflammation, thrombotic microangiopathy (TMA) is a thrombotic complication observed in acute COVID-19. TMA is a microangiopathic hemolytic anemia (MAHA) that occurs when activated platelets aggregate in small vessels and form clots that mechanically shear red blood cells and lyse them open, causing abrupt anemia. It is a consumptive coagulopathy that also causes platelets and clotting factors to be consumed more rapidly than they can be produced, which results in abnormal coagulation labs (i.e., prolonged bleeding time) in patients with significant disease. Several studies have observed significant clot burden within the lungs by autopsy in COVID-19 patients because of TMA [92, 108, 109]. Like thrombotic thrombocytopenic purpura (TTP), TMA is a result of an acquired deficiency of ADAMTS13, a metalloproteinase synthesized by the liver that is responsible for cleaving vWF complexes to break clots [110]. A deficiency in ADAMTS13 means that preformed clots will not be dissolved as easily and may persist and accumulate in size, which can cause tissue ischemia and multi-organ dysfunction. Low ADAMTS13 levels in COVID-19 perpetuate hypercoagulability. Indeed, decreased ADAMTS13 levels are observed in some COVID-19 patients, and a high ADAMTS13:vWF ratio correlates with disease severity [98, 111]. Low levels of ADAMTS13 may be due to increased consumption of coagulation factors as described above. Curiously, though, some patients with acute COVID-19 develop potentially inhibitory antibodies against ADAMTS13. A study by Doevelaar et al. [112] found that ADAMTS13 autoantibodies were detected in 34.4% (31/90) of COVID-19 patients enrolled in their study, and the presence of these autoantibodies was associated with lower ADAMTS13 activity. Further, the concentration of ADAMTS13 antibodies in COVID-19 patients was correlated with disease severity, suggesting that the duration of illness and infection may correlate with autoantibody production [112]. Decreased ADAMTS13 levels and/or activity ultimately increase the risk of TMA and profuse clotting within the lungs during acute COVID-19. In addition to hypoxia-induced vasoconstriction, it is important to consider diffuse pulmonary thrombosis as this can also increase afterload on the RV and result in acute right heart failure (i.e., cor pulmonale).

Long-COVID and the Pulmonary Vasculature

The Lingering Effects of COVID-19

For many patients, COVID-19 symptoms and physiologic manifestations do not stop with acute illness. Patients can experience potentially debilitating symptoms for several weeks, months, or even years following acute COVID-19 infection. Long-COVID is an ambiguous syndrome that continues to be difficult to characterize because of the breadth of symptoms affecting multiple organ systems that patients report. The United Kingdom National Institute for Health and Care Excellence (NICE) guidelines put forth a definition of long COVID in December 2020 that defined the condition in two phases: an ongoing symptomatic phase 4–12 weeks post-acute COVID-19 infection, and a post-acute sequelae of COVID-19 (PASC) syndrome with symptoms persisting ≥12 weeks post-acute COVID-19 infection [113]. Commonly reported symptoms include fatigue, cough, dyspnea, mood changes, brain fog, and loss of taste and smell.

A study of electronic health records of a large population in England and Whales found that the relative incidence of arterial thromboses (i.e., stroke and MI) and VTE remained elevated for up to 49 weeks post-acute COVID-19 [114]. Specifically, the relative incidence of VTE declined slower than the incidence of arterial thromboses and was twofold higher for up to 49 weeks [114]. Another study [115] of more than 1 million patients in Sweden found that the rate ratio of DVT and PE remained elevated for 70 days and 110 days, respectively, post-acute COVID-19. It is not uncommon for viruses to cause an increase in the incidence of clotting post-acute infection, and the incidence of clotting in post-acute COVID-19 patients is clearly significant. However, it remains unclear what mechanism(s) specifically lead to the increased incidence of VTE and arterial thromboses in post-acute COVID-19 patients, making preventive therapy difficult to devise.

There are several theories regarding the etiology of clotting in post-acute COVID-19 patients. It was previously reported that persistent levels of COVID-19 S protein and viral RNA circulating in the plasma and EVs of patients who reported long COVID symptoms [116, 117]. This could mean that SARS-CoV-2 has a mechanism for hiding out in long-lived cells and may be released intermittently, causing inflammation. It is still unclear if the SARS-CoV-2 S protein and viral RNA that persist in post-COVID patients are from mature virions or are fragments of SARS-CoV-2. If SARS-CoV-2 can self-replicate long term, then according to the study by Joffre et al. [106] there may be repeated infection and damage to endothelial cells of the pulmonary microvasculature, which would increase the risk for PE. Regardless, S protein itself can induce the expression of several proinflammatory cytokines, and viral RNA initiates a proinflammatory response via toll-like receptors (TLRs) [118, 119]. As discussed above, inflammation can lead to endothelial activation which promotes clotting, and pro-inflammatory cytokines can activate the coagulation cascade. Therefore, increased incidence of VTE in post-COVID patients may be a result of persistent circulation of SARS-CoV-2 components and inflammation.

Prolonged clotting of the pulmonary microvasculature causes ischemia, which may lead to damage of blood vessels, angiogenesis, and increased pressures within the pulmonary circulatory system. Microclots that are individually asymptomatic may accumulate and disperse throughout the pulmonary vasculature due to endotheliitis and the suspected pro-coagulative state that may exist within some post-COVID patients. Although rare, this is representative of chronic thromboembolic pulmonary hypertension (CTEPH).

Patients with some preexisting comorbidities, such as chronic heart failure, may also suffer accelerated health deficiencies as a result of acute COVID-19. A multicenter study by Núñez-Gil et al. [120] reported that heart failure patients are more likely to have worse health outcomes and an increased risk of mortality compared to patients without heart failure following acute COVID-19. Another large study by Xie et al. [121] reported an increased 12-month burden of ischemic heart disease and heart failure in patients ≥30 days post-acute COVID-19. The association between SARS-CoV-2 and heart disease is unclear but may involve direct infection of ACE-2 expressing cardiomyocytes by SARS-CoV-2 [121, 122]. Severe acute COVID-19 in patients with preexisting heart failure may lead to lasting consequences and accelerated deterioration. Prolonged dysfunction of the heart may predispose individuals to Group 2 PH, or PH secondary to heart disease. In this scenario, the filling or pumping dysfunction of the heart causes fluid to back up into the pulmonary vasculature and cause increased pressures.

Post-COVID-19 pulmonary fibrosis (PCPF) is also reported to be a lasting challenge for patients who have severe, acute COVID-19 infection. In a meta-analysis conducted by Amin et al. [123], it was reported that 44.9% of post-COVID patients suffer from PCPF. It is unclear why some patients develop PCPF after acute illness, though the authors mention a higher prevalence in patients with preexisting COPD [123]. Additionally, in their analysis of studies, the authors found that PCPF resolved within a few months in some patients but persisted after the study in others. It is unclear what the reason is for these findings. Considering the severe damage to pulmonary parenchymal tissue caused by acute COVID-19 lung injury, it is expected that there would be some residual tissue damage, but this often resolves within 1–2 years. It remains unclear if there will be some patients who never return to their pre-COVID lung function due to PCPF. Therefore, patients with prolonged PCPF might be at increased risk of Group 3 PH, or PH caused by chronic lung disease. Pulmonary fibrosis can cause hypoxemia within pulmonary vascular tissue which, as discussed above, causes constriction and increased pressures within the pulmonary vasculature but these sequelae may not be seen for years after infection and development of fibrosis.

Since the eruption of the COVID-19 pandemic, some researchers and physicians have postulated that acute COVID-19 may increase the risk for chronic pulmonary hypertension (PH) by various mechanisms [124, 125]. Few case studies have reported rare instances of pulmonary hypertension being diagnosed following hospitalization with acute COVID-19 and these were limited by confirmatory hemodynamic measurements [126–128]. However, all of the reported individual patients who were diagnosed with PH post-COVID, to our knowledge, were diagnosed during their hospitalization with acute COVID-19 or within 8 weeks of hospital discharge and many of these cases lacked previous results from testing before infection. Therefore, the increased pressures in the pulmonary vasculature seen acutely are more likely due to damage to pulmonary parenchymal tissue resulting in prolonged dysfunction of blood oxygenation in the lungs. As discussed above, the consequential hypoxemia causes vasoconstriction of pulmonary arteries and increases pulmonary arterial pressure. One case study reported severe PH in a 60-year-old male with a past medical history significant for prior myocardial infarction (timeline not reported) [128]. In this gentleman, prior myocardial infarction probably resulted in scarring of cardiac tissue and decreased systolic and/or diastolic dysfunction of the ventricle. Therefore, the PH in this case is probably secondary to heart failure, or Group 2 PH. It is possible that an acute COVID-19 infection resulted in a severe hyperinflammatory response and reduced blood oxygen levels, which would stress the heart in an attempt to increase cardiac output to maintain tissue perfusion. While the immune response and tissue destruction that occurs during acute COVID-19 may contribute to acute PH, to our knowledge, there is no study to date with convincing evidence suggesting that SARS-COV-2 is directly involved in PH pathophysiology. A review article by Eroume Á Egom et al. [124] suggests that SARS-CoV-2 viral proteins, namely the spike S1 protein, instigate endothelial damage and vascular remodeling that may predispose one to PH. Any forms of PH that occur during the course of acute COVID-19 or the brief weeks that follow acute infection are more likely to be due to secondary effects of the infection, as described in this review article, and probably do not have any long-term consequences unless a patient has another preexisting condition (i.e., heart failure) that is worsened by acute infection.

References

1. Matthay MA, et al. A new global definition of acute respiratory distress syndrome. Am J Respir Crit Care Med. 2023. https://doi.org/10.1164/rccm.202303-0558WS.
2. Force ADT, et al. Acute respiratory distress syndrome: the Berlin Definition. JAMA. 2012;307:2526–33. https://doi.org/10.1001/jama.2012.5669.
3. Ware LB, Matthay MA. The acute respiratory distress syndrome. N Engl J Med. 2000;342:1334–49. https://doi.org/10.1056/NEJM200005043421806.
4. Matthay MA, Zemans RL. The acute respiratory distress syndrome: pathogenesis and treatment. Annu Rev Pathol. 2011;6:147–63. https://doi.org/10.1146/annurev-pathol-011110-130158.
5. Matthay MA, Ware LB, Zimmerman GA. The acute respiratory distress syndrome. J Clin Invest. 2012;122:2731–40. https://doi.org/10.1172/JCI60331.
6. Matthay MA, et al. Acute respiratory distress syndrome. Nat Rev Dis Primers. 2019;5:18. https://doi.org/10.1038/s41572-019-0069-0.
7. Yang SC, Tsai YF, Pan YL, Hwang TL. Understanding the role of neutrophils in acute respiratory distress syndrome. Biomed J. 2021;44:439–46. https://doi.org/10.1016/j.bj.2020.09.001.
8. Williams MC. Alveolar type I cells: molecular phenotype and development. Annu Rev Physiol. 2003;65:669–95. https://doi.org/10.1146/annurev.physiol.65.092101.142446.

9. Chuquimia OD, Petursdottir DH, Periolo N, Fernandez C. Alveolar epithelial cells are critical in protection of the respiratory tract by secretion of factors able to modulate the activity of pulmonary macrophages and directly control bacterial growth. Infect Immun. 2013;81:381–9. https://doi.org/10.1128/IAI.00950-12.
10. Knudsen L, Ochs M. The micromechanics of lung alveoli: structure and function of surfactant and tissue components. Histochem Cell Biol. 2018;150:661–76. https://doi.org/10.1007/s00418-018-1747-9.
11. Bhattacharya J, Matthay MA. Regulation and repair of the alveolar-capillary barrier in acute lung injury. Annu Rev Physiol. 2013;75:593–615. https://doi.org/10.1146/annurev-physiol-030212-183756.
12. Opitz B, van Laak V, Eitel J, Suttorp N. Innate immune recognition in infectious and noninfectious diseases of the lung. Am J Respir Crit Care Med. 2010;181:1294–309. https://doi.org/10.1164/rccm.200909-1427SO.
13. Martines RB, et al. Pathology and pathogenesis of SARS-CoV-2 associated with fatal coronavirus disease, United States. Emerg Infect Dis. 2020;26:2005–15. https://doi.org/10.3201/eid2609.202095.
14. Uiprasertkul M, et al. Apoptosis and pathogenesis of avian influenza A (H5N1) virus in humans. Emerg Infect Dis. 2007;13:708–12. https://doi.org/10.3201/eid1305.060572.
15. Mauad T, et al. Lung pathology in fatal novel human influenza A (H1N1) infection. Am J Respir Crit Care Med. 2010;181:72–9. https://doi.org/10.1164/rccm.200909-1420OC.
16. Kawasaki T, Kawai T. Toll-like receptor signaling pathways. Front Immunol. 2014;5:461. https://doi.org/10.3389/fimmu.2014.00461.
17. Tak PP, Firestein GS. NF-kappaB: a key role in inflammatory diseases. J Clin Invest. 2001;107:7–11. https://doi.org/10.1172/JCI11830.
18. Wittekindt OH. Tight junctions in pulmonary epithelia during lung inflammation. Pflugers Arch. 2017;469:135–47. https://doi.org/10.1007/s00424-016-1917-3.
19. Coyne CB, Vanhook MK, Gambling TM, Carson JL, Boucher RC, Johnson LG. Regulation of airway tight junctions by proinflammatory cytokines. Mol Biol Cell. 2002;13:3218–34. https://doi.org/10.1091/mbc.e02-03-0134.
20. Mazzon E, Cuzzocrea S. Role of TNF-alpha in lung tight junction alteration in mouse model of acute lung inflammation. Respir Res. 2007;8:75. https://doi.org/10.1186/1465-9921-8-75.
21. Pober JS, Sessa WC. Evolving functions of endothelial cells in inflammation. Nat Rev Immunol. 2007;7:803–15. https://doi.org/10.1038/nri2171.
22. Zemans RL, Matthay MA. What drives neutrophils to the alveoli in ARDS? Thorax. 2017;72:1–3. https://doi.org/10.1136/thoraxjnl-2016-209170.
23. Grommes J, Soehnlein O. Contribution of neutrophils to acute lung injury. Mol Med. 2011;17:293–307. https://doi.org/10.2119/molmed.2010.00138.
24. Cesta MC, et al. The role of interleukin-8 in lung inflammation and injury: implications for the management of COVID-19 and hyperinflammatory acute respiratory distress syndrome. Front Pharmacol. 2021;12:808797. https://doi.org/10.3389/fphar.2021.808797.
25. Kiehl MG, Ostermann H, Thomas M, Muller C, Cassens U, Kienast J. Inflammatory mediators in bronchoalveolar lavage fluid and plasma in leukocytopenic patients with septic shock-induced acute respiratory distress syndrome. Crit Care Med. 1998;26:1194–9. https://doi.org/10.1097/00003246-199807000-00019.
26. Pallister I, Dent C, Topley N. Increased neutrophil migratory activity after major trauma: a factor in the etiology of acute respiratory distress syndrome? Crit Care Med. 2002;30:1717–21. https://doi.org/10.1097/00003246-200208000-00007.
27. Fahy RJ, Lichtenberger F, McKeegan CB, Nuovo GJ, Marsh CB, Wewers MD. The acute respiratory distress syndrome: a role for transforming growth factor-beta 1. Am J Respir Cell Mol Biol. 2003;28:499–503. https://doi.org/10.1165/rcmb.2002-0092OC.
28. Fuhrmann DC, Brune B. Mitochondrial composition and function under the control of hypoxia. Redox Biol. 2017;12:208–15. https://doi.org/10.1016/j.redox.2017.02.012.

29. Paclet MH, Laurans S, Dupre-Crochet S. Regulation of neutrophil NADPH oxidase, NOX2: a crucial effector in neutrophil phenotype and function. Front Cell Dev Biol. 2022;10:945749. https://doi.org/10.3389/fcell.2022.945749.
30. Papayannopoulos V. Neutrophil extracellular traps in immunity and disease. Nat Rev Immunol. 2018;18:134–47. https://doi.org/10.1038/nri.2017.105.
31. Voynow JA, Shinbashi M. Neutrophil elastase and chronic lung disease. Biomolecules. 2021;11. https://doi.org/10.3390/biom11081065.
32. Cardinal-Fernandez P, Lorente JA, Ballen-Barragan A, Matute-Bello G. Acute respiratory distress syndrome and diffuse alveolar damage. New insights on a complex relationship. Ann Am Thorac Soc. 2017;14:844–50. https://doi.org/10.1513/AnnalsATS.201609-728PS.
33. Simonneau G, et al. Haemodynamic definitions and updated clinical classification of pulmonary hypertension. Eur Respir J. 2019;53:1801913. https://doi.org/10.1183/13993003.01913-2018.
34. Revercomb L, Hanmandlu A, Wareing N, Akkanti B, Karmouty-Quintana H. Mechanisms of pulmonary hypertension in acute respiratory distress syndrome (ARDS). Front Mol Biosci. 2020;7:624093. https://doi.org/10.3389/fmolb.2020.624093.
35. Calcaianu G, Calcaianu M, Gschwend A, Canuet M, Meziani F, Kessler R. Hemodynamic profile of pulmonary hypertension (PH) in ARDS. Pulm Circ. 2018;8:2045893217753415. https://doi.org/10.1177/2045893217753415.
36. Bull TM, Clark B, McFann K, Moss M. Pulmonary vascular dysfunction is associated with poor outcomes in patients with acute lung injury. Am J Respir Crit Care Med. 2010;182:1123–8. https://doi.org/10.1164/rccm.201002-0250OC.
37. Al Sulaiman K, et al. Evaluation of inhaled nitric oxide (iNO) treatment for moderate-to-severe ARDS in critically ill patients with COVID-19: a multicenter cohort study. Crit Care. 2022;26:304. https://doi.org/10.1186/s13054-022-04158-y.
38. Kallet RH, et al. Severity of hypoxemia and other factors that influence the response to aerosolized prostacyclin in ARDS. Respir Care. 2017;62:1014–22. https://doi.org/10.4187/respcare.05268.
39. Torbic H, Saini A, Harnegie MP, Sadana D, Duggal A. Inhaled prostacyclins for acute respiratory distress syndrome: a systematic review and meta-analysis. Critic Care Explorations. 2023;5:e0931. https://doi.org/10.1097/cce.0000000000000931.
40. Matthay MA, et al. Acute respiratory distress syndrome. Nat Rev Dis Prim. 2019;5:18. https://doi.org/10.1038/s41572-019-0069-0.
41. Squara P, Dhainaut JF, Artigas A, Carlet J. Hemodynamic profile in severe ARDS: results of the European Collaborative ARDS Study. Intensive Care Med. 1998;24:1018–28. https://doi.org/10.1007/s001340050710.
42. Osman D, et al. Incidence and prognostic value of right ventricular failure in acute respiratory distress syndrome. Intensive Care Med. 2009;35:69–76. https://doi.org/10.1007/s00134-008-1307-1.
43. Ryan D, Frohlich S, McLoughlin P. Pulmonary vascular dysfunction in ARDS. Ann Intensive Care. 2014;4:28. https://doi.org/10.1186/s13613-014-0028-6.
44. Hopkins SR. Ventilation/perfusion relationships and gas exchange: measurement approaches. Compr Physiol. 2020;10:1155–205. https://doi.org/10.1002/cphy.c180042.
45. Dunham-Snary KJ, et al. Hypoxic pulmonary vasoconstriction: from molecular mechanisms to medicine. Chest. 2017;151:181–92. https://doi.org/10.1016/j.chest.2016.09.001.
46. Olschewski A, Hong Z, Nelson DP, Weir EK. Graded response of K+ current, membrane potential, and [Ca2+]i to hypoxia in pulmonary arterial smooth muscle. Am J Phys Lung Cell Mol Phys. 2002;283:L1143–50. https://doi.org/10.1152/ajplung.00104.2002.
47. Sweeney M, Yuan JX. Hypoxic pulmonary vasoconstriction: role of voltage-gated potassium channels. Respir Res. 2000;1:40–8. https://doi.org/10.1186/rr11.
48. Ataei Ataabadi E, Golshiri K, Juttner A, Krenning G, Danser AHJ, Roks AJM, Nitric oxide-cGMP signaling in hypertension: current and future options for pharmacotherapy. Hypertension. 2020;76:1055–68. https://doi.org/10.1161/HYPERTENSIONAHA.120.15856.

49. Shen YS, Goncharova EA. TWISTed HIF: revisiting smooth muscle HIF-1alpha signaling in pulmonary hypertension. Am J Phys Lung Cell Mol Phys. 2018;315:L387–9. https://doi.org/10.1152/ajplung.00285.2018.
50. Yu J, Taylor L, Wilson J, Comhair S, Erzurum S, Polgar P. Altered expression and signal transduction of endothelin-1 receptors in heritable and idiopathic pulmonary arterial hypertension. J Cell Physiol. 2013;228:322–9. https://doi.org/10.1002/jcp.24132.
51. Nohria A, Garrett L, Johnson W, Kinlay S, Ganz P, Creager MA. Endothelin-1 and vascular tone in subjects with atherogenic risk factors. Hypertension. 2003;42:43–8. https://doi.org/10.1161/01.HYP.0000074426.71392.D8.
52. Hunt BJ, Jurd KM. Endothelial cell activation. A central pathophysiological process. BMJ. 1998;316:1328–9. https://doi.org/10.1136/bmj.316.7141.1328.
53. Liao JK. Linking endothelial dysfunction with endothelial cell activation. J Clin Invest. 2013;123:540–1. https://doi.org/10.1172/JCI66843.
54. Yang L, Froio RM, Sciuto TE, Dvorak AM, Alon R, Luscinskas FW. ICAM-1 regulates neutrophil adhesion and transcellular migration of TNF-alpha-activated vascular endothelium under flow. Blood. 2005;106:584–92. https://doi.org/10.1182/blood-2004-12-4942.
55. Zarbock A, Ley K. Neutrophil adhesion and activation under flow. Microcirculation. 2009;16:31–42. https://doi.org/10.1080/10739680802350104.
56. Rondaij MG, Bierings R, Kragt A, van Mourik JA, Voorberg J. Dynamics and plasticity of Weibel-Palade bodies in endothelial cells. Arterioscler Thromb Vasc Biol. 2006;26:1002–7. https://doi.org/10.1161/01.ATV.0000209501.56852.6c.
57. Zimmerman GA. Two by two: the pairings of P-selectin and P-selectin glycoprotein ligand 1. Proc Natl Acad Sci USA. 2001;98:10023–4. https://doi.org/10.1073/pnas.191367898.
58. Cui N, et al. Deep vein thrombosis in acute respiratory distress syndrome caused by bacterial pneumonia. BMC Pulm Med. 2021;21:264. https://doi.org/10.1186/s12890-021-01632-1.
59. Marini CP, et al. Incidence and effects of deep vein thrombosis on the outcome of patients with coronavirus disease 2019 infection. J Vasc Surg Venous Lymphat Disord. 2022;10:803–10. https://doi.org/10.1016/j.jvsv.2021.10.013.
60. Wolff B, Burns AR, Middleton J, Rot A. Endothelial cell "memory" of inflammatory stimulation: human venular endothelial cells store interleukin 8 in Weibel-Palade bodies. J Exp Med. 1998;188:1757–62. https://doi.org/10.1084/jem.188.9.1757.
61. Romani de Wit T, et al. Von Willebrand factor targets IL-8 to Weibel-Palade bodies in an endothelial cell line. Exp Cell Res. 2003;286:67–74. https://doi.org/10.1016/s0014-4827(03)00094-6.
62. Denis CV, Andre P, Saffaripour S, Wagner DD. Defect in regulated secretion of P-selectin affects leukocyte recruitment in von Willebrand factor-deficient mice. Proc Natl Acad Sci USA. 2001;98:4072–7. https://doi.org/10.1073/pnas.061307098.
63. Yamamoto K, de Waard V, Fearns C, Loskutoff DJ. Tissue distribution and regulation of murine von Willebrand factor gene expression in vivo. Blood. 1998;92:2791–801.
64. Kaufmann JE, Oksche A, Wollheim CB, Gunther G, Rosenthal W, Vischer UM. Vasopressin-induced von Willebrand factor secretion from endothelial cells involves V2 receptors and cAMP. J Clin Invest. 2000;106:107–16. https://doi.org/10.1172/JCI9516.
65. Doepker BA, Lucarelli MR, Lehman A, Shirk MB. Thromboembolic events during continuous vasopressin infusions: a retrospective evaluation. Ann Pharmacother. 2007;41:1383–9. https://doi.org/10.1345/aph.1H498.
66. Bhatraju PK, et al. Covid-19 in critically ill patients in the Seattle region—case series. N Engl J Med. 2020;382:2012–22. https://doi.org/10.1056/NEJMoa2004500.
67. Grasselli G, et al. Baseline characteristics and outcomes of 1591 patients infected with SARS-CoV-2 admitted to ICUs of the Lombardy Region, Italy. JAMA. 2020;323:1574–81. https://doi.org/10.1001/jama.2020.5394.
68. Jackson CB, Farzan M, Chen B, Choe H. Mechanisms of SARS-CoV-2 entry into cells. Nat Rev Mol Cell Biol. 2022;23:3–20. https://doi.org/10.1038/s41580-021-00418-x.

69. Hamming I, Timens W, Bulthuis ML, Lely AT, Navis G, van Goor H. Tissue distribution of ACE2 protein, the functional receptor for SARS coronavirus. A first step in understanding SARS pathogenesis. J Pathol. 2004;203:631–7. https://doi.org/10.1002/path.1570.
70. Mingote A, et al. Prevalence and clinical consequences of atelectasis in SARS-CoV-2 pneumonia: a computed tomography retrospective cohort study. BMC Pulm Med. 2021;21:267. https://doi.org/10.1186/s12890-021-01638-9.
71. Yang L, Xie X, Tu Z, Fu J, Xu D, Zhou Y. The signal pathways and treatment of cytokine storm in COVID-19. Signal Transduct Target Ther. 2021;6:255. https://doi.org/10.1038/s41392-021-00679-0.
72. Li L, et al. Interleukin-8 as a biomarker for disease prognosis of coronavirus disease-2019 patients. Front Immunol. 2020;11:602395. https://doi.org/10.3389/fimmu.2020.602395.
73. Wu X, et al. Viral mimicry of interleukin-17A by SARS-CoV-2 ORF8. MBio. 2022;13:e0040222. https://doi.org/10.1128/mbio.00402-22.
74. Xie M, Cheng B, Ding Y, Wang C, Chen J. Correlations of IL-17 and NF-kappaB gene polymorphisms with susceptibility and prognosis in acute respiratory distress syndrome in a chinese population. Biosci Rep .2019;39. https://doi.org/10.1042/BSR20181987.
75. Mikacenic C, Hansen EE, Radella F, Gharib SA, Stapleton RD, Wurfel MM. Interleukin-17A is associated with alveolar inflammation and poor outcomes in acute respiratory distress syndrome. Crit Care Med. 2016;44:496–502. https://doi.org/10.1097/CCM.0000000000001409.
76. Myers JM, et al. Cardiac myosin-Th17 responses promote heart failure in human myocarditis. JCI Insight. 2016;1 https://doi.org/10.1172/jci.insight.85851.
77. Numasaki M, et al. Interleukin-17 promotes angiogenesis and tumor growth. Blood. 2003;101:2620–7. https://doi.org/10.1182/blood-2002-05-1461.
78. Beyerstedt S, Casaro EB, Rangel EB. COVID-19: angiotensin-converting enzyme 2 (ACE2) expression and tissue susceptibility to SARS-CoV-2 infection. Eur J Clin Microbiol Infect Dis. 2021;40:905–19. https://doi.org/10.1007/s10096-020-04138-6.
79. Babajani F, et al. COVID-19 and renin angiotensin aldosterone system: pathogenesis and therapy. Health Sci Rep. 2021;4:e440. https://doi.org/10.1002/hsr2.440.
80. Heeneman S, Sluimer JC, Daemen MJ. Angiotensin-converting enzyme and vascular remodeling. Circ Res. 2007;101:441–54. https://doi.org/10.1161/CIRCRESAHA.107.148338.
81. Schnee JM, Hsueh WA. Angiotensin II, adhesion, and cardiac fibrosis. Cardiovasc Res. 2000;46:264–8. https://doi.org/10.1016/s0008-6363(00)00044-4.
82. Di Stefano L, et al. Losartan in hospitalized patients with COVID-19 in North America: an individual participant data meta-analysis. Medicine (Baltimore). 2023;102:e33904. https://doi.org/10.1097/MD.0000000000033904.
83. Gerard L, et al. Increased angiotensin-converting enzyme 2 and loss of alveolar type II cells in COVID-19-related acute respiratory distress syndrome. Am J Respir Crit Care Med. 2021;204:1024–34. https://doi.org/10.1164/rccm.202012-4461OC.
84. Tudoran C, et al. Associations between the severity of the post-acute COVID-19 syndrome and echocardiographic abnormalities in previously healthy outpatients following infection with SARS-CoV-2. Biology (Basel). 2021;10. https://doi.org/10.3390/biology10060469.
85. Deng Q, et al. Suspected myocardial injury in patients with COVID-19: evidence from front-line clinical observation in Wuhan, China. Int J Cardiol. 2020;311:116–21. https://doi.org/10.1016/j.ijcard.2020.03.087.
86. Li Y, et al. Prognostic value of right ventricular longitudinal strain in patients with COVID-19. JACC Cardiovasc Imaging. 2020;13:2287–99. https://doi.org/10.1016/j.jcmg.2020.04.014.
87. Wolters AEP, Wolters AJP, van Kraaij TDA, Kietselaer B. Echocardiographic estimation of pulmonary hypertension in COVID-19 patients. Neth Hear J. 2022;30:510–8. https://doi.org/10.1007/s12471-022-01702-x.
88. Mishra A, Lal A, Sahu KK, George AA, Martin K, Sargent J. An update on pulmonary hypertension in coronavirus disease-19 (COVID-19). Acta Biomed. 2020;91:e2020155. https://doi.org/10.23750/abm.v91i4.10698.

89. Eljilany I, Elzouki AN. D-dimer, fibrinogen, and IL-6 in COVID-19 patients with suspected venous thromboembolism: a narrative review. Vasc Health Risk Manag. 2020;16:455–62. https://doi.org/10.2147/VHRM.S280962.
90. Abou-Ismail MY, Diamond A, Kapoor S, Arafah Y, Nayak L. The hypercoagulable state in COVID-19: incidence, pathophysiology, and management. Thromb Res. 2020;194:101–15. https://doi.org/10.1016/j.thromres.2020.06.029.
91. Kollias A, Kyriakoulis KG, Lagou S, Kontopantelis E, Stergiou GS, Syrigos K. Venous thromboembolism in COVID-19: a systematic review and meta-analysis. Vasc Med. 2021;26:415–25. https://doi.org/10.1177/1358863X21995566.
92. Gasecka A, et al. Thrombotic complications in patients with COVID-19: pathophysiological mechanisms, diagnosis, and treatment. Cardiovasc Drugs Ther. 2021;35:215–29. https://doi.org/10.1007/s10557-020-07084-9.
93. Desai R, et al. Prevalence of pulmonary embolism in COVID-19: a pooled analysis. SN Compr Clin Med. 2020;2:2722–5. https://doi.org/10.1007/s42399-020-00605-5.
94. Klok FA, et al. Incidence of thrombotic complications in critically ill ICU patients with COVID-19. Thromb Res. 2020;191:145–7. https://doi.org/10.1016/j.thromres.2020.04.013.
95. Kushner A, West WP, Khan Suheb MZ, Pillarisetty LS. StatPearls. 2023.
96. Jackson SP, Darbousset R, Schoenwaelder SM. Thromboinflammation: challenges of therapeutically targeting coagulation and other host defense mechanisms. Blood. 2019;133:906–18. https://doi.org/10.1182/blood-2018-11-882993.
97. Subrahmanian S, et al. Tissue factor upregulation is associated with SARS-CoV-2 in the lungs of COVID-19 patients. J Thromb Haemost. 2021;19:2268–74. https://doi.org/10.1111/jth.15451.
98. Krishnamachary B, Cook C, Kumar A, Spikes L, Chalise P, Dhillon NK. Extracellular vesicle-mediated endothelial apoptosis and EV-associated proteins correlate with COVID-19 disease severity. J Extracell Vesicles. 2021;10:e12117. https://doi.org/10.1002/jev2.12117.
99. Levi M, van der Poll T, Buller HR. Bidirectional relation between inflammation and coagulation. Circulation. 2004;109:2698–704. https://doi.org/10.1161/01.CIR.0000131660.51520.9A.
100. Bautista-Vargas M, Bonilla-Abadia F, Canas CA. Potential role for tissue factor in the pathogenesis of hypercoagulability associated with in COVID-19. J Thromb Thrombolysis. 2020;50:479–83. https://doi.org/10.1007/s11239-020-02172-x.
101. Setty BN, Betal SG, Zhang J, Stuart MJ. Heme induces endothelial tissue factor expression: potential role in hemostatic activation in patients with hemolytic anemia. J Thromb Haemost. 2008;6:2202–9. https://doi.org/10.1111/j.1538-7836.2008.03177.x.
102. Solovey A, et al. Endothelial cell expression of tissue factor in sickle mice is augmented by hypoxia/reoxygenation and inhibited by lovastatin. Blood. 2004;104:840–6. https://doi.org/10.1182/blood-2003-10-3719.
103. Machado RF, et al. Severity of pulmonary hypertension during vaso-occlusive pain crisis and exercise in patients with sickle cell disease. Br J Haematol. 2007;136:319–25. https://doi.org/10.1111/j.1365-2141.2006.06417.x.
104. Myers CL, Wertheimer SJ, Schembri-King J, Parks T, Wallace RW. Induction of ICAM-1 by TNF-alpha, IL-1 beta, and LPS in human endothelial cells after downregulation of PKC. Am J Phys. 1992;263:C767–72. https://doi.org/10.1152/ajpcell.1992.263.4.C767.
105. Sur S, Steele R, Isbell TS, Ray R, Ray RB. Circulatory exosomes from COVID-19 patients trigger NLRP3 inflammasome in endothelial cells. MBio. 2022;13:e0095122. https://doi.org/10.1128/mbio.00951-22.
106. Joffre J, et al. COVID-19-associated lung microvascular endotheliopathy: a "from the bench" perspective. Am J Respir Crit Care Med. 2022;206:961–72. https://doi.org/10.1164/rccm.202107-1774OC.
107. Reitsma S, Slaaf DW, Vink H, van Zandvoort MA, oude Egbrink MG. The endothelial glycocalyx: composition, functions, and visualization. Pflugers Arch. 2007;454:345–59. https://doi.org/10.1007/s00424-007-0212-8.

108. Wichmann D, et al. Autopsy findings and venous thromboembolism in patients with COVID-19: a prospective cohort study. Ann Intern Med. 2020;173:268–77. https://doi.org/10.7326/M20-2003.
109. Lodigiani C, et al. Venous and arterial thromboembolic complications in COVID-19 patients admitted to an academic hospital in Milan, Italy. Thromb Res. 2020;191:9–14. https://doi.org/10.1016/j.thromres.2020.04.024.
110. Zheng XL. ADAMTS13 and von Willebrand factor in thrombotic thrombocytopenic purpura. Annu Rev Med. 2015;66:211–25. https://doi.org/10.1146/annurev-med-061813-013241.
111. Mancini I, et al. The ADAMTS13-von Willebrand factor axis in COVID-19 patients. J Thromb Haemost. 2021;19:513–21. https://doi.org/10.1111/jth.15191.
112. Doevelaar AAN, et al. Generation of potentially inhibitory autoantibodies to ADAMTS13 in coronavirus disease 2019. Sci Rep. 2023;13:10501. https://doi.org/10.1038/s41598-023-37405-5.
113. NICE. COVID-19 rapid guideline: managing the long-term effects of COVID-19. NICE guideline [NG188];2020. https://www.nice.org.uk/guidance/ng188.
114. Knight R, et al. Association of COVID-19 With major arterial and venous thrombotic diseases: a population-wide cohort study of 48 million adults in England and Wales. Circulation. 2022;146:892–906. https://doi.org/10.1161/CIRCULATIONAHA.122.060785.
115. Katsoularis I, et al. Risks of deep vein thrombosis, pulmonary embolism, and bleeding after covid-19: nationwide self-controlled cases series and matched cohort study. BMJ. 2022;377:e069590. https://doi.org/10.1136/bmj-2021-069590.
116. Craddock V, et al. Persistent circulation of soluble and extracellular vesicle-linked Spike protein in individuals with postacute sequelae of COVID-19. J Med Virol. 2023;95:e28568. https://doi.org/10.1002/jmv.28568.
117. Swank Z, et al. Persistent circulating severe acute respiratory syndrome coronavirus 2 spike is associated with post-acute coronavirus disease 2019 sequelae. Clin Infect Dis. 2023;76:e487–90. https://doi.org/10.1093/cid/ciac722.
118. Khan S, Shafiei MS, Longoria C, Schoggins JW, Savani RC, Zaki H SARS-CoV-2 spike protein induces inflammation via TLR2-dependent activation of the NF-kappaB pathway. Elife. 2021;10. https://doi.org/10.7554/eLife.68563.
119. Lester SN, Li K. Toll-like receptors in antiviral innate immunity. J Mol Biol. 2014;426:1246–64. https://doi.org/10.1016/j.jmb.2013.11.024.
120. Nunez-Gil IJ, et al. Post-COVID-19 symptoms and heart disease: incidence, prognostic factors, outcomes and vaccination: results from a multi-center international prospective registry (HOPE 2). J Clin Med. 2023;12. https://doi.org/10.3390/jcm12020706.
121. Xie Y, Xu E, Bowe B, Al-Aly Z. Long-term cardiovascular outcomes of COVID-19. Nat Med. 2022;28:583–90. https://doi.org/10.1038/s41591-022-01689-3.
122. Yang Y, Wei Z, Xiong C, Qian H. Direct mechanisms of SARS-CoV-2-induced cardiomyocyte damage: an update. Virol J. 2022;19:108. https://doi.org/10.1186/s12985-022-01833-y.
123. Hama Amin BJ, et al. Post COVID-19 pulmonary fibrosis; a meta-analysis study. Ann Med Surg (Lond). 2022;77:103590. https://doi.org/10.1016/j.amsu.2022.103590.
124. Eroume AEE, Shiwani HA, Nouthe B. From acute SARS-CoV-2 infection to pulmonary hypertension. Front Physiol. 2022;13:1023758. https://doi.org/10.3389/fphys.2022.1023758.
125. Cascino TM, Desai AA, Kanthi Y. At a crossroads: coronavirus disease 2019 recovery and the risk of pulmonary vascular disease. Curr Opin Pulm Med. 2021;27:342–9. https://doi.org/10.1097/MCP.0000000000000792.
126. Khan AW, Ullah I, Khan KS, Tahir MJ, Masyeni S, Harapan H. Pulmonary arterial hypertension post COVID-19: a sequala of SARS-CoV-2 infection? Respir Med Case Rep. 2021;33:101429. https://doi.org/10.1016/j.rmcr.2021.101429.
127. Wang X, et al. Pulmonary vascular endothelial injury and acute pulmonary hypertension caused by COVID-19: the fundamental cause of refractory hypoxemia? Cardiovasc Diagn Ther. 10:892, 2020–7. https://doi.org/10.21037/cdt-20-429.
128. van Dongen CM, et al. Unusually rapid development of pulmonary hypertension and right ventricular failure after COVID-19 pneumonia. Eur J Case Rep Intern Med. 2020;7:001784. https://doi.org/10.12890/2020_001784.

Chapter 12
Pulmonary Vascular Disease Associated with Other Parenchymal Lung Diseases

E. H. Louw, J. K. van Heerden, A. Buckley, and B. W. Allwood

Introduction

Although most available data pertaining to group 3 pulmonary hypertension (PH) stems from PH developing in the setting of COPD, interstitial lung disease (in particular idiopathic pulmonary fibrosis) and combined pulmonary fibrosis and emphysema (CPFE), other less common lung parenchymal diseases contribute to the burden of group 3 PH and are less extensively characterised [1]. In addition, certain multisystem diseases with parenchymal lung manifestations are also associated with precapillary PH (mean pulmonary artery pressure >20 mm Hg; pulmonary artery wedge pressure ≤15 mm Hg; and pulmonary vascular resistance ≥2 Wood units) yet are classified into group 5 PH (heterogeneous conditions with unclear or

E. H. Louw
Division of Pulmonology, Department of Medicine, Stellenbosch University, Cape Town, South Africa

Department of Medicine, Karl Bremer Hospital, Cape Town, South Africa
e-mail: ehlouw@sun.ac.za

J. K. van Heerden
Department of Paediatrics, Medical Sciences Division, University of Oxford, Oxford, UK
e-mail: jennifer.vanheerden@paediatrics.ox.ac.uk

A. Buckley
Division of Pulmonology, Department of Medicine, Stellenbosch University, Cape Town, South Africa

B. W. Allwood (✉)
Division of Pulmonology, Department of Medicine, Stellenbosch University & Tygerberg Hospital, Cape Town, South Africa
e-mail: brianallwood@sun.ac.za

F. N. Rahaghi et al. (eds.), *The Pulmonary Vasculature in Chronic Lung Disease*, Respiratory Medicine, https://doi.org/10.1007/978-3-032-03581-3_12

multifactorial aetiologies), according to the 2022 European Society of Cardiology/European Respiratory Society (ESC/ERS) guidelines [2].

Almost all parenchymal lung diseases may cause PH, which is most commonly characterised by a modest increase in pulmonary arterial pressure caused by pulmonary vasoconstriction and vascular remodelling due to hypoxemia. Less frequently, however, the increase in pulmonary arterial pressure may be out of proportion to the severity of the underlying parenchymal cases, possibly indicating different pulmonary vascular involvement mechanisms. Despite sometimes being under-appreciated in global PH literature, the effect on the pulmonary vasculature by less common parenchymal lung diseases may be substantial and the contribution of PH on the outcome of these diseases is commonly profound. In this chapter, we describe the epidemiology, clinical characteristics, and outcomes of PH due to post-tuberculosis lung disease (PTLD), bronchiectasis, lymphangioleiomyomatosis (LAM), neurofibromatosis, and pulmonary Langerhans cell histiocytosis (PLCH) (Table 12.1).

Pulmonary Hypertension in Post-tuberculosis Lung Disease

Overview

Tuberculosis (TB) remains one of the leading causes of death worldwide with major contribution to global burden of disease [24]. In 2021 alone, there were an estimated 10.6 million incident cases of TB, with approximately 1.6 million deaths directly related to TB [24]. More than 90% of incident cases occur in low- and middle-income countries (LMICs), disproportionately affecting those with lower socio-economic circumstances [24, 25]. Traditionally, the treatment of the incident episode of TB has been the focus of most TB programmes, and recent advancements in the diagnosis and treatment of TB have resulted in the global success rate for people treated for TB rising to approximately 86% [24]. However, the significant morbidity and mortality that may occur long after the microbiological cure of disease has recently started to be appreciated [26]. Improved treatment success results in an increase in the prevalence of TB survivors, estimated to be approximately 155 million people worldwide [3]. This patient population is vulnerable to develop multiple complications after the initial episode of TB has been treated, and pulmonary vascular disease is likely an under-recognised and significant post-TB complication [26–28].

Table 12.1 Overview of the epidemiology, treatment and outcomes for pulmonary hypertension associated with select parenchymal lung diseases

Disease entity	People living with disease	Estimated PH burden	Treatment options	Outcomes
Tuberculosis survivors	155 million people [3]	6–65% [4]	Limited data on treatment options Supportive treatment	Increased mortality Longer hospital stays Increased re-admissions Risk for acute exacerbations of respiratory symptoms
Non-CF bronchiectasis	56.7–121.5 million people (0.7–1.5% of the population) [5–7]	16–48% [8, 9]	Treatment of underlying disease Prevention of exacerbations Varying success with PAH specific therapies Consideration for lung transplantation	Increased mortality 3-year survival 56–83% 5-year survival 63–65%
CF bronchiectasis	162,428 people [10]	15–63% [11, 12]	Treatment of underlying lung disease may delay and prevent progression of PH Aggressive treatment of exacerbations Oxygen therapy PDE inhibitors (limited data) Lung transplantation	PH increases risk for CF exacerbations Increased mortality

(continued)

Table 12.1 (continued)

Disease entity	People living with disease	Estimated PH burden	Treatment options	Outcomes
LAM	Sporadic LAM 8000–21,000 people TSC LAM 80,000–160,000 [13, 14] (3.4–7.8/million women)	7–8% [15]	mTOR inhibitors Specific PAH therapies may play a role (limited data) Lung transplantation in advanced disease	Favourable response to mTOR inhibitors Lung transplantation in advanced cases has good outcomes
Neurofibromatosis NF1 NF2	162,000–2.7 million people 1/3500 [16] 1/50,000 [17]	Extremely rare 0.001% [18]	Supportive management of severe lung disease with oxygen, non-invasive ventilation Limited benefit of PAH therapies Lung transplant in advanced cases	Increased mortality Survival less than 50% at 5 years Post-transplant risk of malignancy
PLCH	1–2/million people [19]	4.5–92% [20, 21]	Smoking cessation may improve PH Oxygen therapy in hypoxic patients PAH therapy may be beneficial Lung transplantation in advanced disease	Outcome affected by response to treatment and relapses PLCH survival affected by contribution of malignancies Increased mortality if PH present
Silicosis	2.65 million people [22]	25–35% [23]	Supportive management of severe lung disease Prevention of further exposure No proven benefit of PAH therapies Lung transplantation in advanced disease	Increased mortality

Abbreviations: *CF* cystic fibrosis, LAM Lymphangioleiomyomatosis, *NF* neurofibromatosis, *PAH* pulmonary arterial hypertension, *PH* pulmonary hypertension, *PLCH* pulmonary Langerhans cell histiocytosis

Prevalence

The development of pulmonary hypertension (PH) appears to be associated with both active and previously treated pulmonary TB. Studies with large numbers of patients with current or prior TB found a significant proportion to have PH (~10%)

[29]. Cross-sectional studies have demonstrated that some patients develop PH several years after initial microbiological cure of TB [30–33]. In high TB prevalence areas, 46–89% of symptomatic patients with post-TB pulmonary sequelae were found to have PH, of which many had cor pulmonale [31, 34]. In a study where non-healthcare-seeking outpatients were considered, 16% were found to have possible or probable PH on screening echocardiography [33]. No other known risk factors for PH were present and active TB was excluded, suggesting a purely post-infectious phenomenon [31, 33].

Previous TB is rarely listed as a predisposing factor for PH. This may be partly explained by the under-diagnosis of PH in LMICs and partly due to most PH literature arising from high-income countries. However, given that approximately 80% of people with PH live in LMICs, TB likely contributes substantially to the global PH burden [35, 36]. The Pan-African PH Cohort Registry demonstrated that previous TB was identified in ~20% of African patients with PH, and TB was the most common cause of PH due to chronic lung disease and/or hypoxia [37]. Similarly, studies from India showed that approximately 12–15% of patients with PH have previous or concurrent TB [38, 39].

Risk Factors

Several risk factors may contribute to the development of PH after TB and more data is needed to determine their significance. Proposed risk factors can be considered in three categories: TB- and post-TB-lung-disease-related, host-related and environment-related factors. These factors will be discussed further, bearing in mind that the overall risk for developing PH is likely multifactorial.

TB-Related and PTLD-Related Factors

TB-Related Factors

Multiple episodes of pulmonary TB with resultant accumulative pulmonary damage and pulmonary functional decline may be a risk factor for the development of post-TB PH [33]. It is plausible that the impact of multiple episodes of TB on the pulmonary vasculature is at least additive if not exponential [40]. In a study where 100 outpatients with previous TB were assessed, there was a significant association between the number of previous episodes of TB and the development of PH, with each episode found to increase the odds of developing PH 2.13 fold (95% CI 1.17–3.88; $p = 0.013$) [33].

Patients who interrupt or do not complete anti-tuberculosis treatment and those where the diagnosis of TB is delayed may also be more likely to develop post-TB PH. Poor adherence to anti-tuberculosis therapy has been associated with ~four-fold increased risk for the development of PH and select studies have shown that 24–43%

of patients with post-TB PH did not complete their treatment [30, 32, 34]. Drug-resistant TB is often associated with treatment delays, recurrent therapy, lengthy regimens with poor adherence and tends to cause more severe pulmonary destruction and functional impairment [41], resulting in an increased risk for post-TB PH. However, data on the association between drug-resistant TB and post-TB PH is scarce and a significant correlation has not yet been confirmed [34].

PTLD-Related Factors

The pattern of PTLD with parenchymal damage in the form of cavitation, parenchymal destruction, and fibrotic changes have been found to be common amongst hospitalised patients with combined PTLD and PH [32, 34, 42]. Fibrocavitation has been reported as the most common radiological abnormality, present in up to 50% of patients, and PTLD-associated fibrotic changes have been found to be significantly more frequent in those with post-TB PH (OR of 3.33; $p = 0.03$) [30, 34, 43]. Many patients (up to 40%) have a combination of different PTLD-related clinical patterns, and those with combined patterns may have a greater risk for post-TB PH [34].

PTLD with more severe and greater extent of structural impairment appears to correlate with the risk for developing post-TB PH. Those with greater lung parenchymal destruction and three or more lobes damaged were at increased risk for having associated PH [42, 44]. This is in keeping with one of the proposed mechanisms for the development of post-TB PH due to the destruction of the pulmonary bed and reduced cross-sectional area of the pulmonary vasculature [30, 45].

The presence of pulmonary functional abnormalities, as measured by lung physiology testing, may be equally important in predicting the onset of PH in PTLD. In outpatients, about two-thirds of those with probable post-TB PH had abnormal spirometry and, in hospitalised patients, the detection of any spirometric abnormality resulted in a statistically significantly increased risk for post-TB PH [33, 34]. A variety of pulmonary functional abnormalities have been reported in post-TB PH, in keeping with the heterogenous nature of PTLD [39]. Restrictive and mixed obstructive/restrictive patterns on spirometry have been reported as the major pattern in patients with post-TB PH in several studies. Those with obstructive patterns on spirometry tend to have a reduced FVC [33, 34, 46]. In patients with PTLD and either small airway obstruction or diffuse parenchymal fibrosis, it was found that those with a restrictive phenotype had higher pulmonary pressures [34, 39]. It is plausible that a combination of functional impairment, with mixed fibrosis and small airway disease in the context of PTLD, particularly increases the risk of post-TB PH.

Venous Thromboembolic Disease During the Episode of TB

TB predisposes to venous thromboembolic (VTE) disease by multiple different mechanisms. Chronic inflammation during acute TB and the associated endothelial activation produces a pro-thrombotic state [47]. Other factors such as reduced mobility, rifamycin-containing antibiotics, and hospitalisation also predispose these patients to VTE [48]. Retrospective studies of patients with VTE in TB-endemic countries found that 12.5–53% of VTE presentations were associated with TB [47, 49]. Acute VTE predisposes to subsequent chronic thromboembolic PH (CTEPH), and a retrospective cohort from Korea of patients diagnosed with CTEPH showed that 5% of the patients had a history of pulmonary TB [50]. Therefore, a history of VTE may increase the likelihood of developing post-TB PH, but more evidence is needed to fully evaluate this relationship.

Host-Related Factors

The most affected and at-risk age category appears to be 40–60 years old [34, 42, 43, 51]. Post-TB PH seems to affect a younger age group compared to other respiratory-related PH, such as COPD. This may indicate a more rapid progressive or aggressive natural history, than the more steady pattern of decline seen in patients with COPD [44]. Males consistently appear to be at a higher risk for post-TB PH and, among patients with post-TB lung disease, males are almost three times more likely to develop PH [30, 32, 34]. This correlation may be multifactorial as males are also more likely to fall ill with TB and may be more likely to have other risk factors such as smoking and occupational exposure [24, 38].

Approximately 7% of those diagnosed with TB are people living with HIV (PLWH), therefore it is important to consider this comorbidity as a possible risk factor for the development of post-TB PH [24]. HIV is an acknowledged cause of Group 1 pulmonary arterial hypertension (PAH) in its own right, and approximately 8% of PLWH are said to have PH [36]. This confounder can make it difficult to distinguish PH developing from previous TB as opposed to HIV itself. However, PLWH have been excluded in many studies of post-TB PH [52], and findings from the PAPUCO study suggest that HIV in the presence of TB should be considered co-morbid and not necessarily causative of PH [37]. Furthermore, in some studies assessing post-TB PH, HIV infection has not been found to be a significant risk factor for the development of post-TB PH [33]. One possible explanation is that HIV-associated TB tends to have a less destructive course and may be protected against extensive/destructive PTLD [53].

The presence of comorbid autoimmune connective tissue diseases (CTD), such as systemic sclerosis and systemic lupus erythematosus (as well as the medications used in the treatment of these diseases), may increase the risk of post-TB PH [54, 55]. PH develops in approximately 20% of patients with systemic sclerosis and patients with systemic sclerosis are more likely to develop TB (IRR 2.81; 95% CI 1.36–5.37; $p = 0.004$) [2, 54, 55]. The associated vasculitis and endarteritis obliterans that may develop due to TB may possibly increase the risk for the development of PAH in these patients. Therefore, previous TB may increase the likelihood of PH in these patients; however, this contribution is largely unknown [56]. TB has also been associated with certain autoimmune vasculitides such as the large vessel vasculitis, Takayasu's arteritis (TA). A retrospective study of 1105 patients with TA found that 10% had previous TB, and pulmonary artery involvement with PH was more frequent in TA associated with TB [57]. Uncontrolled diabetes with added cardiovascular disease and risk for more severe TB may also contribute to a higher risk of post-TB PH [58].

Environment-Related Factors

Environmental risk factors include tobacco products, biomass exposure, and occupational exposure. In one study, all subjects with probable post-TB PH were either current smokers or had a smoking history (OR 3.67; 95%CI 0.77–17.46). Biomass exposure has been reported in up to a quarter of patients with post-TB PH and may heighten the risk of PH in people with PTLD [31]. There is a strong association between certain occupational dust diseases, TB, and increased risk for PTLD [53]. In a retrospective review of the cause of death in patients with pneumoconiosis, done over a period of 28 years, decompensated cor pulmonale was most frequently observed in patients with a combination of tuberculosis and silicosis [59].

Lastly, the negative effect of poor social circumstances on general health and access to good healthcare increases the risk of falling ill with TB, recurrent TB episodes, and environmental exposures, with increasing risk of developing post-TB PH [34, 60].

Clinical Features

Due to the overlapping symptoms of PH with that of underlying lung disease, the diagnosis of PH in these patients is often delayed. Clinical findings of overt right heart failure, such as jugular venous distention, loud second heart sound, split second heart sound, and features of tricuspid valve regurgitation usually, appear at the advanced stages of PH [61]. Symptoms such as dyspnoea are present in more than half of patients with PTLD, making this symptom non-specific for PH. However, the converse is true, and the absence of dyspnoea makes the diagnosis of PH unlikely [33, 62].

Pathophysiology

The pathophysiology of post-TB PH is not well established and is likely multifactorial, probably involving mechanisms from all five WHO PH groups (see Fig. 12.1). As with other chronic lung disease aetiologies of PH, the most likely mechanism postulated is that of destruction of the vascular bed, related to parenchymal destruction, obliterative bronchiolitis, and fibrosis (WHO Group 3 PH) [63].

Chronic hypoxia-induced vasoconstriction can occur in addition to vaso-destruction and vaso-obliteration [64]. As with idiopathic pulmonary fibrosis (IPF), there may also be vascular changes in non-affected lung parenchyma which contributes to the increase in pulmonary vascular resistance [65].

Thrombo-embolic disease is well described in patients with active TB [66]. All three aspects of Virchow's triad may be involved, with acute illness affecting mobility and TB causing chronic inflammation, leading to hypercoagulability and endothelial dysfunction, and vascular stasis due to lymph node compression [67]. The pro-thrombotic state may lead to deep venous thrombosis with embolisation but may also lead to in-situ pulmonary thrombosis at microvascular level [68]. There are no published data on the incidence of thromboembolic disease due to the chronic sequela of tuberculosis; however, acute embolism theoretically increases the risk of chronic thromboembolic disease and subsequent PH (Group 4 PH).

In PTLD, the mechanism of cavitation and fibrosis, where mesenchymal cells transform into fibroblasts leading to fibrotic tissue formation, may predispose to the pathogenesis of PH [69]. Triggered by bone morphogenetic protein receptor type 2 (BMPR-2) and vascular endothelial growth factor (VEGF), it may contribute to pulmonary arteriopathy consisting of medial hypertrophy, intimal thickening, and eccentric intimal fibrosis, as found in PAH (WHO group 1 PH) [70].

Mediastinal fibrosis is a rare cause of PH, developing due to encasement and compression of the mediastinal vascular structures [71]. Tuberculosis has been well described as a cause of mediastinal fibrosis, where the presence of mycobacteria in the respiratory tract results in leakage of antigen from the lymph node, resulting in a cell-mediated hypersensitivity reaction, followed by intense, uncontrolled fibrotic response [72]. The WHO classifies this as group 5 PH.

Lastly, TB increases cardiovascular disease risk by causing chronic systemic inflammation, immune activation, hypercoagulability, promotion of atherogenesis due to cholesterol imbalance and, possibly, direct effects on the myocardium and pericardium [73–75]. Thus, it may also contribute to left heart disease with resulting group 2 PH.

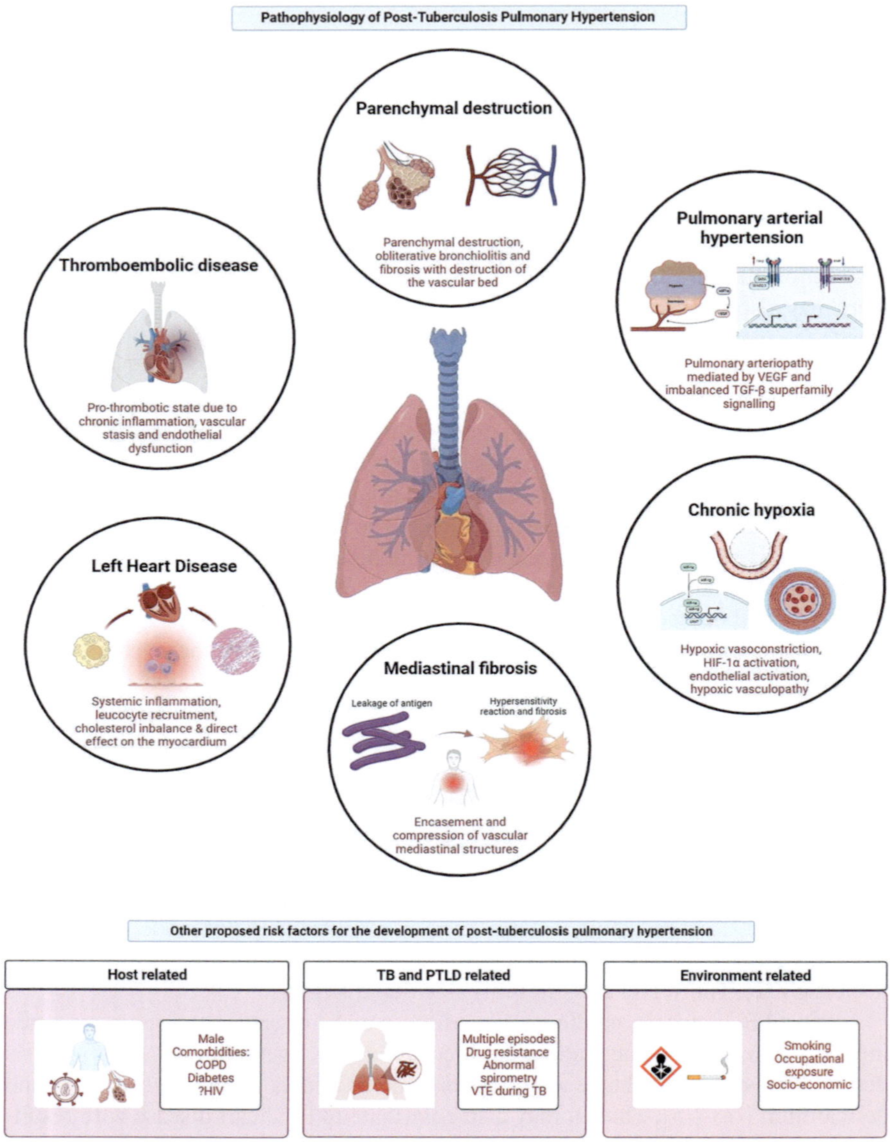

Fig. 12.1 Pathophysiology and risk factors for post-tuberculosis pulmonary hypertensionAbbreviations: *COPD* chronic obstructive pulmonary disease. *HIF-1* hypoxia-inducible factor 1, *HIV* human immunodeficiency virus, *PTLD* post-tuberculosis lung disease, *TB* tuberculosis, *VTE* venous thromboembolism. (Created with BioRender.com)

Screening and Diagnosis

Currently, there is no single investigative test that can accurately predict post-TB PH and a combination of investigations in addition to a high index of suspicion should be used to decide which patients require further confirmative investigations. The gold standard for confirmation of diagnosis of PH is right heart catheterisation (RHC); however, this is not widely available in low-resource settings. Thus, RHC is predominantly reserved for those patients in whom it may affect management, in the evaluation for lung transplantation and in research settings. In the absence of approved treatment, an argument can be made that screening and diagnosis is purely of scientific interest and not of any benefit to the patient. However, there is a drive towards early diagnosis in all classes of PH, not only in scientific interest, because early diagnosis may affect long-term mortality and further phenotyping is important in the development of new treatment strategies, demonstrated with the recently approved therapy for group 3 PH [1, 76].

The symptoms suggestive of PH may overlap with that of the underlying lung disease and as such, the diagnosis of PH may be significantly delayed. In addition, clinical signs of PH and overt right heart failure often appear late in the disease course [61]. Of the available screening modalities, it is important to note that there may be limitations to these tests in the setting of PTLD.

ECG is simple, cheap and readily available, but with a sensitivity of less than 50%. The features of PH on ECG may be obscured due to concealment of the atrial and ventricular electrical forces by the underlying structural lung disease or hyperinflation [77]. Transthoracic echocardiography (TTE) remains the best screening tool, although the sensitivity (81%) and specificity (61%) in patients with structural lung disease are lower than in those without underlying lung disease (sensitivity 93% and specificity 79%) [78, 79]. Poor acoustic windows due to structural lung disease may make the acquisition of an adequate Doppler signal for measuring tricuspid regurgitation impossible in up to 40% of patients [80, 81].

The TTE parameter with the highest sensitivity is the measurement of the pulmonary acceleration time at the right ventricular outflow tract (RVOT AT) and this is usually measurable in more than 90% of patients, with a sensitivity and specificity both reported at 84% [82].

Imaging studies may give information regarding the severity of the underlying structural lung disease and features such as an increased pulmonary artery to aortic ratio (PA:A) and pulmonary artery diameter may point toward PH with reasonable sensitivity and specificity [83]. The severity of the underlying lung damage does not always correlate well with the extend and degree of PH [1]. In PTLD, significant upper lobe fibrosis may also lead to pulmonary artery dilatation in the absence of PH [84, 85]. Therefore, it is uncertain if this can be used in PTLD and further research is needed.

Functional tests like a six-minute walking distance test (6MWD) can be performed with little equipment and used in the risk stratification of patients diagnosed with PH. A value less than 350 m has a sensitivity of 78% and specificity of 90% in predicting PH [61]. Heart rate recovery at 1 min has a poor sensitivity, but a high negative predictive value of 82% for PH [86].

Lung functions are abnormal in at least a third of patients with previous TB and lung function impairment seems to poorly correlate with predicting PH [33, 87]. Diffusion capacity is impaired in almost half of patients with previous TB [88], although values less than 40% predicted have a sensitivity of 72% and specificity of 71% in predicting PH in other parenchymal lung diseases [61].

Elevated pro-BNP levels above 50pg/ml have a sensitivity of 76% and specificity up to 80% in detecting PH, but importantly it can be confounded by co-existing comorbidities and left heart disease [89]. There are no data on the use of cardiopulmonary exercise testing and parameters such as VE/VCO2 slope, oxygen pulse and breathing reserve in detecting post TB PH and further research is needed in this regard.

Treatment

Currently, there is no literature on the proposed treatment of post-TB PH, and treatment is likely similar to that of WHO Group 3 PH, where most of these patients will be categorised. However, the pathogenesis may be multifactorial and each of the five categories possible, with possible different treatment options. Currently, the only FDA registered treatment for group 3 PH, in the setting of interstitial lung disease, is inhaled treprostinil [76]. For most group 3 PH patients, treatment of the underlying lung disease and hypoxia is advised [1]. Hopefully, current and future trials will change the landscape of treatment options; therefore, it is important to have proper phenotyping of these patients (Fig. 12.2).

Outcome

Previous pulmonary TB is associated with an increase in all-cause mortality compared to the general population, with cardiovascular disease being the leading cause [90]. The contribution towards morbidity and mortality of post TB PH in patients with PTLD is currently unknown, but in other chronic lung diseases the development of PH is associated with increased mortality [91, 92].

Patients with PTLD appear to have longer hospital stays, increased re-admission and worse morbidity than their counterparts without PH [31, 93]. Additionally, the presence of PH in patients with PTLD may increase the risk for acute exacerbations of respiratory symptoms and the frequency of exacerbations, further worsening their functional capacity and quality of life [44, 94].

The prognosis of post-TB PH may vary depending on the degree of PH, with a mean survival of 10 months in severe PH [93]. However, even mild PH may contribute to reduced survival [95]. More data is needed regarding which risk factors and

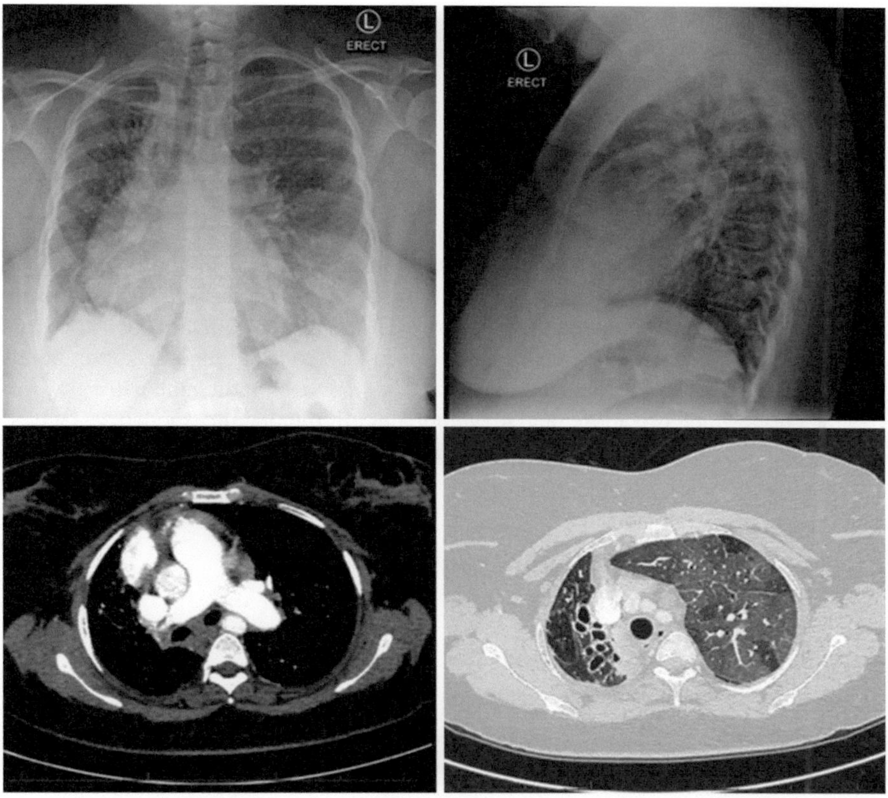

<u>Case description:</u> 30-year-old female with two episodes of multi-drug resistant pulmonary tuberculosis (TB) in 2000 and 2004, complicated by post-TB bronchiectasis. Group 3 pulmonary hypertension confirmed at right heart catherterisation: mPAP 65mmHg, PVR 11.97 WU, RAP 27mmHg and CI 1.67.

Fig. 12.2 Chest radiography and computed tomography imaging in a patient with post-TB lung diseaseAbbreviations: *CI* cardiac index, *mPAP* mean pulmonary arterial pressure, *PVR* pulmonary vascular resistance, *RAP* right atrial pressure, *WU* wood units

clinical parameters or biomarkers can be used to predict survival and for screening purposes.

Future Direction

The exact burden of post-TB PH is unknown; however, due to the significant number of TB survivors, the burden may be substantial. Research should be prioritised to describe the prevalence and emphasis should be placed on methods of diagnosing PH in resource-constrained settings where RHC may not be available. Universal screening is not practical, but a targeted screening approach of high-risk individuals should be considered. Further research is needed in understanding the pathophysiology, accurate categorisation, and development of therapeutic modalities which could prevent or delay the progression of PH in patients with PTLD.

Pulmonary Hypertension in Non-cystic Fibrosis (CF) Bronchiectasis

Overview

Bronchiectasis is characterised by the chronic, progressive, and irreversible dilatation of the bronchial wall and is increasingly recognised as an important and prevalent chronic pulmonary disease [96]. The prevalence of bronchiectasis varies by age and geographic region, but it has been estimated to affect 0.7–1.5% of the population [5–7]. Bronchiectasis is a heterogeneous entity, with multiple aetiologies, variable radiological and pathological morphologies (tubular, saccular or varicose), and differing pulmonary distributions (localised or generalised) [96, 97]. The list of conditions associated with the development of bronchiectasis is extensive, and the frequency of each aetiology varies significantly according to the patient population studied and the specific country or region [7]. Broadly speaking, bronchiectasis may be associated with post-infectious causes (mycobacterial, viral); mucociliary disorders (cystic fibrosis, primary ciliary dyskinesia); airway obstruction (foreign body, tumour); immune dysfunction (primary or secondary immunodeficiency); chronic rheumatic or inflammatory conditions (such as rheumatoid arthritis) and other miscellaneous conditions such as aspiration, asthma, and COPD [98]. It is also notable that a specific aetiological factor is often not identified, and idiopathic bronchiectasis comprises nearly half of all bronchiectasis registries, especially in settings where highly specialised and extensive evaluation is not performed [7, 96]. Bronchiectasis is often divided into cystic fibrosis (CF) and non-cystic fibrosis (non-CF)-related disease and pulmonary hypertension (PH) related to each of these entities will be discussed over the next two sections.

Prevalence

An increased prevalence of non-CF bronchiectasis has been observed over the past few decades, which may be attributable to an aging population with an actual increased prevalence or a perceived increase in prevalence due to increased clinician-identified disease, better diagnostic techniques, and a more thorough appreciation of the multiple aetiologies of bronchiectasis [96, 98]. The prevalence of PH in non-CF bronchiectasis has not been extensively characterised, with particularly few studies reporting right heart catheterisation (RHC) results and therefore confirmation of PH. In studies using echocardiography, however, PH has been detected in approximately 33–48% of participants [8, 9]. This figure may vary between different morphological types of bronchiectasis and in one study the prevalence of PH varied from 16% to 42% in those with cylindrical versus cystic bronchiectasis respectively [8]. Similarly, given the heterogenous nature of non-CF bronchiectasis, it is unsurprising that different aetiological causes of bronchiectasis have different prevalence rates [9].

Risk Factors

Patient-Related Risk Factors

Female sex and older age are associated with both the development of bronchiectasis and the development of PH; however, the precise relationship between age, sex, and non-CF bronchiectasis-related PH has not been determined [92, 96]. Nonetheless, the development of PH in younger patients with bronchiectasis may indicate more severe disease and in a retrospective study, younger patients who presented with PH were more likely to experience severe dyspnoea and more likely to present with right heart failure [99]. Most people with bronchiectasis do not smoke, and those with bronchiectasis-associated PH are no more likely to be smokers than those without PH [92, 96]. However, amongst smokers, those with PH are observed to have a significantly longer duration of smoking [92].

Disease-Related Risk Factors

The risk for developing PH in people with bronchiectasis differs markedly between different non-CF aetiologies. For example, patients with COPD-related bronchiectasis were more likely to develop PH compared to those with post-infectious causes in one cohort [9]. This is likely explained by multiple factors including differing anatomical involvement, alternative pathophysiological mechanisms, and comorbid conditions associated with the patient population.

The radiological extent of disease and morphological differences appear to influence the risk of developing PH in those with bronchiectasis. Bilateral and diffuse bronchiectasis increases the risk of PH, and those with a greater number of involved lobes on high-resolution computed tomography (HRCT) are significantly more likely to develop PH [92]. In addition, cystic and mixed bronchiectasis pose a greater risk for the development of PH compared to cylindrical bronchiectasis [99].

The degree of hypoxaemia and hypercapnia correlates to the risk for PH in individuals with non-CF bronchiectasis, with significant lower arterial partial pressure of oxygen (PaO_2) and O_2 saturations and higher arterial $PaCO_2$ concentrations demonstrated in those with PH [92]. Pulmonary functional impairment is similarly correlated to the development of PH in patients with bronchiectasis and a significant inverse correlation between systolic pulmonary artery pressure and forced expiratory volume in 1 s, forced vital capacity, total lung capacity, and diffusing capacity for carbon monoxide has been demonstrated [9].

Clinical Features

Adult patients with bronchiectasis typically present with chronic cough, daily mucopurulent sputum production, dyspnoea, and recurrent lower respiratory tract infections. The duration between the onset of bronchiectasis and PH may vary significantly. In one small study, the time from onset of dyspnoea to detection of PH varied from 3.5 to 30 years [92]. Rapidly worsening or disproportionate dyspnoea may indicate the development of PH and patients with PH have been found to have worse clinical dyspnoea scores and to perform poorly on functional assessment measured by the six-minute walk test (6MWT) [92]. Clinical features of PH (loud second heart sound, pan-systolic murmur, and right ventricular heave) are often more challenging to elicit in the context of chronic bronchiectasis, although when present are suggestive of PH. It is also notable that in the context of episodes of ventilatory failure, pedal oedema may reflect neuroendocrine abnormalities rather than right heart failure [1].

Pathophysiology

The pathophysiology of bronchiectasis is well described and the "vicious cycle hypothesis", originally described by Cole in 1986, consists of a cycle of impaired mucous clearance, airway inflammation, infection, and airway structural damage. More recently, these elements have been seen to act in a "vortex" where all four components contribute to the pathophysiology of each other with different aetiologies having different entry points into the vortex [100].

The pathophysiology of PH in non-CF bronchiectasis is incompletely understood; however, it is likely complex and highly variable. Mechanisms can be considered in three categories: (1) pathophysiological mechanisms that are shared with other causes of group 3 PH, (2) those specific to non-CF bronchiectasis, and (3) mechanisms that are specific to the underlying aetiology of bronchiectasis.

Similarly to other group 3 PH, chronic hypoxia resulting in vascular smooth muscle contraction and hypoxia-induced endothelial-derived vasoconstrictors likely contributes to PH in bronchiectasis [101]. Resultant pulmonary vasculopathy, characterised by endothelial cell proliferation, pulmonary vascular smooth muscle proliferation, and fibroblast activation with medial hypertrophy and intimal sclerosis, contributes to the development of PH in those with chronic lung disease [1, 64]. Although there is some association between the degree of hypoxia and parenchymal involvement with the presence and severity of PH in chronic lung diseases, this correlation appears to vary significantly [1].

Chronic inflammation is a key feature of bronchiectasis, and chronic cycling of infection and inflammation is likely an important pathway for the development of PH [1, 64]. Inflammation contributes to the development of PH both directly—through release of inflammatory cytokines—and indirectly—via maladaptive parenchymal structural remodelling and subsequent effect on the pulmonary vasculature. In addition, inflammation is worsened by chronic hypoxia (or tobacco exposure in smokers) and the presence of inflammatory cell infiltrate has been shown to be strongly correlated with pulmonary vascular remodelling in other chronic pulmonary conditions [1].

Recently, inflammatory endotypes of bronchiectasis have been described, with a distinction being made between neutrophilic and eosinophilic (type 2 immunity)-driven inflammation [100, 102]. Elevated matrix metalloproteinases are associated with neutrophilic inflammation and mediate extracellular matrix remodelling, contributing to both bronchiectasis progression and, likely, the development of PH [101, 102]. In a murine model of eosinophilic inflammation-induced PH, eosinophils were necessary for pulmonary arterial remodelling and in patients with COPD, those with an eosinophilic endotype were found to have higher mPAP and PVR and increased likelihood of PH [103, 104]. Moreover, bronchiectasis is associated with systemic inflammation, and elevated levels of systemic inflammatory cytokines (such as interleukin-6) may reduce the expression of bone morphogenetic protein receptor type 2 (BMPR-2), a pathogenetic feature of group 1 PH [105].

Lastly, unique features of the underlying aetiology of bronchiectasis may play a role in the pathogenesis of PH. For example, patients with rheumatoid arthritis may have associated vasculitis and a hypercoagulable state which may contribute to the development of PH [106].

Screening and Diagnosis

Specific screening guidelines for PH in non-CF bronchiectasis are not universally defined; however, five important indications to assess patients for PH have been proposed in other chronic lung diseases and should be applied similarly in bronchiectasis. These are (1) unexplained worsening of breathlessness (particularly rapidly worsening and not explained by other causes), (2) breathlessness that is more severe than expected from the extent of lung disease, (3) risk factors for pulmonary arterial hypertension (PAH) or chronic thromboembolic PH exist; (4) during the evaluation for lung surgery; and (5) when lung transplantation is considered [1].

Echocardiography has traditionally been used to estimate pulmonary pressures and is a relatively reliable non-invasive screening test where the probability of PH can be determined as low, intermediate, or high on the basis of tricuspid regurgitation jet velocity and other echocardiographic findings [2]. However, echocardiography is less accurate in patients with lung disease and may overestimate pulmonary artery pressures and RHC remains the investigation of choice for confirmation of suspected PH [107, 108].

More recently, computed tomography (CT) imaging has been proposed as an alternative screening technique, using various measurements for the assessment of PH; however, it has mostly been validated in studies of COPD. A 2022 meta-analysis showed that CT pulmonary angiography, using a pulmonary artery to aorta ratio (PA:A) of greater than one, had an estimated diagnostic sensitivity of 65% and specificity of 83% [83]. Other imaging criteria to suggest the presence of PH include a pulmonary artery diameter greater than 30 mm, right ventricular outflow hypertrophy more than 6 mm, a septal angle of 140 degrees or more, or right ventricle to left ventricle ratio greater than one [109]. Additionally, the use of artificial intelligence may improve the diagnostic accuracy of CT interpretation and therefore its usefulness in predicting PH [110].

Treatment

The treatment of non-CF bronchiectasis requires a personalised and multidimensional approach, including treatment of the underlying cause, improvement of mucociliary clearance and control of infection [111]. Although this will not be detailed here, the prevention of exacerbations and resultant pulmonary decline is particularly important to prevent progression to PH [111].

There is little evidence to support the use of PAH-specific therapies in patients with bronchiectasis; however, PDE-5 inhibitors, endothelin receptor antagonists, and combination therapy have been used in patients with non-CF bronchiectasis with varying success [64, 99].

Lung transplantation for bronchiectasis is rarely indicated (less than 5% of all bilateral lung transplantations recorded in the International Society for Heart and Lung Transplantation Registry); however, the British Thoracic Society bronchiectasis guidelines recommend early consideration for transplantation in patients with poor lung function and (amongst other factors), severe PH [112].

Outcomes

The development of PH has been considered a poor prognostic indicator in patients with bronchiectasis [92, 113]. In a study by Devaraj et al., where CT was used to detect PH, the average right and left main pulmonary artery diameter was the best predictor of mortality (hazard ratio, 1.24; 95% CI, 1.13–1.35; $p < 0.001$) [113]. The three- and 5-year survival rates for patients with bronchiectasis and PH are 56–83% and 63–65% respectively [92, 99]. In a retrospective cross-sectional analysis of 539 patients with non-cystic fibrosis, 10.6% of participants had died at 41 months and the presence of PH was associated with significantly higher mortality rate ($p = 0.01$) [9].

Pulmonary Hypertension in Cystic Fibrosis (CF) Bronchiectasis

Overview

Cystic fibrosis (CF) is an autosomal-recessive monogenetic disease with multisystem involvement, which is estimated to affect more than 100,000 people worldwide [114]. CF typically affects the lungs, with respiratory failure remaining the most significant cause of morbidity and mortality in CF patients [11]. Mutations in the gene encoding for the epithelial ion channel that transports chloride and bicarbonate (CF transmembrane conductance regulator; CFTR) lead to impaired mucus hydration and inadequate mucus clearance causing chronic pulmonary infection and inflammation [114]. This initiates the vicious cycle implicated in the establishment of bronchiectasis, with recurrent infection, inflammation, and aberrant repair leading to abnormal and permanent bronchial dilatation [96].

CF is one of the most important aetiologies of bronchiectasis in developed countries; however, it likely comprises a minority of the overall global burden of bronchiectasis in adult settings [115]. Nevertheless, as the most well-described phenotype of bronchiectasis, many of the treatment modalities for non-CF bronchiectasis are inferred from evidence in CF-bronchiectasis and it remains an important disease entity due to its notable contribution to morbidity in the CF population [115].

Prevalence

Novel treatment options in CF and aggressive antibiotic therapy have resulted in an increased longevity in CF, resulting in patients living for longer periods of time with severe pulmonary disease, and the subsequent development of PH and cor pulmonale is becoming more prevalent [116]. Prevalence estimates of PH developing in the CF population vary from 15% to 63% according to the age-group studied, the severity of the underlying lung disease and screening or diagnostic modality used to determine pulmonary pressures (i.e. estimation by echocardiography or determination at right heart catheterisation (RHC)) [11, 12]. Nonetheless, the prevalence of PH is predictably high in those with CF and advanced lung disease [11]. In CF patients awaiting lung transplantation, the prevalence of PH detected by RHC has been demonstrated to be approximately 57% when large transplant registries are analysed [117].

Risk Factors

Patient-Related Risk Factors

Despite the association between female sex and pulmonary arterial hypertension (PAH), there is insufficient data to indicate whether females with CF-bronchiectasis are more likely to develop PH. In a study where CT imaging of the pulmonary artery was used to indicate pulmonary vascular disease, it was observed that patients with pulmonary artery enlargement were younger than those without enlargement in both cohorts and had elevated sweat chloride concentrations [118]. Lower body mass index (BMI) and poor nutritional state may increase the risk for the development of PH in the context of CF. Malnutrition has been associated with worsening pulmonary decline in patients with CF and a recent systematic review and meta-analysis found that CF patients with a higher BMI had more favourable clinical outcomes including better pulmonary function [119, 120]. Although data is limited on whether malnutrition contributes to the development of PH in CF, malnutrition has been associated with an increased risk for PH in other disease entities and nutritional deficiencies as well as gut dysbiosis have been linked to PH in animal models [121, 122]. There are over 200 mutations in the CFTR gene that have been identified in CF and PH may be more likely to develop in certain CF genotypes; however, specific data are lacking.

Disease-Related Risk Factors

Lower partial pressure of arterial oxygen (PaO_2) on room air and higher oxygen requirements at rest are demonstrated risk factors for the development of PH in patients with CF-bronchiectasis [12, 123]. In addition, higher partial pressure of carbon dioxide has been found to be significantly associated with the development of PH in patients with CF. [12] Functional pulmonary impairment, specifically the finding of a lower forced vital capacity (FVC, %) and a lower forced expiratory volume in 1 s (FEV_1), is associated with the onset of PH in patients with CF. [12]

Recurrent exacerbations in CF-bronchiectasis are related to disease progression and pulmonary functional decline. This results in more severe disease and consequently an increased likelihood of developing PH. In addition, chronic infection coupled with the associated inflammatory response and cytokine release may increase the risk of developing PH, and isolated studies have linked higher pulmonary pressures in people with CF who are chronically infected with *Burkholderia cepacia* (specifically, *B. multivolrans*) [124].

Clinical Features

Clinical features of PH may be difficult to distinguish from the underlying CF lung disease. Dyspnoea which is disproportional to the degree of lung disease may alert clinicians to the development or worsening of PH; however, the 6MWD test appears to poorly distinguish those with or without PH in patients with CF and significant lung disease [92]. Radiologically, CF typically causes diffuse, predominantly upper lobe bronchiectasis. Pulmonary functional abnormality in CF is generally characterised by an obstructive ventilatory pattern; however, a restrictive component caused by pulmonary fibrosis may develop in the final phases of the disease. Pulmonary function tests—specifically FEV_1 and FVC measurements—and oxygen saturations at rest have been correlated with the detection of higher pulmonary pressures [125].

Once detected, PH is a defining feature for advanced CF lung disease; the other features include an $FEV_1 < 40\%$ during a stable period, those awaiting lung transplantation, intensive care unit admission for respiratory failure, hypercarbia, daytime oxygen requirement at rest, and severe functional impairment [126].

Pathophysiology

There are multiple proposed mechanisms in the development of PH in CF, and in most cases, PH is multifactorial [127]. First, similarly to other causes of bronchiectasis, hypoxia due to parenchymal destruction, ventilation-perfusion mismatch, and right-to-left shunting results in hypoxic vasoconstriction with elevated pulmonary pressures and subsequent vascular remodelling. Second, chronic airway inflammation and chronic or recurrent airway infections lead to pulmonary vascular remodelling and PH. On a cellular level, the CFTR has been demonstrated to be expressed in the pulmonary vasculature and epithelia [127]. When CFTR is dysfunctional, this may promote inflammation and angiogenesis in the pulmonary arterial bed. Third, endothelial dysfunction has been reported in patients with CF despite normal oxygen saturation and pulmonary function and this may predispose them to pulmonary arterial hypertension [128].

Furthermore, right ventricular dysfunction has been documented in CF, even in those with mild or minimal pulmonary disease. This phenomenon may be explained by the state of chronic inflammation and immune activation in CF, with an increase in neurohormones and subsequent right ventricular impairment [127]. Additionally, the CFTR's role in cardiomyocyte contraction has been considered and the CFTR appears to interfere in the regulation of cardiomyocyte contraction by altering intracellular calcium. Lastly, other concomitant CF-related complications may contribute to the development or progression of PH in the setting of CF-bronchiectasis [127]. Left ventricular dysfunction and accelerated atherosclerosis have been suggested to occur more frequently within the CF population and may contribute to the development of PH through mechanisms unrelated to pulmonary disease [127, 129]. In addition, CF-related liver disease with portal hypertension, hypothyroidism (more prevalent in CF), and pulmonary thrombosis formation due to chronic inflammation, central venous catheters, and immobility can all cause PH through district mechanisms [11].

Screening and Diagnosis

Many patients with CF are not routinely evaluated for PH, partly because suitable non-invasive diagnostic tests are unavailable. However, the CF foundation consensus guidelines recommend that all patients with advanced CF lung disease undergo routine screening for PH [126].

Echocardiography is often employed in the screening for PH due to its non-invasive nature and due to RHC often not being available. However, echocardiography is often both technically difficult and relatively unreliable in patients with CF due to advanced lung disease and associated hyperinflation. Due to the limitations associated with echocardiography, other screening modalities for the detection of PH in CF have been proposed. Most notably, recently, the use of the pulmonary artery diameter to ascending aorta diameter (PA:A) ratio measured at computed tomography (CT) has been investigated, with a PA:A ratio greater than 1 considered indicative of PH [130].

RHC remains the gold standard for the diagnosis of PH in patients with CF-bronchiectasis. The detection of PH is considered an indication for lung transplant referral, and in those already awaiting transplant, a baseline screening assessment for PH is advised [126]. In addition, if patients' clinical condition deteriorates, it is recommended that evaluation for PH be repeated.

Treatment

Although the comprehensive management of patients with CF in general and with CF-bronchiectasis specifically is beyond the scope of this chapter, it is worth noting that the management of the underlying lung disease including the aggressive treatment of pulmonary exacerbations is important to prevent progressive pulmonary decline, respiratory failure, and the progression to PH.

Over the last two decades, novel CF therapies with the development of drug modulators that target specific CFTR mutations have revolutionised CF medicine and trials using certain combination therapy (such as lumacaftor/ivacaftor) have shown a 2.6–4.0% improvement in FEV_1 and a 30–39% reduction in pulmonary exacerbations compared to placebo. Such therapies likely delay the onset and prevent the progression of PH.

Oxygen therapy has been used in patients with CF-bronchiectasis and PH with some success and small studies have shown a decrease in mean pulmonary arterial pressure (mPAP) and an improvement in right ventricular function with oxygen supplementation [11]. However, larger studies to assess the haemodynamic effects of long-term oxygen therapy in patients with CF-bronchiectasis are needed. Oral phosphodiesterase (PDE) inhibitors appear to be safe and tolerable in patients with CF and appear to improve endothelial function without impeding ventilation; however, limited data exist on their efficacy [126, 127]. In individuals who already have established advanced CF lung disease and PH, the CF Foundation suggests that there is insufficient data to recommend the use of pulmonary vasodilator therapy [126].

Lung transplantation is an important and established treatment for CF patients with advanced lung disease, and current guidelines suggest that those with severe PH should be prioritised for transplantation [131].

Outcomes

PH may increase the rate of pulmonary exacerbation in patients with CF, and a study using CT imaging to screen for PH found that its detection was an independent risk factor for recurrent pulmonary exacerbations [118]. Given that pulmonary exacerbation is a well-established source of progressive lung function decline and increased mortality in patients with CF, this association has significant implications for patients with CF [130]. It also highlights the fact that more attention likely should be directed towards the detection and management of PH in patients with CF [130].

Certain studies have shown an association between higher pulmonary artery pressures and pulmonary vascular resistance and adverse outcomes as well as increased mortality in patients with CF awaiting lung transplantation [132, 133]. In a study by Heynes et al. of CF patients with advanced lung disease, when patients with PH were compared to matched controls, the hazard ratio was 4.2 (95% CI, 1.7–10.2) for those with mPAP $\geq$ 35 mmHg ($p = 0.002$). However, a recent systematic review and meta-analysis found that although the overall survival was lower in CF patients with PH than those without, there was no statistically significant prognostic value of PH on survival outcomes [12]. This finding likely reflects the fact that PH is often mild in patients with CF-related lung disease and that respiratory impairment may hold more prognostic value in these patients. However, it is notable that in the subset of patients with CF and out-of-proportion PH, mortality is predictably higher. Undoubtedly, once right ventricular failure has developed, prognosis is poor and survival without transplantation is limited after the onset of clinical signs of right heart failure.

Pulmonary Hypertension Associated with Lymphangioleiomyomatosis (LAM)

Overview

Lymphangioleiomyomatosis (LAM) is a rare multisystem disease, where constitutive activation of the mechanistic (formerly "mammalian") target of rapamycin (mTOR) signalling results in accumulation of abnormal smooth muscle-like cells (LAM cells) in the lungs, lymphatics, and results in the formation of angiomyolipomas [134]. LAM affects young pre-menopausal women and may occur sporadically or may be associated with tuberous sclerosis complex (TSC). The lungs are primarily affected, with pulmonary infiltration by LAM cells causing parenchymal destruction, with the development of cystic pulmonary lesions [13]. Cystic lung disease leads to recurrent pneumothoraces, airway obstruction, and impairment of gas exchange, and lymphatic disease leads to lymph node enlargement and chylous collections [134].

Prevalence

The prevalence of LAM varies between 3.4 and 7.8/million women with an estimated incidence of 0.23–0.31/million women/per year [14]. Sporadic LAM affects an estimated 8000–21,000 individuals worldwide and TSC-LAM affects approximately 30–60% of women and ~10% of men with TSC, resulting in an estimated 80,000–160,000 individuals living with TSC-LAM worldwide [13].

Data on the prevalence of pulmonary hypertension (PH) in patients with LAM is limited; however, it appears to be relatively infrequent (7–8%) and mild, particularly in an outpatient setting [15]. In a single-centre cross-sectional study, PH was detected in approximately 8% of outpatients with LAM and no patients had mean pulmonary arterial pressures (mPAP) >30 mmHg [15]. Conversely, PH is more prevalent in those with advanced disease and may occur in up to 45–62% of those referred for lung transplantation [135, 136].

PH associated with LAM was previously included in group 5 PH—accounting for the perceived unclear multifactorial mechanisms causing PH [137]. However, the strong association between the detection of pulmonary function alteration and right heart catheterisation (RHC)-confirmed PH has more recently suggested that the rise in mPAP is associated with parenchymal involvement and resulted in this entity being reclassified into group 3 PH in the 2022 ESC/ERS guidelines [2, 138].

Risk Factors and Clinical Features

Although little is known about the risk factors for the development of PH in the context of LAM, PH is usually associated with more severe cystic lung disease and severely altered pulmonary function. In a case series of 20 patients and 72 controls, respiratory symptoms (dyspnoea, New York Heart Association functional class and a history of haemoptysis), an abnormal six-minute walk test, and abnormal pulmonary function tests were the only significant differences between those with PH and controls [139]. In this study, age, smoking, menopausal status or the diagnosis of TSC did not appear to influence the onset of PH in those with LAM. It has also been found that a high $P_{A\text{-}a}O_2$ gradient is a predicter of elevated pulmonary pressures in patients with LAM [140].

Pathophysiology

Two major pathophysiological mechanisms are proposed for the development of PH in patients with LAM [141]. First, a combination of parenchymal destruction and hypoxic vasoconstriction appears to be a significant contributor to disease, and this mechanism has been evidenced by several studies which demonstrate the association of worsening pulmonary haemodynamics with declining lung functions and arterial oxygen tension (PaO_2) both at rest and after exercise [139]. Second, the upregulation of mTOR in the context of hypoxia leads to vascular smooth muscle proliferation resulting in PH [142]. Indeed, the critical role of mTOR signalling, mTOR complex 1 and 2 formation, and the proliferation of pulmonary artery smooth cells has been identified in group 1, 3, and 5 PH.

Screening and Diagnosis

Given the low prevalence of PH in patients with non-severe LAM, screening for PH in this population is not currently recommended, according to the ERS guidelines for the diagnosis and management of LAM [143]. Conversely, in patients with LAM who are under consideration for lung transplantation, estimation of the pulmonary artery pressure should be made [143].Although echocardiography has traditionally been used as the preferred method of screening, a study which used both echocardiography and carbon monoxide diffusion capacity (DLCO) to determine which patients to refer for right heart catheterisation found that using DLCO detected more patients with subsequently confirmed PH [15]. RHC remains the gold standard of PH diagnosis in these patients.

Treatment and Outcomes

Sirolimus, a mTOR inhibitor, has been shown to stabilise lung function, reduce serum vascular endothelial growth factor (VEGF) levels and is associated with a reduction in respiratory symptoms [144]. By improving lung function and hypoxia, sirolimus may improve pulmonary haemodynamics [141]. Additionally, pulmonary arterial hypertension (PAH)-specific therapies may play a role in patients with specific vascular involvement via mTOR signalling; however, evidence for this is currently lacking [141, 142]. Lastly, lung transplantation may be the only option for patients with advanced disease and may be considered for patients with severe PH that persists or progresses on mTOR inhibitors [145]. Outcomes after lung transplantation appear to be favourable in the majority of patients, with survival rates of 94% at 1 year, 73% at 5 years, and 56% at 10 years [145, 146].

Pulmonary Hypertension Associated with Neurofibromatosis (NF)

Overview

Neurofibromatosis type 1 (NF1) is an autosomal dominant condition, caused by mutations in *NF1,* the gene encoding neurofibromin 1, responsible for negative regulation of the Ras signal transduction pathway, which is important for both tumour suppression and cell growth and proliferation. It is characterised by skin features, optic and central nervous system tumours, bony abnormalities, learning disabilities and increased risk for certain cancers. The incidence of NF1 is approximately 1 per 3500 individuals, making this a common inheritable condition [16].

Neurofibromatosis type 2 (NF2) is a different genetic condition, much rarer with approximately 1 in 50,000 affected, where the hallmark thereof is the development of bilateral vestibular schwannomas. The associated skin lesions are less severe than in NF1. It can also be associated with spinal nerve sheath tumours and meningiomas [17].

Prevalence

Pulmonary hypertension (PH) is considered a very rare (exact prevalence unknown) but severe complication of neurofibromatosis 1 (NF1-PH) [147]. NF2-PH is extremely rare, with a brief PubMed search revealing a single case [148], whereas NF1-PH has been limited to case series and large PH registry reports [147, 149]. In the French PH registry only 49 cases were identified over a 15-year period, with an estimated incidence of PH in patients with NF of 1/1000 [18].

Risk Factors

Interestingly, there appears to be a female predominance in NF1-PH (4:1), though NF1 in itself is a disease with equal gender distribution [149]. NF1-PH occurs late in the course of the disease at a mean age of 57 years (50–65 years), at least 10 years later than in other heritable pulmonary arterial hypertension (PAH) conditions [149].

Clinical features

In the cases that were described in literature, most patients presented late in the course of the disease with severe exercise limitation and clinical features of overt right heart failure [149]. In keeping with the proposed pathophysiology, about one-third of patients will have no overt lung features confirmed on HRCT, as well as minimal physiological impairment on lung functions [149]. The other patients with lung disease have mostly cysts or bullae in the upper lobes, diffuse ground-glass opacities sometimes with mosaic attenuation and reticular opacities. Additionally, lung disease is detected only in adulthood, despite the disease being present from birth [149]. Diffusion capacity impairment is an important feature in most patients with NF-PH and should prompt further evaluation for PH, if otherwise unexplained [149].

Pathophysiology

The pathophysiology in NF1-PH is uncertain and likely multifactorial, hence its classification in WHO group 5 PH. Possible mechanisms of NF1-PH include interstitial lung disease, restrictive syndrome due to skeletal abnormalities, left heart disease, vascular remodelling of the capillaries and veins (similar to pulmonary veno-occlusive disease), and vascular remodelling of the small arteries with intimal and medial thickening and plexiform lesions (similar to PAH) [149]. NF1 have been reported to promote smooth muscle proliferation in the pulmonary arteries via activation of the RAS pathway. As only a minority of NF1 patients develop PH, a second genetic hit may be necessary to lead to the development of PH [149]. Pathologic assessment from explanted lungs of NF-PH patients demonstrated intense pulmonary vascular remodelling as well as interstitial remodelling without fibrosis and as such parenchymal disease with hypoxia may be the main mechanism of NF-PH, though the severe vascular remodelling observed favours associated vascular disease and the multifactorial pathophysiological mechanism of PH-NF [149].

The single case report of NF2-PH reports that NF2 have been found to be physiologically expressed in pulmonary endothelial cells, with decreased expression in idiopathic pulmonary arterial hypertension (IPAH). NF2 is also a negative regulator of mTORC1 and NF-kB, which is also one of the pathways activated in pulmonary vascular remodelling in PAH, hence the possible mechanism in NF2-PH [148].

Screening and Diagnosis

There are no recommendations on screening for NF-PH. In patients with severe lung disease and those with severe exercise limitation, certainly investigation is warranted. When PH is suspected on transthoracic echocardiography, further evaluation with RHC is needed to characterise the mechanism as pre- or post-capillary disease, establish the severity, and guide further possible treatment [149].

Treatment

There are no long-term data or recommendations for the use of PAH-approved therapies in NF-PH, though available data suggest limited benefit. In patients with severe lung disease the focus should be on treating the underlying lung disease, including oxygen therapy and non-invasive ventilatory support and treating the right heart failure with appropriate diuretic therapy. In those with severe PH without extensive lung disease, early referral to a PH expert centre with assessment is advised. The limited response to treatment PAH therapy in these patients also makes the early referral and evaluation for lung transplantation necessary. The increased risk of cancers in these patients must be kept in mind with immunosuppression required for transplantation [149].

One case has been described that had mild clinical and haemodynamic improvement with sorafenib, a tyrosine kinase inhibitor (TKI), though theoretically TKI can cause impairment in cardiac output and the second-generation TKIs have been reported to induce pulmonary endothelial dysfunction [150]. Further studies in therapy in the RAS signalling downstream pathways are needed.

Outcome

The average life expectancy of patients with NF1 is reduced by 10–15 years, mostly due to cancer-related death [151]. In those with NF-PH, the outcomes are described as poor with overall survival less than 50% at 5 years [18, 149].

Pulmonary Hypertension Associated with Pulmonary Langerhans Cell Histiocytosis (PLCH)

Overview

Langerhans cell histiocytosis (LCH), an inflammatory myeloid neoplasm previously known as Histiocytosis X, is a rare cause of diffuse parenchymal lung disease, characterised by cysts and nodules, predominantly affecting the upper lobes [152]. The clonal expansion of myeloid precursors differentiating into Langerhans cells infiltrate the lungs and evoke a strong inflammatory response [153]. Pulmonary Langerhans cell histiocytosis (PLCH) primarily affects young adults, with a peak in the 20–40 year old age group, and occurs almost exclusively in smokers [19, 154]. PLCH has an estimated prevalence in adults of 1–2/1,000,000 people and accounts for ±5% of adult diffuse parenchymal lung diseases [19, 155].

Prevalence

Pulmonary hypertension (PH) is uncommon in those with early or mild disease. Conversely, there is a high prevalence of PH in those with advanced disease, and, in patients with PLCH awaiting lung transplantation, PH may be detected in up to 100% of patients [156, 157]. Relative to other chronic lung diseases, PLCH is associated with a higher prevalence of PH [158]. Additionally, in these cases, there is often a marked increase in pulmonary pressures and moderate-to-severe PH appears to be more commonly detected in those awaiting lung transplant for PLCH than those awaiting transplantation for other pulmonary conditions including COPD and IPF [156].

Risk Factors

One of the key factors in the pathogenesis of PLCH is smoking and as such is an important risk factor [159]. There are no other markers or predictors of the occurrence or severity of PLCH PH.

Clinical Features

PLCH can be asymptomatic, associated with dyspnoea, dry cough, chest pain, constitutional symptoms, and recurrent pneumothorax. Pulmonary vascular dysfunction is one of the mechanisms involved in exercise limitation in PLCH patients, in addition to the limitation resulting from dynamic hyperinflation and impaired gas exchange [160]. Severe PH may complicate PLCH, though the degree of lung involvement does not appear to correlate with the degree of PH, except for inverse correlation with FVC [161]. The radiological features of PH are similar to those seen in other forms of PH.

Pathophysiology

The exact pathophysiology of PLCH-associated PH is incompletely understood and is likely multifactorial, as such it is classified as part of the WHO group 5 PH [2]. Proposed mechanisms include invasion of pulmonary arteries by immune cells, immune-mediated pulmonary vasculopathy, hypoxic vasoconstriction and vascular remodelling due to concomitant effects of cigarette smoking exposure [162]. A marked characteristic of PLCH is the bronchiolocentric presence of Langerhans cells and other inflammatory cell types. Interestingly, the observation of Langerhans cells within the vessels is rare and the vascular changes are similar to the changes found in PAH, with involvement of the small and medium-sized pulmonary arteries with intimal fibrosis and medial hypertrophy [1, 156, 158]. This can also be found in areas without parenchymal involvement of Langerhans cells. However, different from PAH, capillary and venular involvement is common in PLCH PH, with veno-occlusive-like disease features found [21].

Screening and Diagnosis

There are no existing protocols on the screening for PLCH PH. Exercise limitation is common in patients with PLCH, especially in those with moderate lung disease [160]. Screening for PH with echocardiography is indicated in patients with unexplained dyspnoea and in those with isolated/disproportionate decrease in diffusing capacity for carbon monoxide (DLCO) [163].

A low FEV_1, DLCO <40% predicted, decreased VO_2 max and oxygen pulse on CPET and oxygen desaturation during 6MWD test are good predictors of PH in PLCH [160]. A study done on the association of the PA:A ratio with PH in diffuse cystic lung diseases found good correlation of mPAP with PA:A ratio, PA diameter, 6MWD oxygen desaturation and echocardiographic variables [164].

Treatment

As part of the management of PLCH in general, smoking cessation is of major importance and can lead to substantial disease regression and at least in case reports also leads to improvement of the vascular component of the disease [21]. As part of managing PLCH refractory to smoking cessation, steroids and chemotherapeutic agents have been used, though with inconsistent results.

Oxygen therapy should be considered in hypoxic patients. PAH-specific therapy success has been described in a case series, where improvement of PH and a trend toward improved survival were found [165]. Theoretically, however, with the involvement of the venules found on histology, the risk of pulmonary oedema in response to PAH-therapy needs to be considered, although it was not found to be a major problem in the small case series described. In patients with severe PLCH lung disease and those with associated PH, lung transplantation should be considered and has similar outcomes to other lung transplant groups [162].

Outcome

The prognosis of PLCH is variable and affected by response to treatment and relapses [20]. Survival of patients with PLCH was found to be shorter compared with individuals of the same sex and age, though other associations like lymphoma, lung cancer and other malignancies may also contribute [163]. The presence of PH in patients with PLCH is associated with marked increased mortality [161].

Pulmonary Hypertension Associated with Silicosis

Overview

Silicosis is a spectrum of fibrosing lung diseases caused by the inhalation of crystalline silica particles from a wide range of occupational and non-occupational sources. The commonest form of crystalline silica is quartz, which occurs naturally in rocks such as granite and sandstone [166]. Despite increasing occupational health measures, silica exposure remains a significant global health concern, especially in the developing world [167, 168]. China has the highest burden of silicosis, but up to 2.3 million workers in the United States are exposed to respiratory crystalline silica with occupational the major risk factor [22, 169].

Beyond silicosis, silica exposure serves as a precipitating factor for other respiratory comorbidities. It increases the risk for tuberculosis (TB), non-tuberculous mycobacterial disease, chronic airflow limitation (even without smoking), chronic renal disease, lung cancer, and various connective tissue diseases, with pulmonary hypertension (PH) as one of the known complications [170].

Prevalence

There is little data known about the epidemiology of silicosis globally, but cases of silicosis increased by 91.4% between 1990 and 2019, with peak rates in persons between 70 and 74 years [22]. Dose and duration of silica exposure contribute significantly to the prevalence of silicosis, the range increasing from 13% to 75% depending on exposed silica levels in hard-rock miners [171].

The prevalence of PH in silicosis varies globally, reflecting differences in the burden of silicosis as well as screening practices for this complication. In India, 34.6% of individuals with chronic simple silicosis had borderline PH (estimated mPAP 20–25 mmHg), and a further 25% had PH (estimated mPAP >25 mmHg) [23].

Risk Factors

Occupational exposure is the primary risk factor for silicosis. High-risk occupations include mining, sandblasting, tunnelling and quarrying as well as foundry work and the production of glass or ceramics and textile workers using sandblasting to create "worn-out" jeans [172]. The duration and intensity of exposure play a critical role in determining the likelihood of developing silicosis, and workplace conditions significantly influence the risk of silicosis.

Regarding PH in silicosis, the incidence of PH increases with increasing disease severity. Patients with more severe silicosis and progressive massive fibrosis (PMF) are at an increased risk for developing right ventricular hypertrophy [173], and more than a third of patients with PMF are found to have PH [174]. Additionally, large and centrally distributed PMF opacities increase PH risk [174]. Pulmonary functional abnormalities may be important in predicting PH in pneumoconiosis. There is a heterogeneity of spirometric patterns in silicosis, but DLCO and PaO_2 when reduced in PMF have been shown to be significantly associated with the development of PH [174].

Silica exposure is associated with autoimmune diseases such as systemic sclerosis, SLE and RA [175], which all have PH as a well-established complication. Additionally, patients with silicosis have an increased risk for TB, which itself may contribute to the development of PH as discussed prior.

There is also a strong and dose-dependent relationship between exposure to silica and the development of chronic airflow limitation independent of smoking, even in the absence of radiographic evidence of silicosis [176]. Smoking in the context of silicosis may potentiate the decline in lung function and severity of chronic airflow limitation in silica-exposed individuals with and without radiological silicosis and thus is a significant contributing risk factor to the development of PH in silicosis [169].

Clinical Features

Silicosis presents as variable clinical courses, from chronic to accelerated and acute forms, with varying disease severity. The CDC categorises silicosis into two forms—either acute (silicoproteinosis) or nodular (includes accelerated and chronic forms) [177]. Silicoproteinosis is an alveolar filling disease, resulting from intense and short-term (<5 years) exposure to high levels of respirable crystalline silica [176]. The hallmark symptom of silicoproteinosis is rapid development of dyspnoea often accompanied by hypoxaemia, reflecting extensive lung damage and is associated with a high mortality rate [169]. Respiratory failure, cor pulmonale and death usually occur within a few months [167]. Nodular silicosis, which is more common, is classified as simple or complicated (progressive massive fibrosis) based on imaging findings [169]. The accelerated form develops within 5–10 years after initial exposure and tends to progress more rapidly than chronic silicosis [175]. Chronic silicosis is characterised by a slow and insidious progression of symptoms, typically manifesting after a latency period of 10–30 years after exposure and can be categorised as either simple or complicated based on imaging [169]. Symptomatology of chronic silicosis is variable, from asymptomatic to severe dyspnoea, fatigue and cough.

On chest imaging, features of simple silicosis consist of multiple upper zone predominant, small, round opacities, which may be calcified. Hilar and mediastinal lymphadenopathy is usually seen and may also be calcified [167]. The opacities may coalesce resulting in progression to complicated silicosis, which is characterised by a conglomerate of mass-like areas of consolidation and fibrosis, often with calcification [175]. With progression of disease, chest imaging may reveal radiographic features of PH, which is a late and often terminal event in accelerated and complicated silicosis. One study found higher pulmonary artery diameter to the aortic diameter (PA/A) ratio in silicosis correlated with disease severity and was a potential indicator for increased mortality [178].

Pathophysiology

Silicosis presents a complex and multifaceted pathophysiology, the details of which are beyond the scope of this text. Respirable silica particles are inhaled and deposited in the alveoli, inducing lung injury, apoptosis and subsequent release of several inflammatory mediators, which initiate and maintain the acute and chronic lung inflammation [179]. Persistent inflammation stimulates fibroblasts leading to the exaggerated production and deposition of extracellular matrix proteins, resulting in the formation of nodules and interstitial fibrosis within the lung parenchyma.

The pathogenesis of PH in silicosis appears multifactorial, arising from the complex interplay of inflammatory cascades, vascular remodelling and altered pulmonary haemodynamics. Inflammatory mediators released in silicosis pass into the pulmonary circulation and cause endothelial damage [180]. Silica particles themselves can also traverse into the pulmonary vascular bed and directly trigger endothelial cell injury and inflammation, producing vascular remodelling as well as inducing thrombosis [179, 180]. The repetitive endothelial injury leads to a proliferative vasculopathy, which ultimately contributes to the development of PH [180].

Other pathogenic mechanisms that may contribute to the development of PH include a combination of parenchymal destruction, reflex hypoxic vasoconstriction and subsequent vascular remodelling. In addition, progressive luminal narrowing may occur due to compression of pulmonary arteries by enlarging silicotic lesions as well as hilar and peribronchial lymph nodes [174, 181, 182].

Screening and Diagnosis

The diagnosis of silicosis encompasses a thorough evaluation of the patient's employment history delineating risk factors of substantial silica exposure together with radiological findings and exclusion of other diseases with a similar presenting profile, such as sarcoidosis, fungal infections, miliary TB, IPF and other ILDs [166, 167]. As with many other lung diseases, there are currently no recommendations for the screening of PH in patients with silicosis. However, a screening methodology for PH in chronic lung disease adapted to silicosis, and using a combination of FEV_1, PaO_2 during exercise, residual volume and airways resistance on body plethysmography, predicted PH with 80% precision [183].

Treatment and Outcomes

There is currently no proven curative treatment for silicosis or no recommendations of PH-approved therapies for PH complicating silicosis.

Management of silicosis primarily revolves around preventing further exposures, alleviating symptoms, slowing disease progression, and improving overall quality of life. Symptomatic management involves addressing airflow limitation with bronchodilators and cough with antitussives, but there is no established benefit for corticosteroid therapy [167], and there is no evidence to suggest survival benefit or improvement of exercise capacity with long-term oxygen therapy in patients with pneumoconiosis [167]. Smoking cessation and vaccination are recommended [167]. Timely identification and management of complications such as cor pulmonale, TB and pneumothorax is integral to preventing further pulmonary function decline. Lung transplantation should be considered in patients with advanced disease.

The development of PH in silicosis is associated with a poor prognosis and high mortality [184], which is predicted by mean pulmonary artery pressure, PVR, arterial oxygen saturation, vital capacity and FEV_1 [184]. Studies have shown a 100% mortality of patients with a PVR higher than 2.55 Wood units and no patients with oxygen saturation less than 89% survived 10 years [184].

References

1. Olsson KM, Corte TJ, Kamp JC, et al. Pulmonary hypertension associated with lung disease: new insights into pathomechanisms, diagnosis, and management. Lancet Respir Med. 2023;11(9):820–35. https://doi.org/10.1016/S2213-2600(23)00259-X.
2. Humbert M, Kovacs G, Hoeper MM, et al. 2022 ESC/ERS Guidelines for the diagnosis and treatment of pulmonary hypertension. Eur Heart J. 2022;43(38):3618–731. https://doi.org/10.1093/eurheartj/ehac237.
3. Dodd PJ, Yuen CM, Jayasooriya SM, van der Zalm MM, Seddon JA. Quantifying the global number of tuberculosis survivors: a modelling study. Lancet Infect Dis. 2021;21(7). https://doi.org/10.1016/S1473-3099(20)30919-1.
4. Van Heerden JK, Louw EH, Thienemann F, Engel M, Allwood B. The prevalence of pulmonary hypertension in post-tuberculosis and active tuberculosis populations: a systematic review and meta-analysis. Eur Resp Rev Published online 2024. https://doi.org/10.1183/16000617.0154-2023.
5. Lin JL, Xu JF, Qu JM. Bronchiectasis in China. Ann Am Thorac Soc. 2016;13(5). https://doi.org/10.1513/AnnalsATS.201511-740PS.
6. Henkle E, Chan B, Curtis JR, Aksamit TR, Daley CL, Winthrop KL. Characteristics and health-care utilization history of patients with bronchiectasis in US medicare enrollees with prescription drug plans, 2006 to 2014. Chest. 2018;154(6):1311–20. https://doi.org/10.1016/j.chest.2018.07.014.
7. Chandrasekaran R, Mac Aogáin M, Chalmers JD, Elborn SJ, Chotirmall SH. Geographic variation in the aetiology, epidemiology and microbiology of bronchiectasis. BMC Pulm Med. 2018;18(1):83. https://doi.org/10.1186/s12890-018-0638-0.
8. Alzeer AH, Al-Mobeirek AF, Al-Otair HAK, Elzamzamy UAF, Joherjy IA, Shaffi AS. Right and left ventricular function and pulmonary artery pressure in patients with bronchiectasis. Chest. 2008;133(2):468–73. https://doi.org/10.1378/chest.07-1639.
9. Goeminne PC, Scheers H, Decraene A, Seys S, Dupont LJ. Risk factors for morbidity and death in non-cystic fibrosis bronchiectasis: a retrospective cross-sectional analysis of CT diagnosed bronchiectatic patients. Respir Res. 2012;13(1). https://doi.org/10.1186/1465-9921-13-21.
10. Guo J, Garratt A, Hill A. Worldwide rates of diagnosis and effective treatment for cystic fibrosis. J Cystic Fibrosis. 2022;21(3). https://doi.org/10.1016/j.jcf.2022.01.009.
11. Tonelli AR. Pulmonary hypertension survival effects and treatment options in cystic fibrosis. Curr Opin Pulm Med. 2013;19(6):652–61. https://doi.org/10.1097/MCP.0b013e3283659e9f.
12. Li D, Wang B, Wang H, Liu Q. Prognostic significance of pulmonary hypertension in patients with cystic fibrosis. Medicine. 2018;97(7):e9708. https://doi.org/10.1097/MD.0000000000009708.
13. McCarthy C, Gupta N, Johnson SR, Yu JJ, McCormack FX. Lymphangioleiomyomatosis: pathogenesis, clinical features, diagnosis, and management. Lancet Respir Med. 2021;9(11):1313–27. https://doi.org/10.1016/S2213-2600(21)00228-9.

14. O'mahony AM, Lynn E, Murphy DJ, Fabre A, McCarthy C. Lymphangioleiomyomatosis: a clinical review. Breathe. 2020;16(2). https://doi.org/10.1183/20734735.0007-2020.
15. Freitas CSG, Baldi BG, Jardim C, et al. Pulmonary hypertension in lymphangioleiomyomatosis: prevalence, severity and the role of carbon monoxide diffusion capacity as a screening method. Orphanet J Rare Dis. 2017;12(1):74. https://doi.org/10.1186/s13023-017-0626-0.
16. Reynolds RM, Browning GGP, Nawroz I, Campbell IW. Von Recklinghausen's neurofibromatosis: neurofibromatosis type 1. Lancet. 2003;361(9368). https://doi.org/10.1016/S0140-6736(03)13166-2.
17. Evans DGR. Neurofibromatosis type 2 (NF2): A clinical and molecular review. Orphanet J Rare Dis. 2009;4(1). https://doi.org/10.1186/1750-1172-4-16.
18. Jutant EM, Jaïs X, Girerd B, et al. Phenotype and outcomes of pulmonary hypertension associated with neurofibromatosis type 1. Am J Respir Crit Care Med. 2020;202(6). https://doi.org/10.1164/rccm.202001-0105OC.
19. Radzikowska E. Update on pulmonary langerhans cell histiocytosis. Front Med (Lausanne). 2021;7. https://doi.org/10.3389/fmed.2020.582581.
20. Benattia A, Bugnet E, Walter-Petrich A, et al. Long-term outcomes of adult pulmonary Langerhans cell histiocytosis: a prospective cohort. Eur Resp J. 2022;59(5). https://doi.org/10.1183/13993003.01017-2021.
21. Parente Y de DM, Fernandes da Silva N, Souza R. Unusual forms of pulmonary hypertension. Heart Fail Clin. 2023;19(1). https://doi.org/10.1016/j.hfc.2022.08.021.
22. Liu X, Jiang Q, Wu P, Han L, Zhou P. Global incidence, prevalence and disease burden of silicosis: 30 years' overview and forecasted trends. BMC Public Health. 2023;23(1). https://doi.org/10.1186/s12889-023-16295-2.
23. Kumari J, Advani M, Purohit G. Prevalence of pulmonary hypertension in chronic simple silicosis patients and its correlation with smoking history, occupation type, age and duration of silica exposure. Monaldi Arch Chest Dis. Published online November 30, 2023. https://doi.org/10.4081/monaldi.2023.2719.
24. World Health Organization (WHO). Global Tuberculosis Report 2022; 2022. Accessed January 5, 2023. https://www.who.int/publications/i/item/9789240061729.
25. Ntoumi F, Nachega JB, Aklillu E, et al. World Tuberculosis Day 2022: aligning COVID-19 and tuberculosis innovations to save lives and to end tuberculosis. Lancet Infect Dis. 2022;22(4). https://doi.org/10.1016/S1473-3099(22)00142-6.
26. Menzies NA, Quaife M, Allwood BW, et al. Lifetime burden of disease due to incident tuberculosis: a global reappraisal including post-tuberculosis sequelae. Lancet Glob Health. 2021;9(12):e1679–87. https://doi.org/10.1016/S2214-109X(21)00367-3.
27. Allwood BW, Maarman GJ, Kyriakakis CG, Doubell AF. Post-pulmonary tuberculosis complications in South Africa and a potential link with pulmonary hypertension: premise for clinical and scientific investigations. S Afr Med J. 2018;108(7). https://doi.org/10.7196/SAMJ.2018.v108i7.13359.
28. Raine R. Screening for pulmonary hypertension secondary to pulmonary tuberculosis. Afr J Thoracic Crit Care Med. 2020;26(4). https://doi.org/10.7196/AJTCCM.2020.v26i4.129.
29. Tiwari M, Gami SP. Pulmonary hypertension in pulmonary tuberculosis- a prognostic indicator. In: Pulmonary circulation and pulmonary vascular disease. European Respiratory Society; 2017. p. PA2432. https://doi.org/10.1183/1393003.congress-2017.PA2432.
30. Ahmed AEH, Ibrahim AS, Elshafie SM. Pulmonary hypertension in patients with treated pulmonary tuberculosis: analysis of 14 consecutive cases. Clin Med Insights Circ Respir Pulm Med. 2011;5(1):CCRPM.S6437. https://doi.org/10.4137/CCRPM.S6437.
31. Jafri S, Jawad N, Ahmed N, Saifullah N, Siddiqui IA. Post pulmonary tuberculosis: the right heart story. Published online 2020. https://doi.org/10.35248/0974-8369.20.12.466.
32. Chordia R. Clinical profile of pulmonary artery hypertension in treated patients of pulmonary tuberculosis at a tertiary hospital. MedPulse Int J Med. 2021;20(1):23–6. https://doi.org/10.26611/10212015.

33. Louw E, Baines N, Maarman G, et al. The prevalence of pulmonary hypertension after successful tuberculosis treatment in a community sample of adult patients. Pulm Circ. Published online January 5, 2023. https://doi.org/10.1002/pul2.12184.
34. Rajeev GS. Pulmonary hypertension in post tuberculosis pulmonary sequelae: attention needed. Chest. 2020;157(6):A406. https://doi.org/10.1016/j.chest.2020.05.454.
35. Walsh KF, Lui JK. Post-tuberculosis pulmonary hypertension: a case of global disparity in health care. Lancet Glob Health. 2022;10(4). https://doi.org/10.1016/S2214-109X(22)00042-0.
36. Maarman GJ, Shaw J, Allwood B. Pulmonary hypertension in majority countries: opportunities amidst challenges. Curr Opin Pulm Med. 2020;26(5):373–83. https://doi.org/10.1097/MCP.0000000000000702.
37. Thienemann F, Dzudie A, Mocumbi AO, et al. The causes, treatment, and outcome of pulmonary hypertension in Africa: Insights from the Pan African Pulmonary Hypertension Cohort (PAPUCO) Registry. Int J Cardiol. 2016;221:205–11. https://doi.org/10.1016/j.ijcard.2016.06.242.
38. Patel V, Khaped K, Solanki B, Patel A, Rathod H, Patel J. Profile of pulmonary hypertension patients coming to civil hospital, Ahmedabad. Int J Res Med. 2013;2(1).
39. Bhattacharyya P, Saha D, Bhattacherjee P, Das S, Bhattacharyya P, Dey R. Tuberculosis associated pulmonary hypertension: the revelation of a clinical observation. Lung India. 2016;33(2):135. https://doi.org/10.4103/0970-2113.177433.
40. Hnizdo E, Singh T, Churchyard G. Chronic pulmonary function impairment caused by initial and recurrent pulmonary tuberculosis following treatment. Thorax. 2000;55(1):32–8. https://doi.org/10.1136/thorax.55.1.32.
41. di Naso FC, Pereira JS, Schuh SJ, Unis G. Functional evaluation in patients with pulmonary tuberculosis sequelae. Rev Portuguesa Pneumol (English Edition). 2011;17(5). https://doi.org/10.1016/j.rppnen.2011.06.005.
42. Kapoor SC. Cor pulmonale in pulmonary tuberculosis. A preliminary report on 66 patients. Indian JTuberc. 1959;6(2).
43. Parekh A, Patel A, Patel K, Adalja M. Clinicoradiological and cardiac profile of pulmonary artery hypertension in treated patients of pulmonary tuberculosis in a tertiary center. Indian J Resp Care. 2020;9(1):62. https://doi.org/10.4103/ijrc.ijrc_26_19.
44. Jo YS, Park JH, Lee JK, Heo EY, Chung HS, Kim DK. Risk factors for pulmonary arterial hypertension in patients with tuberculosis-destroyed lungs and their clinical characteristics compared with patients with chronic obstructive pulmonary disease. Int J COPD. 2017;12. https://doi.org/10.2147/COPD.S136304.
45. Verma A. Tuberculosis and pulmonary hypertension: commentary. Lung India. 2016;33(2):232. https://doi.org/10.4103/0970-2113.177455.
46. Vikram Singh G, Kumar S, Pratap Pandey B, et al. Pulmonary arterial hypertension in patients of healed pulmonary tuberculosis and it's association with quality of life. Med Res Chronicles. 2021;8(4). https://doi.org/10.26838/MEDRECH.2021.8.4.546.
47. Moodley P, Martinson NA, Joyimbana W, et al. Venous thromboembolic disease in adults admitted to hospital in a setting with a high burden of HIV and TB. Afr J Thoracic Crit Care Med. 2021;27(3):99. https://doi.org/10.7196/AJTCCM.2021.v27i3.155.
48. Saluja M, Swami YK, Chittora S, Vimlani H. Rifampicin containing ATT regimen as an emerging cause of thromboembolic complications. J Evid Based Med Healthc. 2018;5(45). https://doi.org/10.18410/jebmh/2018/644.
49. Marjani M, Tabarsi P, Baghaei P, et al. Incidence of thromboembolism in hospitalized patients with tuberculosis and associated risk factors. Arch Clin Infect Dis. 2012;7(2). https://doi.org/10.5812/archcid.13950.
50. Park SY, Lee SM, Shin JW, et al. Epidemiology of chronic thromboembolic pulmonary hypertension in Korea: results from the Korean registry. Korean J Intern Med. 2016;31(2). https://doi.org/10.3904/kjim.2014.122.

51. Kumar Reddy D. Study of prevalence of Corpulmonale in patients with pulmonary tuberculosis with reference to ECG, echocardiographic changes and radiological extent of the disease. IOSR J Dental Med Sci (IOSR-JDMS) e-ISSN. 2019;18:26–9. https://doi.org/10.9790/0853-1808102629.
52. Miri A, Kalla I, Seedat F. Occult pulmonary arterial hypertension in patients with previous pulmonary tuberculosis. Afr J Thoracic Crit Care Med. 2020;26(4):133. https://doi.org/10.7196/AJTCCM.2020.v26i4.110.
53. Allwood BW, Byrne A, Meghji J, Rachow A, Van Der Zalm MM, Schoch OD. Post-tuberculosis lung disease: clinical review of an under-recognised global challenge. Respiration. 2021;100(8). https://doi.org/10.1159/000512531.
54. Fei Y, Shi X, Gan F, et al. Death causes and pathogens analysis of systemic lupus erythematosus during the past 26 years. Clin Rheumatol. 2014;33(1).
55. de Rezende RPV, Gismondi RA, Maleh HC, et al. Distinct mortality profile in systemic sclerosis: a death certificate study in Rio de Janeiro, Brazil (2006–2015) using a multiple causes of death analysis. Clin Rheumatol. 2019;38(1). https://doi.org/10.1007/s10067-017-3951-8.
56. Ou SM, Fan WC, Cho KT, et al. Systemic sclerosis and the risk of tuberculosis. J Rheumat. 2014;41(8). https://doi.org/10.3899/jrheum.131125.
57. Zhang Y, Fan P, Luo F, et al. Tuberculosis in Takayasu arteritis: a retrospective study in 1105 Chinese patients. J Geriat Cardiol. 2019;16(8). https://doi.org/10.11909/j.issn.1671-5411.2019.08.003.
58. Ugarte-Gil C, Alisjahbana B, Ronacher K, et al. Diabetes mellitus among pulmonary tuberculosis patients from 4 tuberculosis-endemic countries: the tandem study. Clin Infect Dis. 2020;70(5). https://doi.org/10.1093/cid/ciz284.
59. Kohout J, Motanova A, Bilek M, Sefrna F. Have the causes of death in patients with pneumoconiosis changed? Prac Lek. 1994;46(4).
60. Bloomfield GS, Lagat DK, Akwanalo OC, et al. Conditions that predispose to pulmonary hypertension and right heart failure in persons exposed to household air pollution in LMIC. Glob Heart. 2012;7(3). https://doi.org/10.1016/j.gheart.2012.06.015.
61. Parikh R, Konstantinidis I, O'Sullivan DM, Farber HW. Pulmonary hypertension in patients with interstitial lung disease: a tool for early detection. Pulm Circ. 2022;12(4). https://doi.org/10.1002/pul2.12141.
62. Thoker ZA, Madan K, Mittal S, et al. Clinical profile and quality of life of patients with post-pulmonary tuberculosis sequelae presenting to a tertiary care hospital. Cureus. Published online 2023. https://doi.org/10.7759/cureus.36354.
63. Klinger JR. Group III pulmonary hypertension: pulmonary hypertension associated with lung disease: epidemiology, pathophysiology, and treatments. Cardiol Clin. 2016;34(3). https://doi.org/10.1016/j.ccl.2016.04.003.
64. Nathan SD, Barbera JA, Gaine SP, et al. Pulmonary hypertension in chronic lung disease and hypoxia. Eur Respir J. 2019;53(1):1801914. https://doi.org/10.1183/13993003.01914-2018.
65. Colombat M, Mal H, Groussard O, et al. Pulmonary vascular lesions in end-stage idiopathic pulmonary fibrosis: histopathologic study on lung explant specimens and correlations with pulmonary hemodynamics. Hum Pathol. 2007;38(1). https://doi.org/10.1016/j.humpath.2006.06.007.
66. Dentan C, Epaulard O, Seynaeve D, Genty C, Bosson JL. Active tuberculosis and venous thromboembolism: association according to international classification of diseases, ninth revision hospital discharge diagnosis codes. Clin Infect Dis. 2014;58(4). https://doi.org/10.1093/cid/cit780.
67. Turken O, Kunter E, Sezer M, et al. Hemostatic changes in active pulmonary tuberculosis. Int J Tuberculosis Lung Dis. 2002;6(10).
68. Lang IM, Mackman N, Kriett JM, Moser KM, Schleef RR. Prothrombotic activation of pulmonary arterial endothelial cells in a patient with tuberculosis. Hum Pathol. 1996;27(4). https://doi.org/10.1016/S0046-8177(96)90118-5.

69. Ruffenach G, Hong J, Vaillancourt M, Medzikovic L, Eghbali M. Pulmonary hypertension secondary to pulmonary fibrosis: clinical data, histopathology and molecular insights. Respir Res. 2020;21(1). https://doi.org/10.1186/s12931-020-01570-2.
70. Dickinson MG, Bartelds B, Borgdorff MAJ, Berger RMF. The role of disturbed blood flow in the development of pulmonary arterial hypertension: Lessons from preclinical animal models. Am J Physiol Lung Cell Mol Physiol. 2013;305(1). https://doi.org/10.1152/ajplung.00031.2013.
71. Wang A, Su H, Duan Y, et al. Pulmonary hypertension caused by fibrosing mediastinitis. JACC: Asia. 2022;2(3). https://doi.org/10.1016/j.jacasi.2021.11.016.
72. Wu Z, Jarvis H, Howard LS, Wright C, Kon OM. Post-tuberculous fibrosing mediastinitis: a review of the literature. BMJ Open Respir Res. 2017;4(1). https://doi.org/10.1136/bmjresp-2016-000174.
73. Salindri AD, Wang JY, Lin HH, Magee MJ. Post-tuberculosis incidence of diabetes, myocardial infarction, and stroke: retrospective cohort analysis of patients formerly treated for tuberculosis in Taiwan, 2002–2013. Int J Infect Dis. 2019;84. https://doi.org/10.1016/j.ijid.2019.05.015.
74. Magee MJ, Salindri AD, Gujral UP, et al. Convergence of non-communicable diseases and tuberculosis: a two-way street? Int J Tuberculosis Lung Dis. 2018;22(11). https://doi.org/10.5588/ijtld.18.0045.
75. Lim K, Yang JH, Miranda WR, et al. Clinical significance of pulmonary hypertension in patients with constrictive pericarditis. Heart. 2021;107(20). https://doi.org/10.1136/heartjnl-2021-319149.
76. Waxman A, Restrepo-Jaramillo R, Thenappan T, et al. Inhaled treprostinil in pulmonary hypertension due to interstitial lung disease. New Engl J Med. 2021;384(4). https://doi.org/10.1056/nejmoa2008470.
77. Al-Naamani K, Hijal T, Nguyen V, Andrew S, Nguyen T, Huynh T. Predictive values of the electrocardiogram in diagnosing pulmonary hypertension. Int J Cardiol. 2008;127(2). https://doi.org/10.1016/j.ijcard.2007.06.005.
78. Ni JR, Yan PJ, Liu SD, et al. Diagnostic accuracy of transthoracic echocardiography for pulmonary hypertension: a systematic review and meta-analysis. BMJ Open. 2019;9(12):e033084. https://doi.org/10.1136/bmjopen-2019-033084.
79. D'Alto M, Bossone E, Opotowsky AR, Ghio S, Rudski LG, Naeije R. Strengths and weaknesses of echocardiography for the diagnosis of pulmonary hypertension. Int J Cardiol. 2018;263. https://doi.org/10.1016/j.ijcard.2018.04.024.
80. Mutlak D, Aronson D, Lessick J, Reisner SA, Dabbah S, Agmon Y. Functional tricuspid regurgitation in patients with pulmonary hypertension: Is pulmonary artery pressure the only determinant of regurgitation severity? Chest. 2009;135(1). https://doi.org/10.1378/chest.08-0277.
81. Soliman D, Bolliger D, Skarvan K, Kaufmann BA, Lurati Buse G, Seeberger MD. Intraoperative assessment of pulmonary artery pressure by transoesophageal echocardiography. Anaesthesia. 2015;70(3). https://doi.org/10.1111/anae.12920.
82. Wang YC, Huang CH, Tu YK. Pulmonary hypertension and pulmonary artery acceleration time: a systematic review and meta-analysis. J Am Soc Echocardiogr. 2018;31(2). https://doi.org/10.1016/j.echo.2017.10.016.
83. Chen R, Liao H, Deng Z, et al. Efficacy of computed tomography in diagnosing pulmonary hypertension: a systematic review and meta-analysis. Front Cardiovasc Med. 2022;9. https://doi.org/10.3389/fcvm.2022.966257.
84. Devaraj A, Wells AU, Meister MG, Corte TJ, Wort SJ, Hansell DM. Detection of pulmonary hypertension with multidetector CT and echocardiography alone and in combination. Radiology. 2010;254(2). https://doi.org/10.1148/radiol.09090548.
85. Devaraj A, Hansell DM. Computed tomography signs of pulmonary hypertension: old and new observations. Clin Radiol. 2009;64(8). https://doi.org/10.1016/j.crad.2008.12.005.

86. Swigris JJ, Olson AL, Shlobin OA, Ahmad S, Brown KK, Nathan SD. Heart rate recovery after six-minute walk test predicts pulmonary hypertension in patients with idiopathic pulmonary fibrosis. Respirology. 2011;16(3). https://doi.org/10.1111/j.1440-1843.2010.01877.x.
87. Meghji J, Lesosky M, Joekes E, et al. Patient outcomes associated with post-tuberculosis lung damage in Malawi: a prospective cohort study. Thorax. 2020;75(3). https://doi.org/10.1136/thoraxjnl-2019-213808.
88. Muñoz-Torrico M, Cid-Juárez S, Gochicoa-Rangel L, et al. Functional impact of sequelae in drug-susceptible and multidrug-resistant tuberculosis. Int J Tuberculosis Lung Dis. 2020;24(7). https://doi.org/10.5588/ijtld.19.0809.
89. Ruocco G, Cekorja B, Rottoli P, et al. Role of BNP and echo measurement for pulmonary hypertension recognition in patients with interstitial lung disease: an algorithm application model. Respir Med. 2015;109(3). https://doi.org/10.1016/j.rmed.2014.12.011.
90. Romanowski K, Baumann B, Basham CA, Ahmad Khan F, Fox GJ, Johnston JC. Long-term all-cause mortality in people treated for tuberculosis: a systematic review and meta-analysis. Lancet Infect Dis. 2019;19(10). https://doi.org/10.1016/S1473-3099(19)30309-3.
91. Corte TJ, Wort SJ, Gatzoulis MA, Macdonald P, Hansell DM, Wells AU. Pulmonary vascular resistance predicts early mortality in patients with diffuse fibrotic lung disease and suspected pulmonary hypertension. Thorax. 2009;64(10) https://doi.org/10.1136/thx.2008.112847.
92. Öcal S, Portakal O, Öcal A, Demir AU, Topeli A, Çöplü L. Factors associated with pulmonary hypertension and long-term survival in bronchiectasis subjects. Respir Med. 2016;119:109–14. https://doi.org/10.1016/j.rmed.2016.08.027.
93. Park SY, Lee CY, Kim C, et al. One-year prognosis and the role of brain natriuretic peptide levels in patients with chronic cor pulmonale. J Korean Med Sci. 2015;30(4):442. https://doi.org/10.3346/jkms.2015.30.4.442.
94. Septiyanti D, Sari AP, Aniwidyaningsih W, Antariksa B, Siswanto BB. The prevalence of pulmonary hypertension in destroyed lung due to post pulmonary tuberculosis and its relation to exercise capacity. J Resp Indonesia. 2019;38(4). https://doi.org/10.36497/jri.v38i4.24.
95. Huston JH, Maron BA, French J, et al. Association of mild echocardiographic pulmonary hypertension with mortality and right ventricular function. JAMA Cardiol. 2019;4(11). https://doi.org/10.1001/jamacardio.2019.3345.
96. O'Donnell AE. Bronchiectasis—a clinical review. N Engl J Med. 2022;387(6):533–45. https://doi.org/10.1056/NEJMra2202819.
97. Neves PC, Guerra M, Ponce P, Miranda J, Vouga L. Non-cystic fibrosis bronchiectasis. Interact Cardiovasc Thorac Surg. 2011;13(6):619–25. https://doi.org/10.1510/icvts.2011.284208.
98. Chalmers JD, Chang AB, Chotirmall SH, Dhar R, McShane PJ. Bronchiectasis. Nat Rev Dis Primers. 2018;4(1):45. https://doi.org/10.1038/s41572-018-0042-3.
99. Wang L, Jiang S, Shi J, et al. Clinical characteristics of pulmonary hypertension in bronchiectasis. Front Med. 2016;10(3). https://doi.org/10.1007/s11684-016-0461-z.
100. Flume PA, Chalmers JD, Olivier KN. Advances in bronchiectasis: endotyping, genetics, microbiome, and disease heterogeneity. The Lancet. 2018;392(10150). https://doi.org/10.1016/S0140-6736(18)31767-7.
101. Ghigna MR, Mooi WJ, Grünberg K. Pulmonary hypertensive vasculopathy in parenchymal lung diseases and/or hypoxia. Eur Resp Rev. 2017;26(144). https://doi.org/10.1183/16000617.0003-2017.
102. Martins M, Keir HR, Chalmers JD. Endotypes in bronchiectasis: moving towards precision medicine. A narrative review. Pulmonology. 2023;29(6). https://doi.org/10.1016/j.pulmoe.2023.03.004.
103. Alzghoul BN, Sayaideh MA, Moreno BF, et al. Pulmonary hypertension in eosinophilic versus noneosinophilic copd. ERJ Open Res. 2021;7(1). https://doi.org/10.1183/23120541.00772-2020.
104. Weng M, Baron DM, Bloch KD, Luster AD, Lee JJ, Medoff BD. Eosinophils are necessary for pulmonary arterial remodeling in a mouse model of eosinophilic inflammation-induced

pulmonary hypertension. Am J Physiol Lung Cell Mol Physiol. 2011;301(6). https://doi.org/10.1152/ajplung.00049.2011.
105. Brock M, Trenkmann M, Gay RE, et al. Interleukin-6 modulates the expression of the bone morphogenic protein receptor type ii through a novel STAT3-microRNA cluster 17/92 pathway. Circ Res. 2009;104(10). https://doi.org/10.1161/CIRCRESAHA.109.197491.
106. Shahane A. Pulmonary hypertension in rheumatic diseases: epidemiology and pathogenesis. Rheumatol Int. 2013;33(7). https://doi.org/10.1007/s00296-012-2659-y.
107. Nathan SD, Shlobin OA, Barnett SD, et al. Right ventricular systolic pressure by echocardiography as a predictor of pulmonary hypertension in idiopathic pulmonary fibrosis. Respir Med. 2008;102(9):1305–10. https://doi.org/10.1016/j.rmed.2008.03.022.
108. Fisher MR, Criner GJ, Fishman AP, et al. Estimating pulmonary artery pressures by echocardiography in patients with emphysema. Eur Respir J. 2007;30(5):914–21. https://doi.org/10.1183/09031936.00033007.
109. Swift AJ, Dwivedi K, Johns C, et al. Diagnostic accuracy of CT pulmonary angiography in suspected pulmonary hypertension. Eur Radiol. 2020;30(9). https://doi.org/10.1007/s00330-020-06846-1.
110. Charters PFP, Rossdale J, Brown W, et al. Diagnostic accuracy of an automated artificial intelligence derived right ventricular to left ventricular diameter ratio tool on CT pulmonary angiography to predict pulmonary hypertension at right heart catheterisation. Clin Radiol. 2022;77(7). https://doi.org/10.1016/j.crad.2022.03.009.
111. Chalmers JD, Elborn S, Greene CM. Basic, translational and clinical aspects of bronchiectasis in adults. Eur Resp Rev. 2023;32(168). https://doi.org/10.1183/16000617.0015-2023.
112. Hill A, Sullivan A, Chalmers J, et al. British Thoracic Society Guideline for bronchiectasis in adults. Thorax. 2019;74(Suppl 1):1–69. https://doi.org/10.1136/thoraxjnl-2018-212463.
113. Devaraj A, Wells AU, Meister MG, Loebinger MR, Wilson R, Hansell DM. Pulmonary hypertension in patients with bronchiectasis: prognostic significance of CT signs. Am J Roentgenol. 2011;196(6). https://doi.org/10.2214/AJR.10.5221.
114. Shteinberg M, Haq IJ, Polineni D, Davies JC. Cystic fibrosis. Lancet. 2021;397(10290):2195–211. https://doi.org/10.1016/S0140-6736(20)32542-3.
115. Redondo M, Keyt H, Dhar R, Chalmers JD. Global impact of bronchiectasis and cystic fibrosis. Breathe. 2016;12(3). https://doi.org/10.1183/20734735.007516.
116. Eckles M, Anderson P. Cor pulmonale in cystic fibrosis. Semin Respir Crit Care Med. 2003;24(3):323–30. https://doi.org/10.1055/s-2003-41093.
117. Hayes D, Higgins RS, Kirkby S, et al. Impact of pulmonary hypertension on survival in patients with cystic fibrosis undergoing lung transplantation: an analysis of the UNOS registry. J Cystic Fibrosis. 2014;13(4). https://doi.org/10.1016/j.jcf.2013.12.004.
118. Wells JM, Farris RF, Gosdin TA, et al. Pulmonary artery enlargement and cystic fibrosis pulmonary exacerbations: a cohort study. Lancet Respir Med. 2016;4(8):636–45. https://doi.org/10.1016/S2213-2600(16)30105-9.
119. Nagy R, Gede N, Ocskay K, et al. Association of body mass index with clinical outcomes in patients with cystic fibrosis. JAMA Netw Open. 2022;5(3):e220740. https://doi.org/10.1001/jamanetworkopen.2022.0740.
120. Milla CE. Nutrition and lung disease in cystic fibrosis. Clin Chest Med. 2007;28(2):319–30. https://doi.org/10.1016/j.ccm.2007.02.006.
121. Genctoy G, Arikan S, Eldem O. Pulmonary hypertension associates with malnutrition and body composition hemodialysis patients. Ren Fail. 2015;37(2):273–9. https://doi.org/10.3109/0886022X.2014.986705.
122. Callejo M, Barberá JA, Duarte J, Perez-Vizcaino F. Impact of nutrition on pulmonary arterial hypertension. Nutrients. 2020;12(1):169. https://doi.org/10.3390/nu12010169.
123. Tonelli AR, Fernandez-Bussy S, Lodhi S, et al. Prevalence of pulmonary hypertension in end-stage cystic fibrosis and correlation with survival. J Heart Lung Transplant. 2010;29(8):865–72. https://doi.org/10.1016/j.healun.2010.04.006.

124. Fauroux B, Hart N, Belfar S, et al. Burkholderia cepacia is associated with pulmonary hypertension and increased mortality among cystic fibrosis patients. J Clin Microbiol. 2004;42(12) https://doi.org/10.1128/JCM.42.12.5537-5541.2004.
125. Rovedder PME, Ziegler B, Pasin LR, et al. Doppler echocardiogram, oxygen saturation and submaximum capacity of exercise in patients with cystic fibrosis. J Cyst Fibros. 2007;6(4):277–83. https://doi.org/10.1016/j.jcf.2006.10.009.
126. Kapnadak SG, Dimango E, Hadjiliadis D, et al. Cystic Fibrosis Foundation consensus guidelines for the care of individuals with advanced cystic fibrosis lung disease. J Cyst Fibros. 2020;19(3):344–54. https://doi.org/10.1016/j.jcf.2020.02.015.
127. Poore TS, Taylor-Cousar JL, Zemanick ET. Cardiovascular complications in cystic fibrosis: a review of the literature. J Cyst Fibros. 2022;21(1):18–25. https://doi.org/10.1016/j.jcf.2021.04.016.
128. Poore S, Berry B, Eidson D, McKie KT, Harris RA. Evidence of vascular endothelial dysfunction in young patients with cystic fibrosis. Chest. 2013;143(4):939–45. https://doi.org/10.1378/chest.12-1934.
129. Shah PH, Lee JH, Salvi DJ, Rabbani R, Gavini DR, Hamid P. Cardiovascular system involvement in cystic fibrosis. Cureus. Published online July 29, 2021. https://doi.org/10.7759/cureus.16723.
130. Ratjen F. Pulmonary artery hypertension: an underrated disease manifestation in cystic fibrosis? Lancet Respir Med. 2016;4(8):596–8. https://doi.org/10.1016/S2213-2600(16)30107-2.
131. Castellani C, Duff AJA, Bell SC, et al. ECFS best practice guidelines: the 2018 revision. J Cystic Fibrosis. 2018;17(2). https://doi.org/10.1016/j.jcf.2018.02.006.
132. Selimovic N, Andersson B, Bergh CH, et al. Pulmonary hemodynamics as predictors of mortality in patients awaiting lung transplantation. Transpl Int. 2008;21(4):314–9. https://doi.org/10.1111/j.1432-2277.2007.00605.x.
133. Hayes D, Tobias JD, Mansour HM, et al. Pulmonary hypertension in cystic fibrosis with advanced lung disease. Am J Respir Crit Care Med. 2014;190(8):898–905. https://doi.org/10.1164/rccm.201407-1382OC.
134. Johnson SR. Lymphangioleiomyomatosis. In: Orphan lung diseases. Springer; 2023. p. 335–51. https://doi.org/10.1007/978-3-031-12950-6_19.
135. Ussavarungsi K, Hu X, Scott JP, et al. Mayo clinic experience of lung transplantation in pulmonary lymphangioleiomyomatosis. Respir Med. 2015;109(10):1354–9. https://doi.org/10.1016/j.rmed.2015.08.014.
136. Reynaud-Gaubert M, Mornex JF, Mal H, et al. Lung transplantation for lymphangioleiomyomatosis: the French experience. Transplantation. 2008;86(4). https://doi.org/10.1097/TP.0b013e31817c15df.
137. Simonneau G, Gatzoulis MA, Adatia I, et al. Updated clinical classification of pulmonary hypertension. J Am Coll Cardiol. 2013;62(25):D34–41. https://doi.org/10.1016/j.jacc.2013.10.029.
138. Simonneau G, Montani D, Celermajer DS, et al. Haemodynamic definitions and updated clinical classification of pulmonary hypertension. Eur Respir J. 2019;53(1):1801913. https://doi.org/10.1183/13993003.01913-2018.
139. Cottin V, Harari S, Humbert M, et al. Pulmonary hypertension in lymphangioleiomyomatosis: characteristics in 20 patients. Eur Respir J. 2012;40(3):630–40. https://doi.org/10.1183/09031936.00093111.
140. Wu X, Xu W, Wang J, Tian X, Tian Z, Xu K. Clinical characteristics in lymphangioleiomyomatosis-related pulmonary hypertension: an observation on 50 patients. Front Med. 2019;13(2). https://doi.org/10.1007/s11684-018-0634-z.
141. Cottin V, Brown K, Richeldi L, Mccormack FX. Orphan lung diseases: a clinical guide to rare lung disease, 2nd ed.
142. Krymskaya VP, Snow J, Cesarone G, et al. mTOR is required for pulmonary arterial vascular smooth muscle cell proliferation under chronic hypoxia. FASEB J. 2011;25(6):1922–33. https://doi.org/10.1096/fj.10-175018.

143. Johnson SR, Cordier JF, Lazor R, et al. European Respiratory Society guidelines for the diagnosis and management of lymphangioleiomyomatosis. Eur Respir J. 2010;35(1):14–26. https://doi.org/10.1183/09031936.00076209.
144. McCormack FX, Inoue Y, Moss J, et al. Efficacy and safety of sirolimus in lymphangioleiomyomatosis. N Engl J Med. 2011;364(17):1595–606. https://doi.org/10.1056/NEJMoa1100391.
145. Warrior K, Dilling DF. Lung transplantation for lymphangioleiomyomatosis. J Heart Lung Transplant. 2023;42(1):40–52. https://doi.org/10.1016/j.healun.2022.09.021.
146. Khawar MU, Yazdani D, Zhu Z, Jandarov R, Dilling DF, Gupta N. Clinical outcomes and survival following lung transplantation in patients with lymphangioleiomyomatosis. J Heart Lung Transplant. 2019;38(9):949–55. https://doi.org/10.1016/j.healun.2019.06.015.
147. Santos MR, Pereira AM. Neurofibromatosis type 1 and pulmonary arterial hypertension: a case report. Rev Portuguesa Cardiol. 2022;41(6). https://doi.org/10.1016/j.repc.2019.05.018.
148. Taniguchi H, Takashima T, Tu L, et al. Pulmonary hypertension associated with neurofibromatosis type 2. Pulm Circ. 2021;11(3). https://doi.org/10.1177/20458940211029550.
149. Jutant EM, Girerd B, Jaïs X, et al. Pulmonary hypertension associated with neurofibromatosis type 1. Eur Resp Rev 2018;27(149). https://doi.org/10.1183/16000617.0053-2018.
150. Tamura Y, Ono T, Sano M, Fukuda K, Kataoka M, Satoh T. Favorable effect of sorafenib in a patient with neurofibromatosis- associated pulmonary hypertension. Am J Respir Crit Care Med. 2012;186(3). https://doi.org/10.1164/ajrccm.186.3.291.
151. Rasmussen SA, Friedman JM. NF1 gene and neurofibromatosis 1. Am J Epidemiol. 2000;151(1). https://doi.org/10.1093/oxfordjournals.aje.a010118.
152. Emile JF, Abla O, Fraitag S, et al. Revised classification of histiocytoses and neoplasms of the macrophage-dendritic cell lineages. Blood. 2016;127(22):2672–81. https://doi.org/10.1182/blood-2016-01-690636.
153. Rodriguez-Galindo C, Allen CE. Langerhans cell histiocytosis. Blood. 2020;135(16):1319–31. https://doi.org/10.1182/blood.2019000934.
154. Tazi A. Adult pulmonary Langerhans' cell histiocytosis. Eur Respir J. 2006;27(6):1272–85. https://doi.org/10.1183/09031936.06.00024004.
155. Thomeer M, Demedts M, Vandeurzen K. Registration of interstitial lung diseases by 20 centres of respiratory medicine in flanders. Acta Clin Belg. 2001;56(3):163–72. https://doi.org/10.1179/acb.2001.026.
156. Fartoukh M, Humbert M, Capron F, et al. Severe pulmonary hypertension in histiocytosis X. Am J Respir Crit Care Med. 2000;161(1):216–23. https://doi.org/10.1164/ajrccm.161.1.9807024.
157. Dauriat G, Mal H, Thabut G, et al. Lung transplantation for pulmonary langerhans' cell histiocytosis: a multicenter analysis. Transplantation. 2006;81(5):746–50. https://doi.org/10.1097/01.tp.0000200304.64613.af.
158. Al-Qadi M, LeVarge B, Ford HJ. Epidemiology, pathogenesis, and clinical approach in group 5 pulmonary hypertension. Front Med (Lausanne). 2021;7. https://doi.org/10.3389/fmed.2020.616720.
159. Tazi A, De Margerie C, Naccache JM, et al. The natural history of adult pulmonary Langerhans cell histiocytosis: a prospective multicentre study. Orphanet J Rare Dis. 2015;10(1). https://doi.org/10.1186/s13023-015-0249-2.
160. Heiden GI, Sobral JB, Freitas CSG, et al. Mechanisms of exercise limitation and prevalence of pulmonary hypertension in pulmonary langerhans cell histiocytosis. Chest. 2020;158. https://doi.org/10.1016/j.chest.2020.05.609.
161. Chaowalit N, Pellikka PA, Decker PA, et al. Echocardiographic and clinical characteristics of pulmonary hypertension complicating pulmonary langerhans cell histiocytosis. Mayo Clin Proc. 2004;79(10). https://doi.org/10.4065/79.10.1269.
162. Wajda N, Zhu Z, Jandarov R, Dilling DF, Gupta N. Clinical outcomes and survival following lung transplantation in patients with pulmonary Langerhans cell histiocytosis. Respirology. 2020;25(6). https://doi.org/10.1111/resp.13671.

163. Lorillon G, Tazi A. How I manage pulmonary langerhans cell histiocytosis. Eur Resp Rev. 2017;26(145). https://doi.org/10.1183/16000617.0070-2017.
164. Baldi BG, Fernandes CJCDS, Heiden GI, et al. Association between pulmonary artery to aorta diameter ratio with pulmonary hypertension and outcomes in diffuse cystic lung diseases. Medicine (United States). 2021;100(25). https://doi.org/10.1097/MD.0000000000026483.
165. Le Pavec J, Lorillon G, Jaïs X, et al. Pulmonary langerhans cell histiocytosis-associated pulmonary hypertension: clinical characteristics and impact of pulmonary arterial hypertension therapies. Chest. 2012;142(5). https://doi.org/10.1378/chest.11-2490.
166. Greenberg MI, Waksman J, Curtis J. Silicosis: a review. Disease-a-Month. 2007;53(8). https://doi.org/10.1016/j.disamonth.2007.09.020.
167. Leung CC, Yu ITS, Chen W. Silicosis. Lancet. 2012;379(9830):2008–18. https://doi.org/10.1016/S0140-6736(12)60235-9.
168. Bhagia L. Non-occupational exposure to silica dust. Indian J Occup Environ Med. 2012;16(3). https://doi.org/10.4103/0019-5278.111744.
169. Krefft S, Wolff J, Rose C. Silicosis: an update and guide for clinicians. Clin Chest Med. 2020;41(4). https://doi.org/10.1016/j.ccm.2020.08.012.
170. Murray J, Reid G, Kielkowski D, De Beer M. Cor pulmonale and silicosis: a necropsy based case-control study. Br J Ind Med. 1993;50(6). https://doi.org/10.1136/oem.50.6.544.
171. Cohen RAC, Patel A, Green FHY. Lung disease caused by exposure to coal mine and silica dust. Semin Respir Crit Care Med. 2008;29(6). https://doi.org/10.1055/s-0028-1101275.
172. Akgun M, Araz O, Akkurt I, et al. An epidemic of silicosis among former denim sandblasters. Eur Resp J. 2008;32(5). https://doi.org/10.1183/09031936.00093507.
173. Fernie JM, Douglas AN, Lamb D, Ruckley VA. Right ventricular hypertrophy in a group of coalworkers. Thorax. 1983;38(6):436–42. https://doi.org/10.1136/thx.38.6.436.
174. Yu S, Wang Y, Fan Y, Ma R, Wang Y, Ye Q. Pulmonary hypertension in patients with pneumoconiosis with progressive massive fibrosis. Occup Environ Med. 2022;79(11). https://doi.org/10.1136/oemed-2021-108095.
175. Churg A, Muller NL. Update on silicosis. Surg Pathol Clin. Published online December 2023. https://doi.org/10.1016/j.path.2023.11.005.
176. Adverse effects of crystalline silica exposure. Am J Respir Crit Care Med. 1997;155(2). https://doi.org/10.1164/ajrccm.155.2.9032226.
177. U.S. Department of Health and Human Services. Silicosis 2010 Case definition. Centers for Disease Control and Prevention.
178. Çankaya BY, Karaman A, Albez FS, Polat G, Alper F, Akgün M. The association of silicosis severity with pectoralis major muscle and subcutaneous fat volumes and the pulmonary artery/aorta ratio evaluated by CT. Diagnostic and Interventional Radiology. 2021;27(1). https://doi.org/10.5152/dir.2020.19534.
179. Huaux F. New developments in the understanding of immunology in silicosis. Curr Opin Allergy Clin Immunol. 2007;7(2). https://doi.org/10.1097/ACI.0b013e32802bf8a5.
180. Zelko IN, Zhu J, Ritzenthaler JD, Roman J. Pulmonary hypertension and vascular remodeling in mice exposed to crystalline silica. Respir Res. 2016;17(1). https://doi.org/10.1186/s12931-016-0478-5.
181. Ye Q, Yu S, Wang Y. Progressive massive fibrosis contributes to pulmonary hypertension in silicosis. 2019. https://doi.org/10.1164/ajrccm-conference.2019.199.1_meetingabstracts.a1176.
182. Zhang R, Ma G, Xu X, Liang L. Percutaneous treatment for silicosis-induced pulmonary artery stenosis: a case report and review of the literature. Medicine (United States). 2018;97(2). https://doi.org/10.1097/MD.0000000000009469.
183. Evers H, Liehs F, Harzbecker K, et al. Screening of pulmonary hypertension in chronic obstructive pulmonary disease and silicosis by discriminant functions. Eur Resp J 1992;5(4). https://doi.org/10.1183/09031936.93.05040444.
184. Jandova R, Widimsky J, Eisler L, Navratil M. Long-term prognosis of pulmonary hypertension in silicosis. Cor Vasa. 1980;22(4).

Chapter 13
Pulmonary Vascular Disease Associated with Hypoxemia and High Altitude

Lindsay M. Forbes and Kurt R. Stenmark

Introduction

Hypoxemia elicits complex short- and long-term responses in the pulmonary circulation. In many individuals, isolated hypoxemia such as that experienced at high altitude is well-tolerated through acute and chronic adaptive responses [1–3]. However, a minority of individuals exposed to hypobaric hypoxia develop significant pulmonary vascular pathobiology manifesting as disease states including high-altitude pulmonary edema (HAPE) and high-altitude pulmonary hypertension. The pathobiology of these diseases provides insight into both health risks to individuals living or traveling to high altitude as well as those exposed for other reasons to acute and chronic hypoxemia.

Pulmonary Vascular Diseases Associated with Hypoxemia

HAPE is an acute and life-threatening disease characterized by hypoxic pulmonary vasoconstriction resulting in a significant increase in pulmonary artery pressure [4]. Vascular permeability is increased in alveolar capillaries resulting in

L. M. Forbes (✉)
Division of Pulmonary, Allergy and Critical Care Medicine, University of Colorado, Denver, CO, USA
e-mail: lindsay.forbes@cuanschutz.edu

K. R. Stenmark
Cardiovascular and Pulmonary Research Laboratory, Departments of Pediatrics and Medicine, University of Colorado School of Medicine, Denver, CO, USA
e-mail: kurt.stenmark@cuanschutz.edu

F. N. Rahaghi et al. (eds.), *The Pulmonary Vasculature in Chronic Lung Disease*, Respiratory Medicine, https://doi.org/10.1007/978-3-032-03581-3_13

noncardiogenic pulmonary edema [5]. HAPE has been reported to occur in as many as 6–15% of individuals undergoing rapid ascent to high altitude [4]. Cases have been identified of patients diagnosed with pulmonary arterial hypertension years following HAPE episodes [4], suggesting underlying shared pulmonary vascular abnormalities between acute HAPE and chronic pulmonary arterial hypertension.

High-altitude pulmonary hypertension is a disease state observed in individuals residing chronically at high altitude >2500 m (approximately 8000 ft) [6]. While hypoxic pulmonary vasoconstriction results in pulmonary artery pressure elevation even in healthy individuals at high altitude [2], in a minority of high-altitude dwellers chronic hypoxia results in pulmonary vascular remodeling and pathologic pulmonary hypertension [7]. High-altitude pulmonary hypertension is commonly defined by a resting mean pulmonary artery pressure> 30 mmHg or pulmonary artery systolic pressure >50 mmHg at residence >2500 m [6]. The reported prevalence of high-altitude pulmonary hypertension ranges from <1% to 18% [8–13]. Prevalence varies across populations, with lower disease prevalence among Tibetans and greater disease prevalence among populations with fewer generations of high-altitude dwelling [4, 11, 14, 15].

In addition to HAPE and high-altitude pulmonary hypertension, chronic exposure to hypobaric hypoxia is associated with pulmonary vascular disease in the setting of chronic mountain sickness, a maladaptation disorder characterized by excessive erythrocytosis and pulmonary hypertension [16]. Outside of high-altitude-related illnesses, chronic hypoxia in the setting of lung diseases, such as pulmonary fibrosis and chronic obstructive pulmonary disease, contributes to pathobiology underlying pulmonary vascular remodeling and World Symposium of Pulmonary Hypertension Group III pulmonary hypertension [17, 18].

Pathologic Findings and Experimental Models of Hypoxic Pulmonary Vascular Disease

The correlation between chronic hypoxia and pulmonary vascular remodeling was first recognized through the study of cattle afflicted with brisket disease [19]. Brisket disease was recognized as a heart failure syndrome provoked by high altitude [19]. It was first studied in the early 1900s by George Glover and Issac Newsom, who recognized that lowland cattle transported to higher altitudes were susceptible to heart failure and that genetic adaptation conferred through breeding with native highland bulls was protective [19]. In the 1960s, collaborative work by Rue Jensen, Archibald Alexander, Donald Will, John Reeves, and Robert Grover elucidated that the heart failure syndrome observed in cattle at high altitude in fact reflected the effects of chronic hypoxia mediating pulmonary vascular remodeling and pulmonary hypertension [19]. In particular, cattle exposed to chronic hypoxia demonstrated a significant and progressive increase in mean pulmonary artery pressure which was directly related to the degree of medial hypertrophy of small muscular pulmonary arteries [19].

Since the connection between hypoxia and pulmonary vascular remodeling was first identified, further pathologic evaluations in both animals and humans have provided additional clarity. Characteristic findings of hypoxic pulmonary vascular remodeling include muscularization of arterioles, medial hypertrophy of muscular pulmonary arteries, and slight medial hypertrophy of veins [20, 21]. In high-altitude dwellers, increased expression of α-smooth muscle actin (α-SMA) is observed in small pulmonary arteries which normally lack smooth muscle [22]. This "distal extension of smooth muscle" is a sine qua non of hypoxic pulmonary vascular remodeling [22]. Necroscopic studies of infants and children suggest that some of the remodeling observed in children may reflect a persistence of fetal pulmonary vascular characteristics [2, 21]. Whereas at sea level distal pulmonary arterial muscularization and right ventricular hypertrophy subside within the first few months of life, in children living at high altitude the fetal pattern can persist through the first decade [21, 23]. On the other hand, the hypertrophy of the more proximal arteries appears to be a secondary change in response to hypoxemia which is not observed in young children [21]. Experimental models support the hypothesis that neonatal hypoxia during critical periods of lung development may contribute to pulmonary vascular remodeling, though this is difficult to confirm in humans [23, 24]. Unlike in primary pulmonary arterial hypertension, intimal changes and plexiform lesions are not observed [20].

The pathognomonic pulmonary arterial medial thickening observed in response to hypoxia results from some combination of smooth muscle proliferation and smooth muscle cell hypertrophy and deposition of extracellular matrix proteins, depending upon the species and the smooth muscle cell populations evaluated [25, 26]. There is substantial heterogeneity in cell populations, with smooth muscle cells arising from endothelial cells, fibroblasts, resident or circulating progenitors [26]. Additionally, developmental stage and the vascular site including both the cellular composition and local environment factors influence hypoxic remodeling responses [22]. Cell population heterogeneity contributes to complex responses to hypoxia which are time- and location-specific [26]. Additionally, responses are dynamic and change over time, reflecting cellular plasticity [26]. Among relevant factors, smooth muscle cells demonstrate variable changes in proliferation, extracellular matrix protein production, expression of growth factors, cytokines, and receptors [22, 26].

For example, in humans, smooth muscle cell proliferation occurs in both large, proximal and distal pulmonary arteries [25]. In a neonatal calf model exposed to hypoxia, distal pulmonary artery medial compartment cells demonstrate early (days 4–7) but not late (day 14) proliferation [25]. The distal smooth muscle cells are comprised of two populations, one which is well-differentiated and resistant to proliferation (α-SMA+, smooth muscle-myosin heavy chain [SM-MHC]+) and one which is highly proliferative and apoptosis-resistant (low α-SMA expression and no SM-MHC) [25]. The latter express hematopoietic and progenitor cell markers suggesting a circulating, nonresident origin, and they release factors including S100A4 and platelet-derived growth factor (PDGF)-β which stimulate proproliferative signaling pathways [25]. Similarly, hyperproliferative smooth muscle-like cells have been identified in distal pulmonary arteries of patients with chronic obstructive pulmonary disease [27]. Thus, it appears that nonresident smooth muscle-like cells are recruited in response to hypoxia to the distal medial compartment, where they promote proliferation and remodeling [27].

Interestingly, there is high variability in the degree of hypoxic pulmonary vascular response both within and between species. Native high-altitude species like yaks, llamas, and guinea pigs tend to demonstrate little vascular remodeling and pulmonary hypertension [28]. Some low-altitude animals like dogs and sheep are observed to be "hypo-responsive," with altitude inducing only modest thickening of pulmonary vessels with mild pulmonary hypertension and right ventricular hypertrophy [28]. On the other hand, "hyper-responsive" low-altitude animals like cows and swine develop significant pulmonary arterial thickening with moderate to severe pulmonary hypertension and right ventricular hypertrophy [28]. Rodents are commonly used in experimental models of pulmonary hypertension [20]. In response to hypoxic exposure, mice demonstrate relatively mild vascular and perivascular remodeling, while rats demonstrate moderate remodeling [20].

The factors accounting for inter-species variability are a topic of interest. Differences in collateral ventilation have been implicated in inter-species variability in hypoxic pulmonary vascular response [19]. Species including dogs, sheep, and humans demonstrate collateral ventilation which can participate in maintaining ventilation-perfusion balance, while "hyper-responsive" species like pigs and cattle lack collateral ventilation and therefore may rely primarily on hypoxic pulmonary vasoconstriction in response to regional hypoxia [19]. Additionally, variations in inflammatory cell profiles have been reported, with increased perivascular peripheral blood mononuclear cell accumulation being observed in rats compared to mice and correlating with perivascular remodeling [20]. Gene expression of major histocompatibility antigen class II and osteopontin and phosphoinositide-3 kinase, which function in part as immune modulators, is upregulated in rats' lungs compared to mice in response to hypoxia [20]. Additionally, higher tryptase-positive mast cells and transforming growth factor (TGF)-β1-positive neutrophils and mononuclear cells in the perivascular sheath of small pulmonary artery cells in Wistar rats exposed to 4300 m compared to pika indigenous to 4300 m, which are relatively resistant to vascular remodeling and pulmonary hypertension [19]. Such changes may promote the differentiation of vascular fibroblasts into myofibroblasts in hypoxia-induced vascular remodeling [19].

Genetic Variation in Hypoxic Pulmonary Vascular Disease

Importantly, genetic adaptations contribute to intra- and inter-species variability. For example, cattle appear to be born with either a "susceptible" or "resistant" phenotype according to whether their parents demonstrated brisket disease [29, 30]. In cattle with brisket disease, increased prevalence of an *EPAS1* variant has been observed [31]. *EPAS1* encodes the transcription factor hypoxia inducible factor (HIF)-2α which upregulates hypoxia-sensitive target genes [31]. Through HIF and other mechanisms, endothelial mediators such as endothelial nitric oxide synthase (eNOS) and its regulator asymmetric dimethylarginine impact hypoxic pulmonary vascular response by modifying the bioavailability of the endogenous pulmonary vasodilator, nitric oxide [32–35]. However, variants in genes encoding endothelial mediators like *eNOS*, *TGIF2* (encoding TG-interacting factor 2), and *BMPR2* (encoding bone morphogenetic protein receptor 2) do not appear to be directly implicated in genetic susceptibility to brisket disease in cattle [36]. Meanwhile, a number of genes that are implicated, including those associated with interleukin-6 (IL6), triggering receptors expressed on myeloid cells (TREM), and nuclear factor-κB (NF-kB) signaling, fall in pathways of inflammation [36].

Genetic variation in susceptibility to high-altitude pulmonary hypertension is also observed in humans. There are four primary regions where populations live at high altitude: the Tibetan Plateau, Ethiopian Plateau, Andean Plateau, and Rocky Mountains [37]. Tibetans demonstrate minimal pulmonary artery pressure elevation relative to Colorado high-altitude dwellers, presumably related to significantly greater duration of genetic adaptation in oxygen delivery and metabolism [38–40]. Andeans and Amhara Ethiopians demonstrate intermediate values [41]. Genomic studies have suggested >1000 genes involved in high-altitude adaptation to hypoxia, summarized in Table 13.1 [42–49]. Of note, there is substantial overlap with inflammatory pathways with the majority of genes mentioned serving roles in regulation of inflammation.

Similarly, epigenetic modifications via DNA methylation and other methods may both regulate proinflammatory pathways and hypoxic pulmonary vascular remodeling [49–52]. Global changes in histone acetylation and DNA methylation are observed in response to hypoxia and are mediated in part by HIF-1α [49]. DNA

Table 13.1 Examples of pathways and genes implicated in circulatory system adaptation to hypoxia

Pathway	Genes
Renin-angiotensin-aldosterone system	*ACE, AGT, AGTR1*
Endothelin pathway	*EDNRA, EDNRB*
Nitric oxide signaling	*NOS1, NOS2, NOS3*
Adrenergic signaling	*ADRA1A, ADRA1B*
Transcription factors mediating response to hypoxia	*EPAS1, PPARα, PPARϒ, PHD3, PIK3CA*
Angiogenesis	*VEGFB, VEGFC*
Tissue repair	*TMOD3*
Endothelial cell function	*VCAM1*
Protein serine/threonine kinase activity	*PIK3CB, PIK3CG*
BMP signaling	*MTMR4*
Plasma membrane gradient maintenance	*ATP1A1, ATP2A1*

methyltransferase 3 beta (DNMT3B), an enzyme involved in DNA methylation, increases during hypoxia and both regulates proinflammatory pathways including chemokine Ccl5 and modifies hypoxic pulmonary vascular remodeling [49, 53]. DNM3TB expression can in turn be modulated by microRNAs such as miR-29, which decreases in hypoxic conditions [49]. Variation in epigenetic patterns across populations have been reported, including decreased *EPAS1* methylation in Andeans [49]. Such modification may allow for increased *EPAS1* expression and confer adaptive benefits [49]. Neonatal hypoxia increases global DNA methylation in the lungs including around the Insulin-like growth factor 1 (IGF-1) promoter region, and histone deacetylation inhibition can reduce IGF-1/protein kinase B (AKT) signaling, attenuating pulmonary vascular remodeling [49]. Exosomes, which are released by cells and contribute to cell-cell communication, increase and their composition including cargo of epigenetic modifiers like microRNAs is changed by hypoxia [49]. For example, microRNA (miR)-210 is highly prevalent in hypoxic exosomes in cancer cells and results in changes to metabolism, angiogenesis, cell proliferation, migration, invasion, and apoptosis [49]. In the future, investigation of exosomes may provide insight into epigenetic mechanisms underlying pulmonary vascular adaptation and maladaptation to hypoxia.

Mechanisms of the Pulmonary Vascular Response to Hypoxia

Hypoxia triggers a complex array of local, regional, and systemic responses. Carotid body chemoreceptors are responsible for sensing hypoxia and triggering the hypoxic ventilatory response, which increases ventilation to partially compensate for low inspired pressure of oxygen [23]. Oxygen sensors in the pulmonary vasculature trigger hypoxic pulmonary vasoconstriction, which is a conserved adaptive response that in the case of regional alveolar hypoxia serves to preserve ventilation-perfusion matching, but in the setting of global alveolar hypoxia results in increased pulmonary artery pressure [23]. Finally, oxygen sensors in other tissues result in the activation of vascular endothelial growth factor (VEGF) in the heart and brain and erythropoietin expression in the kidney and liver [23]. Finally, tissue-level metabolic reprogramming results from the activation of hypoxia-sensitive signaling pathways and influences inflammatory and vascular remodeling responses to hypoxia [18, 23].

Within the pulmonary vasculature, oxygen-sensitive potassium channels are inhibited by hypoxia [16, 54, 55]. The resulting depolarization of pulmonary artery smooth muscle cells and activation of voltage-gated calcium channels causes calcium influx and Rho kinase-mediated pulmonary artery smooth muscle cell vasoconstriction [17, 54, 55]. Pulmonary vascular endothelial cells respond to hypoxia with production of vasoactive and mitogenic factors that affect pulmonary artery smooth muscle cell function, proliferation, and apoptosis [25, 56]. Those factors include endothelin, thromboxane A2, and other vasoconstrictive substances. [10, 38, 57, 58] Variations in the signaling response to hypoxia impact pulmonary vascular disease susceptibility. For example, Kyrgyz highlanders with high-altitude pulmonary hypertension demonstrate higher levels of endothelin-1 relative to healthy highlanders [48]. During acute ascent to high altitude, mountaineers demonstrate a "transpulmonary gain" of endothelin-1 which correlates with pulmonary artery systolic pressure increase [58]. While vasoconstrictors are increased, the endogenous pulmonary vasodilator nitric oxide is decreased (less so in the Tibetan population with corresponding lower incidence of high-altitude pulmonary hypertension) [38–40]. Among HAPE-susceptible individuals compared to HAPE-resistant individuals, a greater reduction in exhaled nitric oxide levels is observed in response to hypoxia, and exhaled nitric oxide levels are inversely correlated with pulmonary artery pressure elevation [16]. The decrease in nitric oxide may in part result from the increased action of asymmetric dimethylarginine, a competitive inhibitor of nitric oxide synthase [59]. Individuals with chronic intermittent high-altitude exposure (such as miners) demonstrate increased asymmetric dimethylarginine levels that correlate with mean pulmonary artery pressure [9, 60]. Additionally, reactive oxygen species produced by mitochondria under conditions of hypoxia contribute to hypoxic pulmonary vasoconstriction, potentially by directly stimulating pulmonary artery smooth muscle cell intracellular calcium increase as well as interactions with other mediators [16]. In mountaineers ascending to high altitude, increased reactive oxygen species correlate with increased pulmonary artery pressure and are more pronounced in individuals who develop HAPE [61].

One of the central mechanisms by which hypoxia mediates cellular responses is through the actions of the transcription factors HIF-1 and HIF-2. The HIF family directly or indirectly regulates the expression of several hundred genes [62]. Among those recognized as central in mediating responses to hypoxia are those encoding erythropoietin, transferrin, VEGF, nitric oxide synthase, and endothelin 1 [63]. Mice deficient in HIF-1α (HIF-1α +/−) demonstrate less pulmonary vascular remodeling, pulmonary hypertension, and right ventricular hypertrophy in response to chronic hypoxia compared to mice without HIF-1α deficiency (HIF-1α +/+) [63]. HIF proteolysis by prolyl hydroxylase enzymes depends upon iron as a cofactor, and manipulation of iron levels impacts the acute hypoxic pulmonary vasoconstrictive response in humans [62]. Finally, pathologically increased HIF-mediated gene activation in the genetic disease of Chuvash polycythemia is associated with pulmonary hypertension [62]. The magnitude of hypoxic stimulus correlates with HIF-1α expression as well as HIF-1α-mediated gene transcription and physiological responses [63].

Hypoxia impacts additional pathways beyond HIF-mediated genes with direct effects on pulmonary vascular remodeling. For example, hypoxia increases TGF-β expression, which regulates collagen synthesis in fibroblasts and contributes to extracellular matrix protein accumulation in pulmonary artery media and adventitia [22]. A negative mutation in the TGF-β receptor abrogates pulmonary vascular remodeling in response to chronic hypoxia in rats [22]. In addition, TGF-β promotes the Nox4 isoform of nicotinamide adenine dinucleotide phosphate (NADPH) oxidase, contributing to the production of endogenous reactive oxygen species which reduces nitric oxide availability and promotes pulmonary artery smooth muscle cell proliferation [61].

Central Role of Inflammation in the Pulmonary Vascular Response to Hypoxia

Inflammatory pathways play a central role in the pulmonary vascular response to hypoxia [17]. Pathologically, perivascular inflammation with accumulation of peripheral blood mononuclear cells in pulmonary artery adventitia and media is observed in hypoxia-induced vascular and perivascular remodeling in mice, rats and calves [20, 22]. In remodeled pulmonary arteries, there is an imbalance of cellular proliferation and apoptosis [18]. Increased proliferation and apoptosis resistance are observed in adventitial mesenchymal cells in combination with activation of immune cells in both experimental hypoxic pulmonary hypertension models as well as humans with pulmonary hypertension [18]. Specifically, mononuclear cells are critical to hypoxia-induced vascular remodeling [25]. Depletion of circulating mononuclear phagocytes results in absence of pulmonary vascular remodeling in response to chronic hypoxia [25]. Mononuclear cells are recruited by activated fibroblasts [18]. In response to hypoxia, adventitial fibroblasts secrete chemokines, cytokines, and glycolytic metabolites including IL-6 and lactate which contribute to the recruitment, retention, and activation of naïve macrophages to a pro-inflammatory/pro-remodeling phenotype [18]. In particular, cytoplasmic and mitochondrial metabolic alterations contribute to the pro-inflammatory, apoptosis-resistant smooth muscle cell phenotype [26]. This pro-inflammatory/pro-remodeling phenotype promotes chronic, ongoing inflammation and vascular remodeling [25]. Pathways implicated in maintaining a pro-inflammatory fibroblast phenotype include HIF and NF-kB, as well as epigenetic modifications including changes in micro-RNAs, increased histone deacetylase activity, and increased DNA methylation [25]. Additionally, the involvement of glycolytic metabolites in macrophage activation suggests that proinflammatory activation occurs in concert with metabolic reprogramming [18], with metabolites contributing to the induction and maintenance of signaling networks that increase cellular proliferation and an inflammatory phenotype [18]. Additionally, activated macrophages are characterized by signal transducer and activator of transcription 3 (STAT-3)-HIF-1-CCAAT/enhancer-binding protein-β and NF-κB signaling, as well as aerobic glycolysis [25]. The activity of these signaling and metabolic processes within activated macrophages serve to induce further monocyte recruitment, macrophage activation, and smooth muscle cell proliferation and fibroblast activation [25]. Thus, crosstalk between fibroblasts and macrophages including inflammatory signaling and metabolic reprogramming perpetuate ongoing hypoxic pulmonary vascular remodeling [18, 25].

While the adventitia appears to be central to the coordinated inflammatory and proliferative pulmonary vascular response to hypoxia, inflammatory pathways directly impact medial and intimal remodeling [25]. Specifically, medial pulmonary artery smooth muscle cell recruitment and activation of progenitor cells are observed in concert with activation of inflammatory pathways under hypoxic conditions [25]. Macrophage migration inhibitor factor (MIF) increases in response to hypoxia and contributes to the release of inflammatory mediators and stimulation of pulmonary artery smooth muscle cell proliferation [64, 65]. Deletion of phosphatase and tensin homolog (PTEN) in smooth muscle in mice resulted in increased whole-lung expression of the inflammatory mediators of stromal cell-derived factor 1 and IL-6 with increased perivascular macrophage recruitment, and simultaneously severe pulmonary hypertension in response to chronic hypoxia [25]. IL-6 increases in pulmonary artery smooth muscle cells in response to hypoxia and activates inflammatory responses and remodeling [66, 67]. For example, IL-6-deficient mice exposed to hypoxia demonstrate less macrophage recruitment and correspondingly experience less pulmonary vascular remodeling and pulmonary hypertension [66, 67]. Finally, abnormal BMPR2 signaling in response to chronic hypoxia may contribute to pro-inflammatory smooth muscle cells [25]. Recruited pro-inflammatory cells can then exert mitogenic effects on pulmonary artery smooth muscle cells [25].

Pulmonary artery endothelial cells likewise contribute to pro-inflammatory signaling pathways [25]. In addition to secreting vasoactive mediators [25, 56], endothelial cells respond to hypoxia with the synthesis and release of pro-inflammatory mediators including IL-1, IL-6, and IL-8 and increased expression of inflammatory cell adhesion molecules [22, 25]. Thus, endothelial cells secrete both vasoactive and inflammatory mediators which both directly contribute to intimal thickening as well as interact with circulating cells to contribute to medial remodeling [22, 25]. Pro-inflammatory interactions with circulating cells facilitate recruitment of progenitor cells into the pulmonary artery walls [22].

Inflammatory pathways are central to the pulmonary vascular response in HAPE as well [22]. In mice and rats, acute hypoxia increases lung vascular permeability in conjunction with increases in macrophage and neutrophil numbers [22]. Inflammation-related genes including *MMP8* (encoding matrix metallopeptidase 8), *MMP9*, *IL-17β*, and TIMP metallopeptidase inhibitor 1 (*Timp1*) are upregulated in rats exposed to acute hypoxia [5]. In humans with HAPE, increased neutrophils and macrophages are observed in bronchoalveolar lavage fluid [68]. Additionally, increased levels of tumor necrosis factor (TNF)-α, IL-1-β, IL-6, and IL-8 are observed [68]. Patients with HAPE also demonstrate increased TNF-α and IL-6 levels in the serum, which may further contribute to lung permeability [5]. Additionally, proinflammatory chemokines including macrophage inhibitory protein (MIP)-1α and monocyte chemoattractant protein (MCP)-1 and the inflammatory biomarker soluble urokinase-type plasminogen activator receptor (suPAR) are increased in HAPE-susceptible humans, suggesting that inflammatory mediators may modulate the response to acute hypoxia and confer susceptibility to HAPE [5].

Importantly, there is also interaction between HIF and inflammatory molecules. For example, HIF-1α is stabilized by IL-1-β, NF-κB, and TNF-α [5]. NF-κB may play a particularly important role in regulating inflammation under hypoxic conditions [5]. Additionally, crosstalk between reactive oxygen species and inflammation may contribute to hypoxic responses [5]. Finally, various pro-inflammatory markers of endoplasmic reticulum stress including G protein-coupled receptor 78 (GRP78), protein kinase R-like endoplasmic reticulum kinase (PERK), inositol-requiring enzyme (IRE)1, activating transcription factor (ATF)4, ATF6, C/EBP homologous protein (CHOP) and caspase-12 are observed in subacute to chronic hypoxia, again highlighting the potential role for pro-inflammatory pathways in the development of hypoxic pulmonary vascular remodeling [69]. Thus, inflammatory pathways may mediate both acute and chronic responses to hypoxia both directly and in concert with other hypoxia-responsive mechanisms.

Time Course of Hypoxic Pulmonary Vascular Response

As suggested earlier, pathologic pulmonary vascular responses to hypoxia include acute and chronic responses. Acute hypoxia causes biphasic hypoxic pulmonary vasoconstriction, with an immediate transient vasoconstriction peaking in the first 10–15 min followed after approximately 40 min by a more gradual, progressive increase that plateaus after 2 h and persists for 8 h [16]. In animal models, the onset of neomuscularization of small pulmonary arteries is rapid, appearing within hours of hypoxic exposure and peaking at 1 week [70]. Thus, in humans the second phase of the acute hypoxic pulmonary vasoconstriction effect may actually reflect in part the effects of pulmonary vascular remodeling [71]. Notably, there is significant variation in the acute hypoxic pulmonary vasoconstrictive response between individuals, which contributes to susceptibility to diagnoses such as HAPE [16, 72]. With progressive hypoxic exposure over a period of weeks as studied in Operation Everest II, the degree of pulmonary artery pressure elevation gradually increases [3, 16]. However, after prolonged acclimatization of 1 year, the elevation in pulmonary artery pressure is less than that observed at 24 h [16]. Similarly, chronic high-altitude dwellers demonstrate a lower degree of pulmonary artery pressure elevation when exposed to acute hypoxia than do sea level dwellers [16], suggesting a preserved adaptive response to acute hypoxic exposure. However, chronic pulmonary artery pressure elevation among high-altitude dwellers does not appear to differ significantly from sea level dwellers who have undergone acclimatization to high altitude [16].

The effect of removing a hypoxic stimulus on the pulmonary vascular system is a point of particular interest. In acute hypoxic pulmonary vasoconstriction as observed in HAPE, removing the individual from hypoxia appears to lead to rapid reduction in pulmonary artery pressure elevation [16, 72]. However, when evaluated after 2–3 weeks of high-altitude exposure, the administration of supplemental oxygen failed to fully reverse the elevation in pulmonary vascular resistance [3]. Similarly, in animal models, following weeks of hypoxia the removal of the hypoxic stimulus results in reduction but not normalization of pulmonary artery pressure [73]. Additionally, while after weeks of exposure to normoxia the neomuscularized arterioles dedifferentiated, residual structural changes persist [70, 73, 74]. There are important sex and age differences in pulmonary vascular remodeling due to hypoxia in rats, with males and infants experiencing greater muscularization of small and peripheral intra-acinar arteries and more significant elevation in pulmonary artery pressure in response to hypoxia [73, 75]. Similarly, persistence of remodeling and pulmonary arterial pressure elevation after return to normoxia is greatest in infants [73]. Thus, some studies suggest that in animal models the pulmonary vascular remodeling that is observed in response to sustained hypoxia appears to partially but not completely reverse with removal of hypoxia. However, other observations suggest more complete resolution of hypoxic pulmonary hypertension in animals with sustained normoxia [20]. In humans, moving to sea level residence in many individuals with high-altitude pulmonary hypertension appears to improve symptoms of pulmonary hypertension within months to years, but in a minority of patients such a move does not resolve the disease [16]. Among the few reports of high-altitude dwellers who have moved to sea level, results suggest that resting pulmonary artery pressure tends to normalize at an evaluation time of 1–2 years after leaving high altitude, but that an abnormal pulmonary vascular response to exercise is observed [76–78]. The latter may reflect the effects of residual, persistent pulmonary vascular remodeling.

Therapies for Hypoxic Pulmonary Vascular Diseases

Most of the therapies trialed in hypoxic pulmonary vascular disease are based on therapies used in pulmonary arterial hypertension. A significant limitation to many studies is the investigation of pulmonary arterial pressure in healthy lowlanders exposed to high altitude, rather than in individuals with pathologic high-altitude pulmonary hypertension. With that caveat, perhaps the most data exists regarding phosphodiesterase-5 inhibitors. Increased levels of phosphodiesterase 5 are observed in the muscular coat of remodeled pulmonary arteries of individuals with high-altitude pulmonary hypertension [79]. In a randomized controlled trial of 22 individuals with high-altitude pulmonary hypertension, 3 months of sildenafil 25 mg three times daily reduced mean pulmonary arterial pressure (−6.9 mmHg, 95% CI −12.4 to −1.3) and improved six-minute walk distance (45.4 m; 95% CI 11.5 to 79.4, $p = 0.011$) [79]. Separate randomized controlled trials of sildenafil administered to healthy individuals exposed to high altitude suggest reduced echocardiographic pulmonary artery systolic pressure and improved maximal oxygen consumption and workload with exercise [80–82]. Additionally, tadalafil has demonstrated efficacy in reducing the pulmonary artery pressure increase and HAPE incidence among individuals with prior episodes of HAPE [16]. However, other randomized controlled trials of sildenafil suggest no benefit of sildenafil in healthy individuals exposed to high altitude on pulmonary arterial pressure or exercise performance [83, 84]. Meta-analyses of the use of sildenafil at high altitude suggest a benefit in reducing pulmonary artery systolic pressure acutely with more conflicting results with longer-term therapy [85, 86].

Endothelin receptor antagonists have also been evaluated. In preclinical data, macitentan administered to rats exposed to hypobaric hypoxia appears to reduce pulmonary arterial pressures and right ventricular remodeling [87, 88]. The data is more limited in humans. In Kyrgyz highlanders, a single dose of bosentan 125 mg reduced pulmonary artery systolic pressure and increased pulmonary artery acceleration time [48]. However, in healthy lowlanders 5 days of bosentan 125 mg twice daily prior to ascent to 3800 m did not improve pulmonary artery systolic pressure or time to complete a cycle ergometer time trial and in fact was associated with worsened oxygen saturation during exercise, possibly related to fluid retention and interstitial pulmonary edema [89]. Prostacyclin receptor agonists like selexipag and soluble guanylate cyclase stimulators like riociguat have been studied in animal models, with selexipag but not riociguat suggesting benefit [88]. Among individuals with non-altitude-mediated hypoxic pulmonary hypertension (e.g., Group 3 pulmonary hypertension), only the inhaled prostacyclin treprostinil has demonstrated efficacy in improving clinical outcomes associated with pulmonary hypertension [90]. Finally, calcium channel blockers, effective in pulmonary arterial hypertension with positive vasodilator response, were associated with decreased pulmonary artery pressure in a non-randomized trial of 31 asymptomatic high-altitude dwellers [91]. Among HAPE-susceptible individuals, nifedipine has been demonstrated to reduce pulmonary artery pressure and reduce the incidence of HAPE, and calcium channel blockers are the recommended agents for both prophylaxis and treatment in HAPE-susceptible individuals [16, 72].

Finally, a number of therapies not derived from approved pulmonary arterial hypertension therapies have been tested. Fasudil, a RhoA/Rho kinase (ROCK) inhibitor, was studied in 19 Kyrgyz patients with high-altitude pulmonary hypertension in a randomized double-blind study [92]. Fasudil significantly decreased echocardiographic pulmonary artery systolic pressure (−10.37 +/− 0.97 mmHg), reduced pulmonary vascular resistance (−0.39 +/− 0.05 WU), and increased pulmonary artery acceleration time (0.015 +/− 0.001 ms) [92]. Irbesartan, an angiotensin receptor blocker, reduced pulmonary artery pressure in rats with high-altitude pulmonary hypertension [93, 94]. In humans with high-altitude pulmonary hypertension and systemic hypertension, the angiotensin-converting enzyme inhibitor captopril was associated with reduced pulmonary artery pressure [95]. Acetazolamide, a carbonic anhydrase inhibitor which triggers increased ventilation by causing metabolic acidosis, has been studied in various conditions in part due to its positive effect in chronic mountain sickness [96, 97]. Acetazolamide may inhibit hypoxic pulmonary vasoconstriction [16, 98], thus reducing the risk of HAPE. However, while it has been associated with a higher minute ventilation, arterial oxygenation, and maximal oxygen consumption during hypoxic peak exercise [99], definitive evidence of an effect in high-altitude pulmonary hypertension remains to be demonstrated. As mentioned earlier, intravenous iron has been demonstrated to modulate pulmonary vascular response to acute hypoxia [62, 100]. Its effect may arise from its role as a cofactor for prolyl hydroxylase, which degrades HIF [101]. In healthy individuals, iron infusion administered before or during hypoxic exposure greatly reduced the elevation in pulmonary artery systolic pressure [62, 100]. Similarly, intravenous iron reduced echocardiographic pulmonary artery systolic pressure during hypoxia in both healthy high-altitude Andeans and partially acclimatized lowlanders at 4300 m [102].

Anti-inflammatory approaches have been evaluated in animal models. Cerium oxide nanoparticles administered prior to hypoxia exposure (7620 m; 6 h) ameliorated cytokine increase and neutrophil infiltration [5]. Netrine-1 pretreatment prior to acute hypoxic exposure in mice reduced neutrophil infiltration in the lungs and attenuated the increase in MIP-2 [5]. Additional anti-inflammatory therapies that have been demonstrated in animal models to reduce inflammatory signaling and pulmonary vascular effects of acute hypoxic exposure include cobalt, curcumin, nanocurcumin, quercetin, and *Potentilla anserina* L. polysaccharide [5]. In humans, the potent anti-inflammatory glucocorticosteroid dexamethasone has demonstrated efficacy in HAPE prophylaxis and other acute high-altitude illnesses [5]. Dexamethasone's efficacy in preventing HAPE may relate to its ability to increase the expression and activity of nitric oxide synthase, as well as increasing alveolar fluid clearance through effect on membrane sodium channels and sodium-potassium ATPase [16].

Additional non-pharmacologic interventions have been considered particularly for HAPE in the form of ischemic preconditioning, i.e., provoking local ischemia through mechanisms like intermittent thigh cuff inflation, or intermittent hypoxia or reoxygenation. Local limb ischemia via thigh cuff has produced variable effects [16]. Intermittent reoxygenation appears to reduce pulmonary artery remodeling and pulmonary hypertension [103–105]. The effect of the latter may be related to reduced cytokine production in the setting of oxygen enrichment as well as modulated expression of HIF-1α and HIF-2α related pathways [103–105]. Perhaps the most effective therapy for HAPE is prophylaxis through careful acclimatization. Reducing the rapidity of ascent particularly in sleeping altitude as well as reducing strenuous physical activity during the early acclimatization process appears to reduce the incidence and severity of hypoxic pulmonary vascular response [16]. The treatment for HAPE once it develops is rapid reoxygenation through supplemental oxygen administration and descent [16, 72].

In summary, the greatest amount of interest has historically been in applying pulmonary arterial hypertension therapies to hypoxic pulmonary vascular diseases, though there have been smaller targeted trials of alternative agents. However, the vast majority of therapeutic trials in this area are limited by the use of healthy populations rather than those with clinical high-altitude pulmonary hypertension. Further investigations of therapies directed at hypoxia-induced pulmonary vascular diseases in individuals with clinical disease are necessary.

Conclusion

Hypoxia causes complex responses both systemically and within the pulmonary vasculature. While many of these responses appear to serve adaptive purposes in the majority of humans, complex pathobiology can emerge both in acute and chronic hypoxic exposure. Genetic susceptibility to maladaptive responses underlies differences observed between different populations as well as between individuals. In particular, hypoxic pulmonary vascular remodeling appears to result from crosstalk between inflammatory and metabolic pathways. Elucidation and ultimately intervention upon the pathobiological mechanisms underlying maladaptive pulmonary vascular response to hypoxia in high-altitude disorders such as HAPE and high-altitude pulmonary hypertension will likewise provide insights into pulmonary vascular maladaptation in other disorders characterized by acute and chronic hypoxia.

References

1. Forbes LM, Bull TM, Lahm T, Lawley JS, Hunter K, Levine BD, et al. Right ventricular response to acute hypoxia among healthy humans. Am J Respir Crit Care Med. 2023;208(3):333–6.
2. Penaloza D, Arias-Stella J. The heart and pulmonary circulation at high altitudes: healthy highlanders and chronic mountain sickness. Circulation. 2007;115(9):1132–46.
3. Groves BM, Reeves JT, Sutton JR, Wagner PD, Cymerman A, Malconian MK, et al. Operation Everest II: elevated high-altitude pulmonary resistance unresponsive to oxygen. J Appl Physiol (1985). 1987;63(2):521–30.
4. Eichstaedt CA, Benjamin N, Grünig E. Genetics of pulmonary hypertension and high-altitude pulmonary edema. J Appl Physiol (1985). 2020;128(5):1432–8.
5. El Alam S, Pena E, Aguilera D, Siques P, Brito J. Inflammation in pulmonary hypertension and edema induced by hypobaric hypoxia exposure. Int J Mol Sci. 2022;23(20).
6. León-Velarde F, Maggiorini M, Reeves JT, Aldashev A, Asmus I, Bernardi L, et al. Consensus statement on chronic and subacute high altitude diseases. High Alt Med Biol. 2005;6(2):147–57.
7. León-Velarde F, Villafuerte FC, Richalet JP. Chronic mountain sickness and the heart. Prog Cardiovasc Dis. 2010;52(6):540–9.
8. Soria R, Egger M, Scherrer U, Bender N, Rimoldi SF. Pulmonary artery pressure and arterial oxygen saturation in people living at high or low altitude: systematic review and meta-analysis. J Appl Physiol (1985). 2016;121(5):1151–9.
9. Brito J, Siques P, López R, Romero R, León-Velarde F, Flores K, et al. Long-term intermittent work at high altitude: right heart functional and morphological status and associated cardiometabolic factors. Front Physiol. 2018;9:248.
10. Brito J, Siques P, Pena E. Long-term chronic intermittent hypoxia: a particular form of chronic high-altitude pulmonary hypertension. Pulm Circ. 2020;10(1 Suppl):5–12.
11. Gou Q, Shi R, Zhang X, Meng Q, Li X, Rong X, et al. The prevalence and risk factors of high-altitude pulmonary hypertension among native Tibetans in Sichuan Province, China. High Alt Med Biol. 2020;21(4):327–35.
12. Negi PC, Marwaha R, Asotra S, Kandoria A, Ganju N, Sharma R, et al. Prevalence of high altitude pulmonary hypertension among the natives of Spiti Valley—a high altitude region in Himachal Pradesh, India. High Alt Med Biol. 2014;15(4):504–10.

13. Lichtblau M, Saxer S, Furian M, Mayer L, Bader PR, Scheiwiller PM, et al. Cardiac function and pulmonary hypertension in Central Asian highlanders at 3250 m. Eur Respir J. 2020;56(2).
14. Groves BM, Droma T, Sutton JR, McCullough RG, McCullough RE, Zhuang J, et al. Minimal hypoxic pulmonary hypertension in normal Tibetans at 3,658 m. J Appl Physiol (1985). 1993;74(1):312–8.
15. Maggiorini M, Léon-Velarde F. High-altitude pulmonary hypertension: a pathophysiological entity to different diseases. Eur Respir J. 2003;22(6):1019–25.
16. Sydykov A, Mamazhakypov A, Maripov A, Kosanovic D, Weissmann N, Ghofrani HA, et al. Pulmonary hypertension in acute and chronic high altitude maladaptation disorders. Int J Environ Res Public Health. 2021;18(4).
17. Gu S, Goel K, Forbes LM, Kheyfets VO, Yu YA, Tuder RM, Stenmark KR. Tensions in taxonomies: current understanding and future directions in the pathobiologic basis and treatment of group 1 and group 3 pulmonary hypertension. Compr Physiol. 2023;13(1):4295–319.
18. Stenmark KR, Tuder RM, El Kasmi KC. Metabolic reprogramming and inflammation act in concert to control vascular remodeling in hypoxic pulmonary hypertension. J Appl Physiol (1985). 2015;119(10):1164–72.
19. Rhodes J. Comparative physiology of hypoxic pulmonary hypertension: historical clues from brisket disease. J Appl Physiol (1985). 2005;98(3):1092–100.
20. Stenmark KR, Meyrick B, Galie N, Mooi WJ, McMurtry IF. Animal models of pulmonary arterial hypertension: the hope for etiological discovery and pharmacological cure. Am J Phys Lung Cell Mol Phys. 2009;297(6):L1013–32.
21. Arias-Stella J, Saldana M. The terminal portion of the pulmonary arterial tree in people native to high altitudes. Circulation. 1963;28:915–25.
22. Stenmark KR, Fagan KA, Frid MG. Hypoxia-induced pulmonary vascular remodeling: cellular and molecular mechanisms. Circ Res. 2006;99(7):675–91.
23. Huicho L. Postnatal cardiopulmonary adaptations to high altitude. Respir Physiol Neurobiol 2007;158(2-3):190-203.
24. Niermeyer S, Andrade MM, Vargas E, Moore LG. Neonatal oxygenation, pulmonary hypertension, and evolutionary adaptation to high altitude (2013 Grover Conference series). Pulm Circ. 2015;5(1):48–62.
25. Pugliese SC, Poth JM, Fini MA, Olschewski A, El Kasmi KC, Stenmark KR. The role of inflammation in hypoxic pulmonary hypertension: from cellular mechanisms to clinical phenotypes. Am J Phys Lung Cell Mol Phys. 2015;308(3):L229–52.
26. Stenmark KR, Frid MG, Graham BB, Tuder RM. Dynamic and diverse changes in the functional properties of vascular smooth muscle cells in pulmonary hypertension. Cardiovasc Res. 2018;114(4):551–64.
27. Howard LS, Crosby A, Vaughan P, Sobolewski A, Southwood M, Foster ML, et al. Distinct responses to hypoxia in subpopulations of distal pulmonary artery cells contribute to pulmonary vascular remodeling in emphysema. Pulm Circ. 2012;2(2):241–9.
28. Tucker A, Rhodes J. Role of vascular smooth muscle in the development of high altitude pulmonary hypertension: an interspecies evaluation. High Alt Med Biol. 2001;2(2):173–89.
29. Will DH, Hicks JL, Card CS, Alexander AF. Inherited susceptibility of cattle to high-altitude pulmonary hypertension. J Appl Physiol. 1975;38(3):491–4.
30. Will DH, Hicks JL, Card CS, Reeves JT, Alexander AF. Correlation of acute with chronic hypoxic pulmonary hypertension in cattle. J Appl Physiol. 1975;38(3):495–8.
31. Newman JH, Holt TN, Cogan JD, Womack B, Phillips JA 3rd, Li C, et al. Increased prevalence of EPAS1 variant in cattle with high-altitude pulmonary hypertension. Nat Commun. 2015;6:6863.
32. Lüneburg N, Siques P, Brito J, Arriaza K, Pena E, Klose H, et al. Long-term chronic intermittent hypobaric hypoxia in rats causes an imbalance in the asymmetric dimethylarginine/nitric oxide pathway and ROS activity: a possible synergistic mechanism for altitude pulmonary hypertension? Pulm Med. 2016;2016:6578578.

33. Mizuno S, Ishizaki T, Toga H, Sakai A, Isakova J, Taalaibekova E, et al. Endogenous asymmetric dimethylarginine pathway in high altitude adapted yaks. Biomed Res Int. 2015;2015:196904.
34. Siques P, López de Pablo AL, Brito J, Arribas SM, Flores K, Arriaza K, et al. Nitric oxide and superoxide anion balance in rats exposed to chronic and long term intermittent hypoxia. Biomed Res Int. 2014;2014:610474.
35. Rodriguez-Miguelez P, Lima-Cabello E, Martínez-Flórez S, Almar M, Cuevas MJ, González-Gallego J. Hypoxia-inducible factor-1 modulates the expression of vascular endothelial growth factor and endothelial nitric oxide synthase induced by eccentric exercise. J Appl Physiol (1985). 2015;118(8):1075–83.
36. Newman JH, Holt TN, Hedges LK, Womack B, Memon SS, Willers ED, et al. High-altitude pulmonary hypertension in cattle (brisket disease): candidate genes and gene expression profiling of peripheral blood mononuclear cells. Pulm Circ. 2011;1(4):462–9.
37. Moore LG. Measuring high-altitude adaptation. J Appl Physiol (1985). 2017;123(5):1371–85.
38. Sylvester JT, Shimoda LA, Aaronson PI, Ward JP. Hypoxic pulmonary vasoconstriction. Physiol Rev. 2012;92(1):367–520.
39. Beall CM, Laskowski D, Strohl KP, Soria R, Villena M, Vargas E, et al. Pulmonary nitric oxide in mountain dwellers. Nature. 2001;414(6862):411–2.
40. Hoit BD, Dalton ND, Erzurum SC, Laskowski D, Strohl KP, Beall CM. Nitric oxide and cardiopulmonary hemodynamics in Tibetan highlanders. J Appl Physiol (1985). 2005;99(5):1796–801.
41. Crawford JE, Amaru R, Song J, Julian CG, Racimo F, Cheng JY, et al. Natural selection on genes related to cardiovascular health in high-altitude adapted andeans. Am J Hum Genet. 2017;101(5):752–67.
42. Azad P, Stobdan T, Zhou D, Hartley I, Akbari A, Bafna V, Haddad GG. High-altitude adaptation in humans: from genomics to integrative physiology. J Mol Med (Berl). 2017;95(12):1269–82.
43. Droma Y, Hanaoka M, Basnyat B, Arjyal A, Neupane P, Pandit A, et al. Genetic contribution of the endothelial nitric oxide synthase gene to high altitude adaptation in sherpas. High Alt Med Biol. 2006;7(3):209–20.
44. Wilkins MR, Aldashev AA, Wharton J, Rhodes CJ, Vandrovcova J, Kasperaviciute D, et al. α1-A680T variant in GUCY1A3 as a candidate conferring protection from pulmonary hypertension among Kyrgyz highlanders. Circ Cardiovasc Genet. 2014;7(6):920–9.
45. Aldashev AA, Sarybaev AS, Sydykov AS, Kalmyrzaev BB, Kim EV, Mamanova LB, et al. Characterization of high-altitude pulmonary hypertension in the Kyrgyz: association with angiotensin-converting enzyme genotype. Am J Respir Crit Care Med. 2002;166(10):1396–402.
46. Iranmehr A, Stobdan T, Zhou D, Poulsen O, Strohl KP, Aldashev A, et al. Novel insight into the genetic basis of high-altitude pulmonary hypertension in Kyrgyz highlanders. Eur J Hum Genet. 2019;27(1):150–9.
47. León-Velarde F, Mejía O. Gene expression in chronic high altitude diseases. High Alt Med Biol. 2008;9(2):130–9.
48. Kojonazarov B, Isakova J, Imanov B, Sovkhozova N, Sooronbaev T, Ishizaki T, Aldashev AA. Bosentan reduces pulmonary artery pressure in high altitude residents. High Alt Med Biol. 2012;13(3):217–23.
49. Padmasekar M, Savai R, Seeger W, Pullamsetti SS. Exposomes to exosomes: exosomes as tools to study epigenetic adaptive mechanisms in high-altitude humans. Int J Environ Res Public Health. 2021;18(16).
50. Yang Q, Sun M, Ramchandran R, Raj JU. IGF-1 signaling in neonatal hypoxia-induced pulmonary hypertension: Role of epigenetic regulation. Vasc Pharmacol. 2015;73:20–31.
51. Yang Q, Lu Z, Ramchandran R, Longo LD, Raj JU. Pulmonary artery smooth muscle cell proliferation and migration in fetal lambs acclimatized to high-altitude long-term hypoxia: role of histone acetylation. Am J Phys Lung Cell Mol Phys. 2012;303(11):L1001–10.

52. Wang D, Zhang H, Li M, Frid MG, Flockton AR, McKeon BA, et al. MicroRNA-124 controls the proliferative, migratory, and inflammatory phenotype of pulmonary vascular fibroblasts. Circ Res. 2014;114(1):67–78.
53. Yan Y, He YY, Jiang X, Wang Y, Chen JW, Zhao JH, et al. DNA methyltransferase 3B deficiency unveils a new pathological mechanism of pulmonary hypertension. Sci Adv. 2020;6(50).
54. Hainsworth R, Drinkhill MJ. Cardiovascular adjustments for life at high altitude. Respir Physiol Neurobiol. 2007;158(2–3):204–11.
55. Moudgil R, Michelakis ED, Archer SL. Hypoxic pulmonary vasoconstriction. J Appl Physiol (1985). 2005;98(1):390–403.
56. Remillard CV, Yuan JX. High altitude pulmonary hypertension: role of K+ and Ca2+ channels. High Alt Med Biol. 2005;6(2):133–46.
57. Firth AL, Remillard CV, Platoshyn O, Fantozzi I, Ko EA, Yuan JX. Functional ion channels in human pulmonary artery smooth muscle cells: voltage-dependent cation channels. Pulm Circ. 2011;1(1):48–71.
58. Berger MM, Dehnert C, Bailey DM, Luks AM, Menold E, Castell C, et al. Transpulmonary plasma ET-1 and nitrite differences in high altitude pulmonary hypertension. High Alt Med Biol. 2009;10(1):17–24.
59. Hannemann J, Zummack J, Hillig J, Böger R. Metabolism of asymmetric dimethylarginine in hypoxia: from bench to bedside. Pulm Circ. 2020;10(2):2045894020918846.
60. Siques P, Brito J, Schwedhelm E, Pena E, León-Velarde F, De La Cruz JJ, et al. Asymmetric dimethylarginine at sea level is a predictive marker of hypoxic pulmonary arterial hypertension at high altitude. Front Physiol. 2019;10:651.
61. Bailey DM, Dehnert C, Luks AM, Menold E, Castell C, Schendler G, et al. High-altitude pulmonary hypertension is associated with a free radical-mediated reduction in pulmonary nitric oxide bioavailability. J Physiol. 2010;588(Pt 23):4837–47.
62. Smith TG, Balanos GM, Croft QP, Talbot NP, Dorrington KL, Ratcliffe PJ, Robbins PA. The increase in pulmonary arterial pressure caused by hypoxia depends on iron status. J Physiol. 2008;586(24):5999–6005.
63. Yu AY, Shimoda LA, Iyer NV, Huso DL, Sun X, McWilliams R, et al. Impaired physiological responses to chronic hypoxia in mice partially deficient for hypoxia-inducible factor 1alpha. J Clin Invest. 1999;103(5):691–6.
64. Siques P, Pena E, Brito J, El Alam S. Oxidative stress, kinase activation, and inflammatory pathways involved in effects on smooth muscle cells during pulmonary artery hypertension under hypobaric hypoxia exposure. Front Physiol. 2021;12:690341.
65. Zhang Y, Talwar A, Tsang D, Bruchfeld A, Sadoughi A, Hu M, et al. Macrophage migration inhibitory factor mediates hypoxia-induced pulmonary hypertension. Mol Med. 2012;18(1):215–23.
66. Maston LD, Jones DT, Giermakowska W, Resta TC, Ramiro-Diaz J, Howard TA, et al. Interleukin-6 trans-signaling contributes to chronic hypoxia-induced pulmonary hypertension. Pulm Circ. 2018;8(3):2045894018780734.
67. Savale L, Tu L, Rideau D, Izziki M, Maitre B, Adnot S, Eddahibi S. Impact of interleukin-6 on hypoxia-induced pulmonary hypertension and lung inflammation in mice. Respir Res. 2009;10(1):6.
68. Schoene RB, Swenson ER, Pizzo CJ, Hackett PH, Roach RC, Mills WJ Jr, et al. The lung at high altitude: bronchoalveolar lavage in acute mountain sickness and pulmonary edema. J Appl Physiol (1985). 1988;64(6):2605–13.
69. Pu X, Lin X, Duan X, Wang J, Shang J, Yun H, Chen Z. Oxidative and endoplasmic reticulum stress responses to chronic high-altitude exposure during the development of high-altitude pulmonary hypertension. High Alt Med Biol. 2020;21(4):378–87.
70. Sobin SS, Tremer HM, Hardy JD, Chiodi HP. Changes in arteriole in acute and chronic hypoxic pulmonary hypertension and recovery in rat. J Appl Physiol Respir Environ Exerc Physiol. 1983;55(5):1445–55.

71. Talbot NP, Balanos GM, Dorrington KL, Robbins PA. Two temporal components within the human pulmonary vascular response to approximately 2 h of isocapnic hypoxia. J Appl Physiol (1985). 2005;98(3):1125–39.
72. Hackett PH, Roach RC. High-altitude illness. N Engl J Med. 2001;345(2):107–14.
73. Rabinovitch M, Gamble WJ, Miettinen OS, Reid L. Age and sex influence on pulmonary hypertension of chronic hypoxia and on recovery. Am J Phys. 1981;240(1):H62–72.
74. Fried R, Reid LM. Early recovery from hypoxic pulmonary hypertension: a structural and functional study. J Appl Physiol Respir Environ Exerc Physiol. 1984;57(4):1247–53.
75. Ou LC, Sardella GL, Leiter JC, Brinck-Johnsen T, Smith RP. Role of sex hormones in development of chronic mountain sickness in rats. J Appl Physiol (1985). 1994;77(1):427–33.
76. Sime F, Peñaloza D, Ruiz L. Bradycardia, increased cardiac output, and reversal of pulmonary hypertension in altitude natives living at sea level. Br Heart J. 1971;33(5):647–57.
77. Robinson JC, Abbott C, Meadows CA, Roach RC, Honigman B, Bull TM. Long-term health outcomes in high-altitude pulmonary hypertension. High Alt Med Biol. 2017;18(1):61–6.
78. Grover RF, Vogel JH, Voigt GC, Blount SG Jr. Reversal of high altitude pulmonary hypertension. Am J Cardiol. 1966;18(6):928–32.
79. Aldashev AA, Kojonazarov BK, Amatov TA, Sooronbaev TM, Mirrakhimov MM, Morrell NW, et al. Phosphodiesterase type 5 and high altitude pulmonary hypertension. Thorax. 2005;60(8):683–7.
80. Richalet JP, Gratadour P, Robach P, Pham I, Déchaux M, Joncquiert-Latarjet A, et al. Sildenafil inhibits altitude-induced hypoxemia and pulmonary hypertension. Am J Respir Crit Care Med. 2005;171(3):275–81.
81. Ghofrani HA, Reichenberger F, Kohstall MG, Mrosek EH, Seeger T, Olschewski H, et al. Sildenafil increased exercise capacity during hypoxia at low altitudes and at Mount Everest base camp: a randomized, double-blind, placebo-controlled crossover trial. Ann Intern Med. 2004;141(3):169–77.
82. Reichenberger F, Kohstall MG, Seeger T, Olschewski H, Grimminger F, Seeger W, Ghofrani HA. Effect of sildenafil on hypoxia-induced changes in pulmonary circulation and right ventricular function. Respir Physiol Neurobiol. 2007;159(2):196–201.
83. Bates MG, Thompson AA, Baillie JK, Sutherland AI, Irving JB, Hirani N, Webb DJ. Sildenafil citrate for the prevention of high altitude hypoxic pulmonary hypertension: double blind, randomized, placebo-controlled trial. High Alt Med Biol. 2011;12(3):207–14.
84. Faoro V, Lamotte M, Deboeck G, Pavelescu A, Huez S, Guenard H, et al. Effects of sildenafil on exercise capacity in hypoxic normal subjects. High Alt Med Biol. 2007;8(2):155–63.
85. Jin B, Luo XP, Ni HC, Shi HM. Phosphodiesterase type 5 inhibitors for high-altitude pulmonary hypertension: a meta-analysis. Clin Drug Investig. 2010;30(4):259–65.
86. Xu Y, Liu Y, Liu J, Qian G. Meta-analysis of clinical efficacy of sildenafil, a phosphodiesterase type-5 inhibitor on high altitude hypoxia and its complications. High Alt Med Biol. 2014;15(1):46–51.
87. Gao X, Zhang Z, Li X, Li C, Hao J, Luo Y, et al. Macitentan attenuates chronic mountain sickness in rats by regulating arginine and purine metabolism. J Proteome Res. 2020;19(8):3302–14.
88. Xu X, Li H, Wei Q, Li X, Shen Y, Guo G, et al. Novel targets in a high-altitude pulmonary hypertension rat model based on RNA-seq and proteomics. Front Med (Lausanne). 2021;8:742436.
89. Seheult RD, Ruh K, Foster GP, Anholm JD. Prophylactic bosentan does not improve exercise capacity or lower pulmonary artery systolic pressure at high altitude. Respir Physiol Neurobiol. 2009;165(2–3):123–30.
90. Waxman A, Restrepo-Jaramillo R, Thenappan T, Ravichandran A, Engel P, Bajwa A, et al. Inhaled treprostinil in pulmonary hypertension due to interstitial lung disease. N Engl J Med. 2021;384(4):325–34.

91. Antezana AM, Antezana G, Aparicio O, Noriega I, Velarde FL, Richalet JP. Pulmonary hypertension in high-altitude chronic hypoxia: response to nifedipine. Eur Respir J. 1998;12(5):1181–5.
92. Kojonazarov B, Myrzaakhmatova A, Sooronbaev T, Ishizaki T, Aldashev A. Effects of fasudil in patients with high-altitude pulmonary hypertension. Eur Respir J. 2012;39(2):496–8.
93. Nijiati Y, Maimaitiyiming D, Yang T, Li H, Aikemu A. Research on the improvement of oxidative stress in rats with high-altitude pulmonary hypertension through the participation of irbesartan in regulating intestinal flora. Eur Rev Med Pharmacol Sci. 2021;25(13):4540–53.
94. Nijiati Y, Yang T, Aimaiti M, Maimaitiyiming D, Aikemu A. Irbesartan ameliorates chronic mountain sickness in a rat model via the cholesterol metabolism: an iTRAQ -based proteomics analysis. Biomed Pharmacother. 2021;141:111802.
95. Niazova ZA, Batyraliev TA, Aikimbaev KS, Kudaiberdieva GZ, Akgul F, Soodanbekova YK, Birand A. High-altitude pulmonary hypertension: effects of captopril on pulmonary and systemic arterial pressures. J Hum Hypertens. 1996;10(Suppl 3):S141–2.
96. Richalet JP, Rivera-Ch M, Maignan M, Privat C, Pham I, Macarlupu JL, et al. Acetazolamide for Monge's disease: efficiency and tolerance of 6-month treatment. Am J Respir Crit Care Med. 2008;177(12):1370–6.
97. Pichon A, Connes P, Quidu P, Marchant D, Brunet J, Levy BI, et al. Acetazolamide and chronic hypoxia: effects on haemorheology and pulmonary haemodynamics. Eur Respir J. 2012;40(6):1401–9.
98. Rivera-Ch M, León-Velarde F, Huicho L. Treatment of chronic mountain sickness: critical reappraisal of an old problem. Respir Physiol Neurobiol. 2007;158(2–3):251–65.
99. Schoene RB, Bates PW, Larson EB, Pierson DJ. Effect of acetazolamide on normoxic and hypoxic exercise in humans at sea level. J Appl Physiol Respir Environ Exerc Physiol. 1983;55(6):1772–6.
100. Smith TG, Talbot NP, Privat C, Rivera-Ch M, Nickol AH, Ratcliffe PJ, et al. Effects of iron supplementation and depletion on hypoxic pulmonary hypertension: two randomized controlled trials. JAMA. 2009;302(13):1444–50.
101. Robinson JC, Graham BB, Rouault TC, Tuder RM. The crossroads of iron with hypoxia and cellular metabolism. Implications in the pathobiology of pulmonary hypertension. Am J Respir Cell Mol Biol. 2014;51(6):721–9.
102. Patrician A, Dawkins T, Coombs GB, Stacey B, Gasho C, Gibbons T, et al. GLOBAL REACH 2018: iron infusion at high altitude reduces hypoxic pulmonary vasoconstriction equally in both lowlanders and healthy Andean highlanders. Chest. 2021.
103. Berger MM, Macholz F, Lehmann L, Dankl D, Hochreiter M, Bacher B, et al. Remote ischemic preconditioning does not prevent acute mountain sickness after rapid ascent to 3,450 m. J Appl Physiol (1985). 2017;123(5):1228–34.
104. Lyu Q, Bai Y, Cheng J, Liu H, Li S, Yang J, et al. Intermittent short-duration reoxygenation protects against simulated high altitude-induced pulmonary hypertension in rats. FASEB J. 2021;35(2):e21212.
105. Shao X, Dong X, Cai J, Tang C, Xie K, Yan Z, et al. Oxygen enrichment ameliorates cardiorespiratory alterations induced by chronic high-altitude hypoxia in rats. Front Physiol. 2020;11:616145.

Index

F. N. Rahaghi et al. (eds.), *The Pulmonary Vasculature in Chronic Lung Disease*, Respiratory Medicine, https://doi.org/10.1007/978-3-032-03581-3

N

O

P

Q

R

S

MIX
Papier aus verantwortungsvollen Quellen
Paper from responsible sources
FSC® C105338

If you have any concerns about our products,
you can contact us on
ProductSafety@springernature.com

In case Publisher is established outside the EU,
the EU authorized representative is:
Springer Nature Customer Service Center GmbH
Europaplatz 3, 69115 Heidelberg, Germany

Printed by Libri Plureos GmbH
in Hamburg, Germany